HORMONES AND REPRODUCTIVE BEHAVIOR

Readings from
**SCIENTIFIC
AMERICAN**

HORMONES AND REPRODUCTIVE BEHAVIOR

With Introductions by
Rae Silver
*Barnard College
of Columbia University*

Harvey H. Feder
Rutgers University

W. H. Freeman and Company
San Francisco

Most of the *Scientific American* articles in *Hormones and Reproductive Behavior* are available as separate Offprints. For a complete list of articles now available as Offprints, write W. H. Freeman and Company, 660 Market Street, San Francisco, California 94104.

Library of Congress Cataloging in Publication Data

Main entry under title:

Hormones and reproductive behavior.

   Bibliography: p.
   Includes index.
   1. Hormones, Sex—Addresses, essays, lectures.
2. Reproduction—Addresses, essays, lectures.
3. Sex behavior in animals—Addresses, essays, lectures.
4. Sex—Addresses, essays, lectures.
1. Silver, Rae.   II. Feder, Harvey H., 1940–
III. Scientific American.
QP572.S4H67   599'.05'6   79–1192
ISBN 0-7167-1093-5
ISBN 0-7167-1094-3 pbk.

Printed in the United States of America

1 2 3 4 5 6 7 8 9

PREFACE

Our understanding of the biological roots of behavior is rapidly increasing. The study of sex hormones in relation to reproductive behavior is a particularly active area of research, partly because the relations between sex hormones and sex behavior are often directly observable and highly predictable. The advances made in this area have already wrought enormous philosophical and material changes in our lives. Because research on reproductive hormones has such dramatic consequences, some understanding of the nature of this research is important for each of us.

The relationship between sex hormones and reproductive behavior is an extraordinarily interdisciplinary study. To understand this relationship it is necessary to transcend traditional boundaries and to incorporate knowledge from disciplines as diverse as psychology, neuroanatomy, endocrinology, embryology, and biochemistry. The papers in this collection bring together information from these disciplines in an interesting and highly readable form. Some of the articles provide a general historical perspective, while others present a more detailed picture of particular research areas.

Section I shows some of the ways in which environmental factors influence hormone secretions and behavior. This section points to the many phenomena that need to be analyzed by the methods of various disciplines.

Section II focuses on the ways that hormones are regulated within the body. Physiological mechanisms by which hormones exert their effects are explained and the application of this knowledge to the regulation of fertility is described.

Section III describes the action of hormones on cells of the body. It is at this level of analysis that the interface among diverse disciplines is currently most active. The actions of hormones on the cell's genetic apparatus have received considerable attention. The research has been fruitful and promises to contribute greatly not only to prevention and alleviation of pathologies of the reproductive system but also to the understanding of the cellular bases of hormone effects on behavior and mood.

In Section IV the biochemical consequences of hormone action are explored further. Hormones alter communication among brain cells by influencing the production of neurotransmitters. In this section we see how the system of communication within the body is regulated by a complex interplay between brain cells and hormones.

Finally, in Section V we step back to examine the larger implications of all of these technical advances. The papers in this section evaluate the political, legal, and ethical problems in research on reproduction. These problems are common to all research on the biological bases of behavior.

The subject matter included under the rubric of sex hormones and reproductive behavior is incorporated into various courses at high school and university levels. This collection is designed to serve the requirements of teachers and students at these levels. The introduction to each section outlines the significance of each article and the general problem to which it is addressed. Where appropriate, the papers are presented in historical sequence and in increasing order of complexity. Thus, this collection may serve as a text around which lectures are organized, or it may be used as an accompaniment to other texts in the area.

February 1979   Rae Silver
                                                                                Harvey H. Feder

CONTENTS

Note on cross-references to SCIENTIFIC AMERICAN *articles:* Articles included in this book are referred to by title and page number; articles not included in this book but available as Offprints are referred to by title and offprint number; articles not included in this book and not available as Offprints are referred to by title and date of publication.

HORMONES AND REPRODUCTIVE BEHAVIOR

I

ENVIRONMENTAL REGULATION OF SEX HORMONES

I ENVIRONMENTAL REGULATION OF SEX HORMONES

INTRODUCTION

We are all familiar with the idea that hormones influence our behavior and physiology. We are less familiar with the notion that our perceptions, behavior, and moods influence the production of hormones.

Evidence demonstrating environmental effects on hormone production comes from studies of both humans and animals. These studies show that information from each of our senses, including sight, sound, smell, and touch, can alter hormone levels as well as other bodily functions. For example, blind girls reach puberty earlier than normally sighted girls. A lactating mother may eject milk when she hears or sees her baby. Some effects of environmental stimuli in animals are even more dramatic. For example, many animals come into breeding condition only when days have reached a critical length. Thus, in sheep, the gonads (ovaries and testes) produce high levels of hormones only in the fall, when the days are short. In other animals, such as birds living in temperate zones, the gonads produce high levels of sex hormones only in the spring, when days are long. In both instances, bodily responses to day length allow these species to produce young when food and weather are optimal for survival of the offspring.

Although we could cite examples demonstrating that stimuli from each sensory system influence the production of sex hormones in humans and animals, we will focus on the effects of light and visual stimuli on hormone production. Richard J. Wurtman, in the first article, outlines the effects of light on the human body. The way in which light alters bodily functions has become a major concern in recent years as a result of our exposure to artificial light for artificial durations in our homes and at work. As Wurtman points out, this exposure has many direct and indirect effects throughout the body and can even affect the sex hormones.

In studies of humans it is often difficult to determine precisely where and how stimuli act on the body. By examining a variety of animals, we can find more clear-cut examples of stimulus effects on sex hormones. Also, by studying many different systems in which external stimuli alter hormone production, we can better understand the *mechanisms* by which stimuli affect the brain, hormones, and behavior and the biological functions that are served. The second article, by Michael Menaker, makes the important point that in birds light can act on the brain directly and need not travel via the eyes and visual system. As Menaker points out, however, direct effects of light on the brain have not been demonstrated in mammals.

The stimuli that affect hormone secretion can also come from the behavior of another animal, such as a mate or a competitor. Many investigators have shown that social stimuli alter levels of sex hormones in the body. A classic paper that drew attention to this general phenomenon is Daniel S. Lehrman's article on ring doves. Lehrman shows that changes in behavior which ensure that courtship, mating, and care of young occur at the appropriate times and in the appropriate sequence are governed by complex interactions of outside stimuli, hormones, and the behavior of each mate.

It is tempting to take the view that biological control mechanisms, such as levels of hormones in the blood, represent a fixed constraint on behavior. In reality, many hormone-mediated behaviors remain flexible throughout life. The article by G. Gray Eaton emphasizes the importance of social factors and the ways in which they modify hormone-mediated behavior. As Eaton shows, even though male sex hormones are important for sexual and aggressive behavior, knowledge of levels of hormones in the blood alone does not allow us to predict behavior. Social factors that emerge over the lifetime of an organism, as it interacts with others, are important modifers of hormonally mediated behaviors.

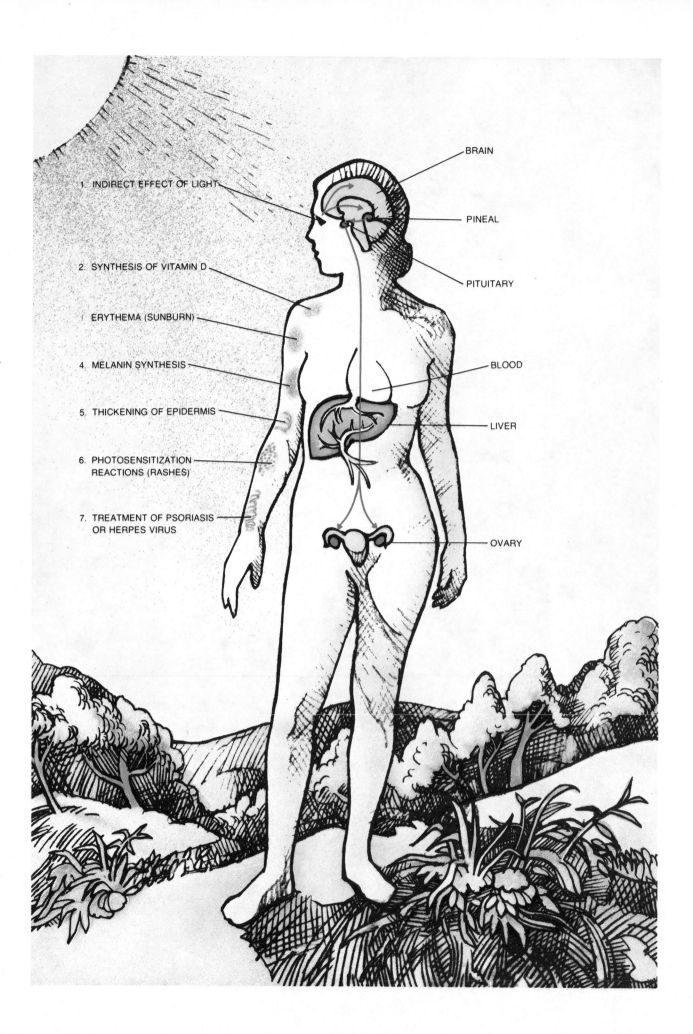

1. INDIRECT EFFECT OF LIGHT

2. SYNTHESIS OF VITAMIN D

3. ERYTHEMA (SUNBURN)

4. MELANIN SYNTHESIS

5. THICKENING OF EPIDERMIS

6. PHOTOSENSITIZATION
   REACTIONS (RASHES)

7. TREATMENT OF PSORIASIS
   OR HERPES VIRUS

BRAIN

PINEAL

PITUITARY

BLOOD

LIVER

OVARY

The Effects of Light on the Human Body

by Richard J. Wurtman
July 1975

Sunlight tans skin, stimulates the formation of vitamin D and sets biological rhythms. Light is also used in the treatment of disease. Such effects now raise questions about the role of artificial light

Since life evolved under the influence of sunlight, it is not surprising that many animals, including man, have developed a variety of physiological responses to the spectral characteristics of solar radiation and to its daily and seasonal variations. With the coming of summer in the Northern Hemisphere millions of people living in the North Temperate Zone will take the opportunity to darken the shade of their skin, even at the risk of being painfully burned. Coincidentally the sunbathers will replenish their body's store of vitamin D, the vitamin that is essential for the proper metabolism of calcium. Skin-tanning and subcutaneous synthesis of vitamin D from its precursors, however, are only the best-known consequences of exposure to sunlight.

Investigators are slowly uncovering subtler physiological and biochemical responses of the human body to solar radiation or its artificial equivalent. Within the past few years, for example, light has been introduced as the standard method of treatment for neonatal jaundice, a sometimes fatal disease that is common among premature infants. More recently light, in conjunction with a sen-sitizing drug, has proved highly effective in the treatment of the common skin inflammation psoriasis. It seems safe to predict that other therapeutic uses for light will be found.

At least equally significant for human well-being is the growing evidence that fundamental biochemical and hormonal rhythms of the body are synchronized, directly or indirectly, by the daily cycle of light and dark. For example, my co-workers at the Massachusetts Institute of Technology and I have recently discovered a pronounced daily rhythm in the rate at which normal human subjects excrete melatonin, a hormone synthesized by the pineal organ of the brain. In experimental animals melatonin induces sleep, inhibits ovulation and modifies the secretion of other hormones. In man the amount of the adrenocortical hormone cortisol in the blood varies with a 24-hour rhythm. Although seasonal rhythms associated with changes in the length of the day have not yet been unequivocally demonstrated in human physiology, they are well known in other animals, and it would be surprising if they were absent in man. The findings already in hand suggest that light has an important influence on human health, and that our exposure to artificial light may have harmful effects of which we are not aware.

The wavelengths of radiation whose physiological effects I shall discuss here are essentially those supplied by the sun after its rays have been filtered by the atmosphere, including the tenuous high-altitude layer of ozone, which removes virtually all ultraviolet radiation with a wavelength shorter than 290 nanometers. The solar radiation that reaches the earth's surface consists chiefly of the ultraviolet (from 290 to 380 nanometers), the visible spectrum (from 380 to 770 nanometers) and the near infrared (from 770 to 1,000 nanometers). About 20 percent of the solar energy that reaches the earth has a wavelength longer than 1,000 nanometers.

The visible spectrum of natural sunlight at sea level is about the same as the spectrum of an ideal incandescent source radiating at a temperature of 5,600 degrees Kelvin (degrees Celsius above absolute zero). The solar spectrum is essentially continuous, lacking only certain narrow wavelengths absorbed by elements in the sun's atmosphere, and at midday it has a peak intensity in the blue-green region from 450 to 500 nanometers [*see upper illustration on next page*]. The amount of ultraviolet radiation that penetrates the atmosphere varies markedly with the season: in the northern third of the U.S. the total amount of erythemal (skin-inflaming) radiation that reaches the ground in December is only about a fifteenth of the amount present in June. Otherwise there is little seasonal change in the spectral composition of the sunlight reaching the ground. The actual number of daylight hours, of course, can vary greatly, depending on the season and the distance north or south of the Equator.

SOME DIRECT AND INDIRECT EFFECTS OF LIGHT on the human body are outlined in the drawing shown on page 127. Indirect effects include the production or entrainment (synchronization) of biological rhythms. Such effects are evidently mediated by photoreceptors in the eye (1) and involve the brain and neuroendocrine organs. For example, excretion of melatonin, a hormone produced by the pineal organ, follows a daily rhythm. In animals melatonin synthesis is regulated by light. The hormone, acting on the pituitary, plays a role in the maturation and the cyclic activity of the sex glands. Ultraviolet radiation acts on the skin to synthesize vitamin D (2). Erythema, or reddening of the skin (3), is caused by ultraviolet wavelengths between 290 and 320 nanometers. In response melanocytes increase their synthesis of melanin (4), a pigment that darkens the skin. Simultaneously the epidermis thickens (5), offering further protection. In some people the interaction of light with photosensitizers circulating in the blood causes a rash (6). In conjunction with selected photosensitizers light can be used to treat psoriasis and other skin disorders (7). In infants with neonatal jaundice light is also used therapeutically to lower the amount of bilirubin circulating in the blood until infant's liver is mature enough to excrete the substance. The therapy prevents the bilirubin from concentrating in the brain and destroying brain tissue.

The most familiar type of artificial light is the incandescent lamp, in which the radiant source is a hot filament of tungsten. The incandescent filament in a typical 100-watt lamp has a temperature of only about 2,850 degrees K., so that its radiation is strongly shifted to the red, or long-wavelength, end of the spectrum. Indeed, about 90 percent of the total emission of an incandescent lamp lies in the infrared.

Fluorescent lamps, unlike the sun and incandescent lamps, generate visible light by a nonthermal mechanism. Within the glass tube of a fluorescent lamp ultraviolet photons are generated by a mercury-vapor arc; the inner surface of the tube is coated with phosphors, luminescent compounds that emit visible radiations of characteristic colors when they are bombarded with ultraviolet photons. The standard "cool white" fluorescent lamp has been designed to achieve maximum brightness for a given energy consumption. Brightness, of course, is a subjective phenomenon that depends on the response of the photoreceptive cells in the retina. Since the photoreceptors are most sensitive to yellow-green light of 555 nanometers, most fluorescent lamps are designed to concentrate much of their output in that wavelength region. It is possible, however, to make fluorescent lamps whose spectral output closely matches that of sunlight [see lower illustration on this page].

Since fluorescent lamps are the most widely used light source in offices, factories and schools, most people in industrial societies spend many of their waking hours bathed in light whose spectral characteristics differ markedly from those of sunlight. Architects and lighting engineers tend to assume that the only significant role of light is to provide adequate illumination for working and reading. The illumination provided at eye level in artificially lighted rooms is commonly from 50 to 100 footcandles, or less than 10 percent of the light normally available outdoors in the shade of a tree on a sunny day.

The decision that 100 footcandles or less is appropriate for indoor purposes seems to be based on economic and technological considerations rather than on any knowledge of man's biological needs. Fluorescent lamps could provide higher light intensities without excessive heat production, but the cost of the electric power needed for substantially higher light levels would probably be prohibitive. Nevertheless, the total amount of light to which a resident of Boston, say, is exposed in a conventionally lighted indoor environment for 16 hours a day is considerably less than would impinge on him if he spent a single hour each day outdoors. If future studies indicate that significant health benefits (for example better bone mineralization) might accrue from increasing the levels of indoor lighting, our society might, in a period of energy shortages, be faced with hard new choices.

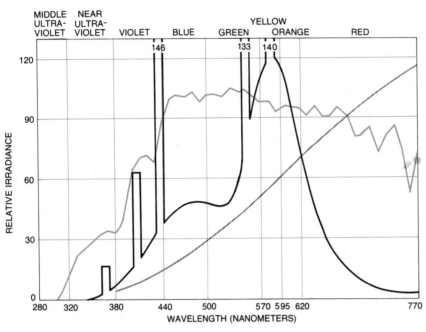

SPECTRUM OF SUN at sea level (color) is compared with the spectra of a typical incandescent lamp (gray curve) and of a standard "cool white" fluorescent lamp (black curve). The visible spectrum lies between the wavelengths of 380 and 770 nanometers. The peak of the sun's radiant energy falls in the blue-green region between 450 and 500 nanometers. Cool-white fluorescent lamps are notably deficient precisely where the sun's emission is strongest. Incandescent lamps are extremely weak in the entire blue-green half of the visible spectrum.

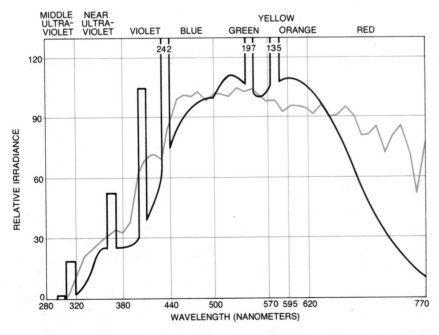

BROAD-SPECTRUM FLUORESCENT LAMP known as Vita-Lite (black curve) closely approximates spectral characteristics of sunlight (color). Wavelengths emitted by fluorescent lamps can be adjusted by selecting phosphors with which inner surface of lamp is coated.

Each of the various effects of light on mammalian tissues can be classified as direct or indirect, depending on whether the immediate cause is a photochemical reaction within the tissue or a neural or neuroendocrine signal generated by a photoreceptor cell. When the effect is direct, the molecule that changes may or may not be the one that actually absorbs the photon. For example, certain molecules can act as photosensitizers: when they are raised to transient high-energy states by the absorption of radiation, they are able to catalyze the oxidation of numerous other compounds before they return to the ground state. Photosensitizers sometimes present in human tissues include constituents of foods and drugs and of toxins produced in excess by some diseases.

In order to prove that a particular chemical change in a tissue is a direct response to light one must show that light energy of the required wavelength does in fact penetrate the body to reach the affected tissue. In addition the photoenergetic and chemical characteristics of the reaction must be fully specified, first in the test tube, then in experimental animals or human beings, by charting the reaction's "action spectrum" (the relative effectiveness of different spectral bands in producing the reaction) and by identifying all its chemical intermediates and products. Visible light is apparently able to penetrate all mammalian tissues to a considerable depth; it has even been detected within the brain of a living sheep.

Ultraviolet radiation, which is far more energetic than visible wavelengths, penetrates tissues less effectively, so that erythemal radiations barely reach the capillaries in the skin. The identification of action spectra for the effects of light on entire organisms presents major technical problems: few action spectra have been defined for chemical responses in tissues other than the skin and the eyes.

The indirect responses of a tissue to light result not from the absorption of light within the tissue but from the actions of chemical signals liberated by neurons or the actions of chemical messengers (hormones) delivered by circulation of the blood. These signals in turn are ultimately the result of the same process as the one that initiates vision: the activation by light of specialized photoreceptive cells. The photoreceptor transduces the incident-light energy to a neural signal, which is then transmitted over neural, or combined neural-endocrine, pathways to the tissue in which the indirect effect is observed. For example, when young rats are kept continuously under light, photoreceptive cells in their retina release neurotransmitters that activate brain neurons; these neurons in turn transmit signals over complex neuroendocrine pathways that reach the anterior pituitary gland,

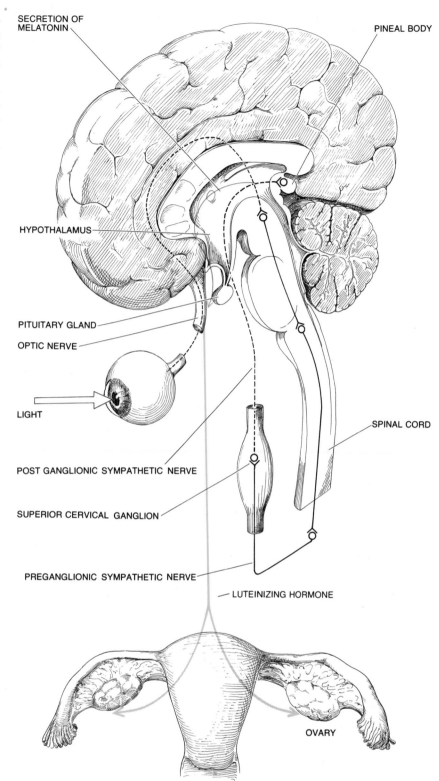

SECRETION OF MELATONIN

PINEAL BODY

HYPOTHALAMUS

PITUITARY GLAND

OPTIC NERVE

LIGHT

POST GANGLIONIC SYMPATHETIC NERVE

SUPERIOR CERVICAL GANGLION

PREGANGLIONIC SYMPATHETIC NERVE

LUTEINIZING HORMONE

SPINAL CORD

OVARY

INDIRECT EFFECT OF LIGHT ON OVARIES OF RATS is shown schematically. Light activates receptors in the retina, giving rise to nerve impulses that travel via a chain of synapses through the brain, the brain stem and the spinal cord, ultimately decreasing the activity of neurons running to the superior cervical ganglion (in the neck) and of the sympathetic nerves that reenter the cranium and travel to the pineal organ. There the decrease in activity reduces both the synthesis and the secretion of melatonin. With less melatonin in blood or cerebrospinal fluid, less reaches brain centers (probably in hypothalamus) on which melatonin acts to suppress secretion of luteinizing hormone from anterior pituitary. Thus more hormone is released, facilitating ovarian growth and presumably ovulation.

where they stimulate the secretion of the gonadotropic hormones that accelerate the maturation of the ovaries [*see illustration on opposite page*].

That the ovaries are not responding directly to light can be shown by removing the eyes or the pituitary gland of the rat before exposing it to continuous light. After either procedure light no longer has any influence on ovarian growth or function. Various studies confirm that the effect of light on the ovaries is mediated by photoreceptive cells in the retina. It has not been possible to show, however, which of the photoreceptors in the eye release the neurotransmitters that ultimately affect the pituitary gland.

Natural sunlight acts directly on the cells of the skin and subcutaneous tissues to generate both pathological and protective responses. The most familiar example of a pathological response is sunburn; in susceptible individuals exposed over many years sunlight also causes a particular variety of skin cancer. The chief protective response is tanning. Ultraviolet wavelengths in the narrow band from 290 to 320 nanometers cause the skin to redden within a few hours of exposure. Investigators generally agree that the inflammatory reaction, which may persist for several days, results either from a direct action of ultraviolet photons on small blood vessels or from the release of toxic compounds from damaged epidermal cells. The toxins presumably diffuse into the dermis, where they damage the capillaries and cause reddening, heat, swelling and pain. A number of compounds have been proposed as the offending toxins, including serotonin, histamine and bradykinin. Sunburn is largely an affliction of industrial civilization. If people were to expose themselves to sunlight for one or two hours every day, weather permitting, their skin's reaction to the gradual increase in erythemal solar radiation that occurs during late winter and spring would provide them with a protective layer of pigmentation for withstanding ultraviolet radiation of summer intensities.

Immediately after exposure to sunlight the amount of pigment in the skin increases, and the skin remains darker for a few hours. The immediate darkening probably results from the photooxidation of a colorless melanin precursor and is evidently caused by all the wavelengths in sunlight. After a day or two, when the initial response to sunlight has subsided, melanocytes in the epidermis begin to divide and to increase their synthesis of melanin granules, which are then extruded and taken up into the adjacent keratinocytes, or skin cells [*see illustration at left*]. Concurrently accelerated cell division thickens the ultraviolet-absorbing layers of the epidermis. The skin remains tan for several weeks and offers considerable protection against further tissue damage by sunlight. Eventually the keratinocytes slough off and the tan slowly fades. (In the U.S.S.R. coal miners are given suberythemal doses of ultraviolet light every day on the theory that the radiation provides protection against the development of black-lung disease. The mechanism of the supposed protective effect is not known.)

In addition to causing sunburn and tanning, sunlight or its equivalent initiates photochemical and photosensitization reactions that affect compounds present in the blood, in the fluid space between the cells or in the cells themselves. A number of widely prescribed drugs (such as the tetracyclines) and constituents of foods (such as riboflavins) are potential photosensitizers. When they are activated within the body by light, they may produce transient intermediates that can damage the tissues in sensitive individuals. A typical response is the appearance of a rash on the parts of the body that are exposed to the sun.

In individuals with the congenital disease known as erythropoietic protoporphyria unusually large amounts of porphyrins (a family of photosensitizing chemicals) are released into the bloodstream as a result of a biochemical ab-

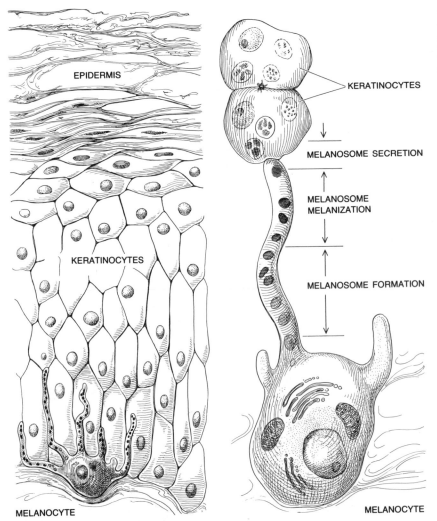

MECHANISM OF SUN-TANNING is an extension of the mechanism responsible for skin pigmentation. After exposure to the sun melanocytes begin to divide and increase their output of melanin granules, produced in the tiny intracellular bodies called melanosomes. The melanosomes are secreted into the adjacent keratinocytes, or skin cells, where the melanin causes the skin to take on a darker appearance. The tan fades as the keratinocytes slough off.

normality. The porphyrins absorb visible radiations and give rise to intermediates that are toxic to tissues. Patients with the disease complain at first of a burning sensation in areas of the skin that are exposed to sunlight; reddening and swelling soon follow.

Investigators can easily induce these typical symptoms without serious consequences in patients suffering from mild forms of erythropoietic protoporphyria, so that the disease is one of the few of its kind where the action spectrum for a direct effect of light has been studied in detail. The skin damage is caused by a fairly narrow band of wavelengths in the region of 400 nanometers. This band has also been shown to coincide with one of the absorption peaks of abnormal porphyrins. The symptoms of the disease can be ameliorated by administering photoprotective agents such as carotenoids, which quench the excited states of oxygen produced as intermediates in the photosensitization reactions.

In the past few years physicians have treated several skin diseases by deliberately inducing photosensitization reactions on the surface of the body or within particular tissues. The intent is to cause selective damage to invading organisms (such as the herpes virus), to excessively proliferating cells (as in psoriasis) or to certain types of malignant cells. The activated photosensitizers appear to be capable of inactivating the DNA in the viruses or in the unwanted cells. In treating herpes infections the photosensitizer (usually a dye, neutral red) is applied directly to the skin or to the mucous membrane under the ruptured blister; the area is then exposed to low-intensity white fluorescent light.

The treatment for psoriasis was devised by John A. Parrish, Thomas B. Fitzpatrick and their colleagues at the Massachusetts General Hospital. They administer a special photosensitizer (8-methoxypsoralen, or methoxalen) by mouth and two hours later expose the afflicted skin areas for about 10 minutes to the radiation from special lamps that emit strongly in the long-wave ultraviolet at about 365 nanometers. The sensitizing agent is present in small amounts in carrots, parsley and limes. It is derived commercially from an Egyptian plant (*Ammi majus* Linn.) that was used in ancient times to treat skin ailments. Scores of patients have responded successfully to the new light treatment, which will soon be generally available.

The formation of vitamin D_3, or cholecalciferol, in the skin and subcutaneous tissue is the most important of the beneficial effects known to follow exposure to sunlight. Vitamin D_3 is formed when ultraviolet radiation is absorbed by a precursor, 7-dehydrocholesterol. A related biologically active compound, vitamin D_2, can be obtained by consuming milk and other foods in which ergosterol, a natural plant sterol, has been converted to vitamin D_2 by exposure to ultraviolet radiation. Although vitamin D_2 can cure rickets in children who are deficient in vitamin D_3, it has not been demonstrated that vitamin D_2 is biologically as effective as the vitamin D_3 formed in the skin.

In a population of normal white adults living in St. Louis, studied by John G. Haddad, Jr., and Theodore J. Hahn of the Washington University School of Medicine, some 70 to 90 percent of the vitamin D activity in blood samples was found to be accountable to vitamin D_3 or its derivatives. The investigators concluded that sunlight was vastly more important than food as a source of vitamin D. (Although vitamin D_3 is also found in fish, seafood is not an important source in most diets.) In Britain and several other European countries the fortification of foods with vitamin D_2 has now been sharply curtailed because of evidence that in large amounts vitamin D_2 can be toxic, causing general weakness, kidney damage and elevated blood levels of calcium and cholesterol.

A direct study of the influence of light on the human body's ability to absorb calcium was undertaken a few years ago by Robert Neer and me and our coworkers. The study, conducted among elderly, apparently normal men at the Chelsea Soldiers' Home near Boston, suggests that a lack of adequate exposure to ultraviolet radiation during the long winter months significantly impairs the body's utilization of calcium, even when there is an adequate supply in the diet. The calcium absorption of a control group and an experimental group was followed for 11 consecutive weeks from the onset of winter to mid-March.

During the first period of seven weeks, representing the severest part of the winter, all the subjects agreed to remain indoors during the hours of daylight. Thus both groups were exposed more or less equally to a typical low level of mixed incandescent and fluorescent lighting (from 10 to 50 footcandles). At the end of the seven weeks the men in both groups were found to absorb only about 40 percent of the calcium they ingested. During the next four-week period, from mid-February to mid-March, the lighting was left unchanged for the control subjects, and their ability to ab-

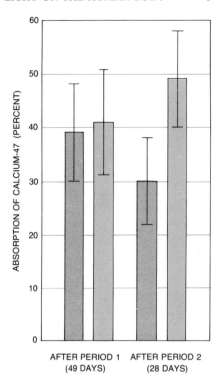

CALCIUM ABSORPTION was increased by a daily eight-hour exposure to broad-spectrum artificial light in a study made by the author and his colleagues at a veterans' home. During the first seven weeks after the beginning of winter, control subjects (*gray bars*) and experimental subjects (*colored bars*) were equally exposed to the same low levels of typical indoor lighting. The bars at the left show their ability to absorb calcium at the end of the initial period. During the next four-week period conditions for the control subjects were unchanged; their ability to absorb calcium fell about 25 percent. The experimental subjects, who were exposed to 500 footcandles of broad-spectrum fluorescent light for eight hours per day for four weeks, showed an average increase of about 15 percent in their calcium absorption.

sorb calcium fell by about 25 percent. The men in the experimental group, however, were exposed for eight hours per day to 500 footcandles of light from special fluorescent (Vita-Lite) lamps, which simulate the solar spectrum in the visible and near-ultraviolet regions. In contrast with the control subjects' loss of 25 percent of their capacity to absorb calcium, the experimental group exhibited an increase of about 15 percent [*see illustration above*]. The additional amount of ultraviolet radiation received by the experimental subects was actually quite small: roughly equivalent to what they would get during a 15-minute lunchtime walk in the summer.

Our study indicates that a certain amount of ultraviolet radiation, whether it is from the sun or from an artificial source, is necessary for adequate calcium metabolism. This hypothesis receives support from a recent study conducted by Jean Aaron of the Mineral Metabolism Unit at the General Infirmary at Leeds in England, who found that undermineralization (osteomalacia) is far more prevalent in autopsy samples collected in England during the winter months than it is in samples collected during the summer. Thus it seems likely that properly designed indoor lighting environments could serve as an important public-health measure to prevent the undermineralization of bones among the elderly and others with limited access to natural sunlight.

Perhaps 25,000 premature American infants were sucessfully treated with light last year as the sole therapy for neonatal jaundice. The rationale for this remarkable treatment is as follows. When red blood cells die, they release hemoglobin, which soon degrades into the yellow compound bilirubin. An increase in the concentration of bilirubin in the blood, due to excessive production of the compound or to failure of the liver to remove it, gives the skin its characteristic jaundiced color.

A potentially dangerous form of hyperbilirubinemia afflicts from 15 to 20 percent of premature infants because their liver is physiologically immature; in some cases the amounts of bilirubin released into the bloodstream are also increased as a result of blood-type incompatibility or concurrent infections. In such infants the bilirubin, which is soluble in fat, becomes concentrated in cer-

tain parts of the brain, where it can destroy neurons, producing the clinical syndrome kernicterus (yellow nuclei). The toxicity of bilirubin is aggravated by other factors, such as anoxia, acidosis, low body temperature, low blood sugar, low blood protein and infection. The brain damage resulting from kernicterus is often irreversible; it can cause various degrees of motor and mental retardation, leading to cerebral palsy and even death.

All current therapies for neonatal hyperbilirubinemia are based on the hope that if the level of bilirubin in the blood plasma can be kept from reaching between 10 and 15 milligrams per 100 milliliters until the maturing liver is able to remove the offending substance, there will be no brain damage. One widely used therapy involves exchange transfusions, in which jaundiced blood from the infant is completely replaced with normal blood from the donor.

Some years ago it was discovered that bilirubin in solution could be bleached by light and thus destroyed; the nature of the photodecomposition products remains unknown. This observation prompted R. J. Cremer, P. W. Perryman and D. H. Richards, who were then working at the General Hospital at Rockford in England, to see if light might be effective in lowering the plasma bilirubin in infants suffering from hyperbilirubinemia. That possibility was supported by informal observations that newborn infants whose crib had been placed near an open window tended to show less evidence of jaundice than infants whose crib was less exposed to light. Perhaps sunlight was accelerating

the destruction of bilirubin. If it was, it should be possible to reproduce the effect with artificial light.

The efficacy of light therapy was fully confirmed in a controlled study conducted by Jerold F. Lucey of the University of Vermont College of Medicine. The treatment consists in exposing jaundiced infants to light for three or four days, or until their liver is able to metabolize bilirubin. Although it was initially assumed that the light converted the bilirubin into nontoxic products that could be excreted, it now turns out that a major fraction of the excreted material is unchanged bilirubin itself. Hence it is at least conceivable that phototherapy has a direct beneficial effect on the liver and the kidneys.

Many questions remain concerning the mechanism of phototherapy for hyperbilirubinemia and the long-term effectiveness of that therapy in protecting infants against brain damage. Blue light is the most effective in decomposing pure solutions of bilirubin. In clinical tests, however, full-spectrum white light in almost any reasonable dosage (continuous, intermittent or in brief strong pulses) has proved effective in lowering plasma-bilirubin levels, regardless of the fraction of the radiant energy that falls in the blue region of the spectrum. Thus the mechanism by which light destroys bilirubin in infants may differ from the simple photochemical reaction that takes place in a test tube. For example, a photosensitization reaction, perhaps mediated by circulating riboflavin, may underlie the desirable effect. Another possibility is that the light may act on the

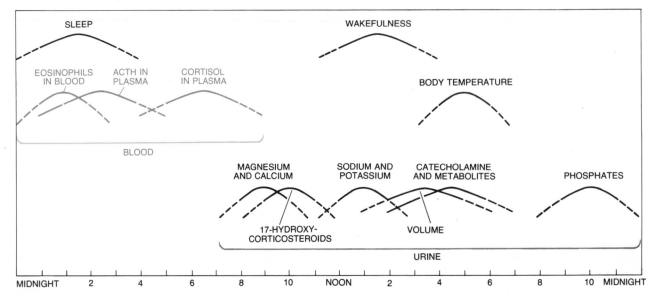

DAILY RHYTHMS are characteristic of many human physiological functions. Whether these 24-hour rhythms are produced by the daily light-dark cycle or are simply entrained by that cycle remains to be unequivocally established. Each curve represents the typical daily peak for a physiological state or for the levels of particular substances that circulate in the blood or are excreted in the urine.

plasma albumin to which most of the circulating bilirubin is bound. Alternatively the physiologically effective wavelength may be not in the blue region at all but in some other region of the spectrum, still to be identified, that is present in all the white-light sources.

The observation that ordinary sunlight or artificial light sources can drastically alter the plasma level of even one body compound (in this case bilirubin) opens a Pandora's box for the student of human biology. It presents the strong possibility that the plasma or tissue levels of many additional compounds are similarly affected by light. Some such responses must be physiologically advantageous, but some may not be.

Let us turn now to the indirect effects of light, those associated in one way or another with biological rhythms. The amount of time that all mammals are exposed to light varies with two cycles: the 24-hour cycle of day and night and the annual cycle of changing day length. (Even at the Equator there are small seasonal variations in the light-dark cycle.) These light cycles appear to be associated with many rhythmic changes in mammalian biological functions. Physical activity, sleep, food consumption, water intake, body temperature and the rates at which many glands secrete hormones all vary with periods that approximate 24 hours.

In human beings, for example, the concentration of cortisol, one of the principal hormones produced by the adrenal cortex, varies with a 24-hour rhythm [see *illustration on opposite page*]. The level is at a maximum in the morning hours, soon after waking, and drops to a minimum in the evening. When people reverse their activity cycle, by working at night and sleeping during the day, the plasma-cortisol rhythm takes from five to 10 days to adapt to the new conditions. When the cortisol level is studied in rats, it is found that the rhythm persists in animals that are blinded but not in animals kept under continuous illumination. Blindness in human beings seems to upset the rhythm, so that the times of the daily peaks and valleys are out of phase with the normal pattern and may even vary from day to day.

Among the rhythmic functions that can be closely studied in one and the same animal (specifically rhythms in sleep, physical activity and food consumption) it has been shown that in the absence of cyclic exposure to light the rhythms become "circadian" (that is, their periods become approximately 24

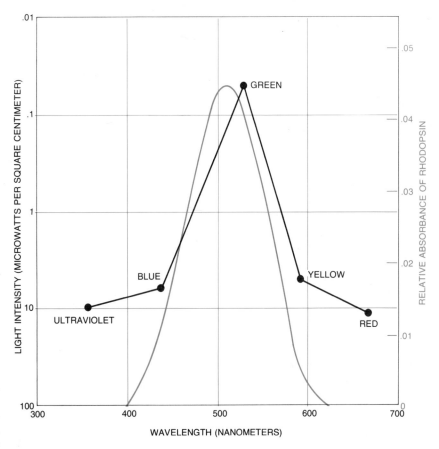

BODY-TEMPERATURE RHYTHM IN RATS, which follows a 24-hour cycle, can be altered by shifting the hours of the light-dark cycle. The author and his colleagues have found that green light is much more effective in establishing a new rhythm than radiation of other wavelengths (red, yellow, blue or ultraviolet). Black curve estimates the wavelength and intensity needed to establish a new 24-hour rhythm in half of an experimental group of rats. It closely follows the relative sensitivity of rhodopsin from rat retinas (*curve in color*).

hours in length rather than exactly). The fact that such rhythms can "free-run" suggests that they are not simply reflex responses to 24-hour cycles of light or some other environmental component. The factors responsible for the rhythms are not yet known; they might include other cyclic inputs such as the consumption of food or the intake of water, which also free-run in the absence of light. Some investigators are convinced that the rhythms are generated by intrinsic oscillators, commonly called biological clocks.

Little is known about the action spectra or the light intensities needed either to generate or to "entrain" (synchronize) daily rhythms in mammals. There is strong presumptive evidence, however, that in most mammals light exerts its effects indirectly through photoreceptors in the eye. It is not known whether the photoreceptors are the same ones (the rods and the cones) that mediate vision, discharging into nonvisual pathways, or

whether they are a distinct family of photoreceptors with their own neural network.

In our laboratory at M.I.T. we have investigated the daily rhythmicity in the body temperature of rats to see what colors of light are most effective in inducing a change in rhythm to a new light-dark cycle and what intensities are needed. The body temperature of rats normally rises by one or two degrees C. at the onset of darkness and falls again at daybreak. We found that green light is the most potent in changing the phase of the temperature cycle and that ultraviolet and red wavelengths are the least potent. The action spectrum plotted from these results closely follows the absorption spectrum for rhodopsin, the photosensitive pigment in the rods of the retina [see *illustration above*]. In separate studies a similar action spectrum, peaking in the green, was found for the wavelengths of light that are most effective in inhibiting the function

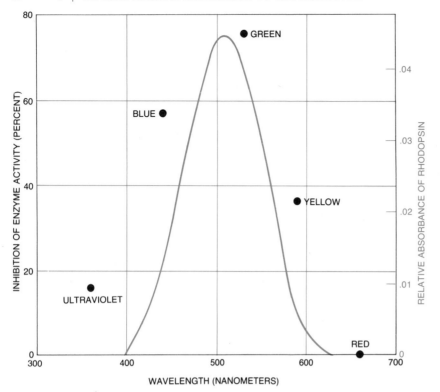

PINEAL ACTIVITY OF RATS can be suppressed by exposing the animals continuously to light. As in the case of the daily temperature rhythm, green light is more effective than light of other spectral colors in suppressing the organ's enzyme activity, as is shown by the labeled dots. The enzyme that is measured is the melatonin-forming enzyme hydroxyindole-O-methyltransferase. Presumably the suppression is mediated by rhodopsin (*curve in color*).

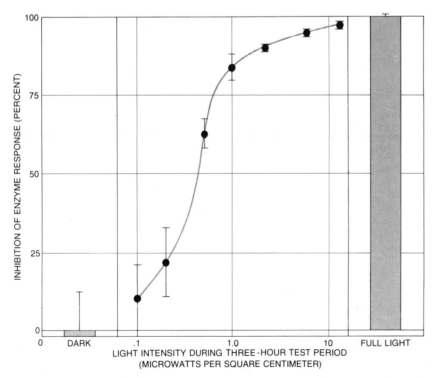

GRADATION IN LIGHT INTENSITY leads to proportional inhibition in the activity of the rat's pineal gland, indicating that light controls synthesis of the pineal hormone, melatonin. Rats that had been kept in constant light for 48 hours were exposed to various light intensities for the next three hours. Their pineals were then analyzed for serotonin-N-acetyltransferase, an enzyme that participates in melatonin synthesis, with the results plotted here.

of the pineal gland of rats [*see top illustration at right*].

Cycles in environmental lighting can interact with biological rhythms in two ways. The light cycle may directly induce the rhythm, in which case either continuous light or darkness should rapidly abolish it, or the cycle may simply entrain the biological rhythm so that all animals of a given species exhibit maximums or minimums at about the same time of day or night. In the latter case the rhythmicity itself may be generated by a cyclic input other than light, either exogenous (for example food intake) or endogenous (a biological clock). If the cycle is simply entrained by light, an environment of continuous light or darkness might not extinguish it. In human beings psychosocial factors are probably of greater importance than light cycles in generating or synchronizing biological rhythms. The biological utility of even so dramatic a rhythm as that of sleep and wakefulness, for example, remains to be discovered.

Annual rhythms in sexual activity, hibernation and migratory behavior are widespread among animals. The rhythms enable members of a species to synchronize their activities with respect to one another and to the exigencies of the environment. For example, sheep ovulate and can be fertilized only in the fall, thus anticipating the spring by many months, when food will be available to the mother for nursing the newborn. In man no annual rhythms have been firmly established, except, of course, those (such as in sun-tanning and vitamin D_3 levels) that are directly correlated with exposure to summer sunlight.

The best-characterized indirect effect of light on any process other than vision is probably the inhibition of melatonin synthesis by the pineal organ of mammals. Although melatonin seems to be the major pineal hormone, its precise role has not yet been established. When melatonin is administered experimentally, it has several effects on the brain: it induces sleep, modifies the electroencephalogram and raises the levels of serotonin, a neurotransmitter. In addition melatonin inhibits ovulation and modifies the secretion of other hormones from such organs as the pituitary, the gonads and the adrenals, probably by acting on neuroendocrine control centers in the brain.

Experiments performed on rats and other small mammals during the past decade provide compelling evidence that the synthesis of melatonin is suppressed by nerve impulses that reach the pineal over pathways of the sympathetic nervous system. These impulses in turn vary inversely with the amount of visible light impinging on the retina. In rats the pineal function is depressed to half its maximum level when the animals are subjected to an amount of white light only slightly greater than that shed by the full moon on a clear night [*see bottom illustration on preceding page*]. A multisynaptic neuronal system mediates the effects of light on the pineal. The pathway involved, which is apparently unique to mammals, differs from the route taken by the nerve impulses responsible for vision.

Quite recently Harry Lynch, Michael Moskowitz and I have found a daily rhythm in the rate at which normal human subjects excrete melatonin. During the third of the day corresponding to the bedtime hours, 11:00 P.M. to 7:00 A.M., the level of melatonin in the urine is much higher than it is in any other eight-hour period [*see illustration at right*]. It remains to be determined whether the rhythm in melatonin excretion in humans is induced by light or is simply entrained by it.

In some birds and reptiles the pineal responds directly to light, thereby serving as a photoreceptive "third eye" that sends messages about light levels to the brain. In the pineal organ of mammals any trace of a direct response to light is lost. Evidently photoreceptors in the retina mediate the control of the pineal by light. Since, as I have noted, the function of the pineal in rats is influenced most strongly by green light, corresponding to the peak sensitivity of the rod pigment rhodopsin, the retinal photoreceptor would seem to be a rod cell, at least in this species.

Light levels and rhythms influence the maturation and subsequent cyclic activity in the gonads of all mammals and birds examined so far. The particular response of each species to light seems to depend on whether the species is monestrous or polyestrous, that is, on whether it normally ovulates once a year (in the spring or fall) or at regular intervals throughout the year. Examples of polyestrous species are rats (ovulation every four or five days), guinea pigs (every 12 to 14 days) and humans (every 21 to 40 days). The gonadal responses also seem to depend on whether the members of the species are physically active during the daylight hours or during the night. Recently Leona Zacharias and I had the opportunity to examine more than a score of girls and women (members of a diurnally active polyestrous species) who had become blind in the

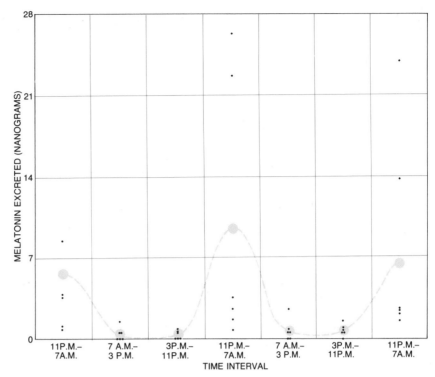

RHYTHM IN MELATONIN SECRETION in human beings has been found by the author and his colleagues. The black dots show the melatonin content of urine samples from six subjects during consecutive eight-hour periods. The colored circles and broken curve correspond to the mean values. High values that were recorded for the 11:00-P.M.-to-7:00-A.M. samples suggest that synthesis of melatonin in man, as in rats, increases with onset of darkness.

first year of life. We observed that gonadal maturation had in general occurred earlier in this group than in normal girls. In contrast, in rats (a polyestrous species that is active at night) blindness delays maturation, and continuous illumination accelerates the maturation of weanlings with normal vision.

The gonads of most birds and of most diurnally active, monestrous animals (the ferret, for instance) mature in the spring, in response to the gradual increase in day length. Ovulation can be accelerated in such animals by exposing them to artificially long days. The annual gonadal activity in domestic sheep, on the other hand, occurs in the fall, in response to the decrease in day length. The mechanisms that cause some species to be monestrous and others polyestrous, or that cause some animals to sleep by day and others by night, are entirely unknown, as are the factors that cause the gonadal responses of various species to light to vary as widely as they do.

The multiple and disparate effects of light I have described support the view that the design of light environments should incorporate considerations of human health as well as visual and aesthetic concerns. We have learned that the chemical constituents of the environment in the form of food, drugs and pollutants must be monitored and regulated by agencies with suitable powers of enforcement. A major part of their responsibility is to see that nothing harmful is put into food or drugs and that nothing essential is left out of food. The food and drug industries, for their part, look to public and private research organizations, including their own laboratories, for intellectual guidance in creating wholesome and beneficial (as well as profitable) products.

In contrast, only minuscule sums have been expended to characterize and exploit the biological effects of light, and very little has been done to protect citizens against potentially harmful or biologically inadequate lighting environments. Both government and industry have been satisfied to allow people who buy electric lamps—first the incandescent ones and now the fluorescent—to serve as the unwitting subjects in a long-term experiment on the effects of artificial lighting environments on human health. We have been lucky, perhaps, in that so far the experiment has had no demonstrably baneful effects. One hopes that this casual attitude will change. Light is potentially too useful an agency of human health not to be more effectively examined and exploited.

2   Nonvisual Light Reception

by Michael Menaker
March 1972

In the brains of some vertebrates are unidentified organs that respond to daylight. Experiments with blinded birds demonstrate that these organs control biological rhythms

Pattern vision, which we regard as being synonymous with seeing, is so important for our conscious perception of the world that we tend to assume that all effects of light are mediated by the retina of the eye and the associated areas of the brain. It may seem surprising, therefore, that the behavior of many animals with image-forming eyes is regulated by light in ways that do not depend on the perception of a visual pattern but only on the organism's ability to distinguish between light and dark.

The behavior that is regulated in this nonvisual manner is of two quite distinct kinds: day-to-day and year-to-year. For example, in most animals the 24-hour cycle of alternating light and darkness serves to synchronize certain physiological activities so that the rhythms of these activities also follow a cycle that is exactly 24 hours in length. Such rhythms are driven by a "biological clock," which, although it is precise in its own way, does not keep a 24-hour schedule. In the absence of cues from the environment, such as the natural daily cycle of light and darkness, the biological clock has a period close to, but not exactly, 24 hours. The rhythms the clock controls are therefore called circadian, from the Latin words for "approximately" and "day." When environmental cues are absent, the circadian cycle is "free-running."

In nature the free-running rhythms are forced by the cycle of night and day to maintain a length of cycle that exactly matches the natural 24-hour cycle. The process that synchronizes circadian rhythms in this precise way is called entrainment.

Many animals also respond to changes in the length of day and night that have a seasonal cycle. For example, the length of the day can serve as a reliable cue for the regulation and timing of reproductive cycles and other physiological processes that must be correlated with different times of the year. This response to seasonal changes in the length of the day is somewhat loosely called photoperiodism. The fact that plants as well as animals exhibit both photoperiodism and entrainment with respect to the daily cycle of light and darkness demonstrates that an organized eye is not essential for coupling an organism to the light cycles of the environment. Nevertheless, the effort to demonstrate a nonretinal photoreceptor in animals, particularly the higher vertebrates, has long been marked by controversy.

It is well established that among fishes, amphibians and reptiles the pineal organ, a small structure embedded in the top of the brain, and such associated structures as the parietal "eye" are sensitive to light. The function of the pineal organ in the life of the lower vertebrates remains uncertain, and it has not been shown that the structure acts as a light detector in either birds or mammals. In 1935 Jacques Benoit, who was then working at the University of Strasbourg Medical School, reported finding a light-sensitive area in the brain of Pekin ducks; direct illumination of the duck's head stimulates the growth of the duck's testes. Testis growth in ducks is a normal response to long days. Benoit's work was the first indication that complex image-forming eyes, in animals that possess them, are not necessarily the exclusive mediator of photoperiodism. Although Benoit and his colleagues have persevered in their study of extraretinal photoreception and have uncovered many fascinating phenomena, the photodetecting structure itself has not been identified.

Until 1967, when we began studying extraretinal photoreception in house sparrows at the University of Texas, Benoit's experiments had not been repeated outside his laboratory. Although ducks have some advantages as experimental animals, they also present certain technical difficulties. They are not only relatively large but also they (and many other birds) will not eat if they are kept in the dark or if they are blind. Because ducks are inconveniently large and because Benoit had to feed his ducks by hand the number he could maintain and study at any one time was limited. The difficulty of working with such animals may have discouraged other physiologists from repeating Benoit's experiments.

My students and I did not set out to repeat Benoit's experiments when we first began working with house sparrows. Our original intention was to investigate photoperiodism: the mechanism that enables birds with normal vision to synchronize their reproductive activities with the changing seasons. Knowing little about birds, we picked the house sparrow (*Passer domesticus*) primarily because of its toughness, adaptability and continuous availability. The house sparrow turned out to be a fortunate choice for quite different reasons.

Our experimental plan called for us to measure both a circadian rhythm and a photoperiodic response simultaneously in the same bird. Although there was a literature on photoperiodism in sparrows, there was no previous work on circadian rhythms. We therefore began to collect baseline data by recording the sparrow's locomotor activity when the ratio of light to darkness was varied artificially.

We used a reliable, automatic and rather inexpensive experimental chamber that had worked well with perching birds in other laboratories. Each bird is

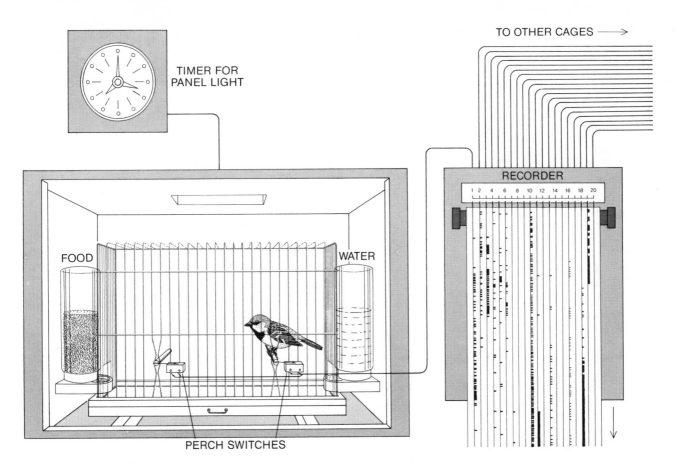

TIMER FOR PANEL LIGHT

TO OTHER CAGES ⟶

RECORDER

1 2 4 6 8 10 12 14 16 18 20

FOOD

WATER

PERCH SWITCHES

RECORDING CAGE housed each of the sparrows used as subjects in the investigation. Movement of the bird from perch to perch or to its supply of food or water closed switch contacts and sent a signal to a recording pen that marked all such activity over a 24-hour period on a revolving drum. When a series of 24-hour records was assembled (*see illustration below*), the bird's near-to-daily, or "circadian," rhythmic pattern of activity and rest was seen to persist over long periods of time. It was also found that the bird's circadian rhythm, although readily shifted, would persist in continuous darkness or when blinded birds were the subjects.

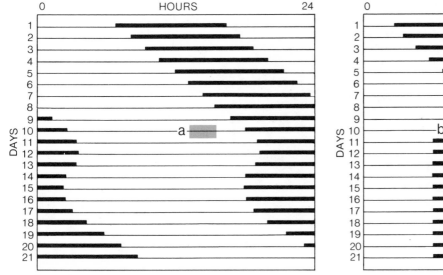
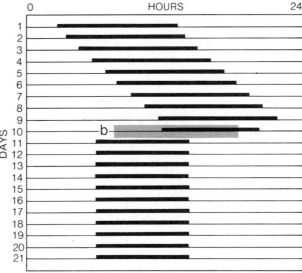

DIFFERING PROPERTIES of circadian rhythms allowed an assessment of the nonretinal response to light by blinded sparrows. If a normal bird is kept in continuous darkness (*left*), its circadian rhythm becomes "free-running"; its daily periods of activity are unchanged in duration but start a little later each day. Even one brief exposure to light (*a*), however, will "reset" a free-running rhythm. The crucial role of light in governing circadian rhythm is further demonstrated (*right*) with respect to "entrainment." When a cage is illuminated for a set time each day (*b*), the occupant's activity develops an equally regular, although not necessarily synchronous, relation with the light cycle: it is entrained. If a blinded, regularly free-running sparrow should react to the cyclic illumination of its cage by exhibiting an entrained pattern of activity, it would be evidence that it is capable of nonretinal light perception.

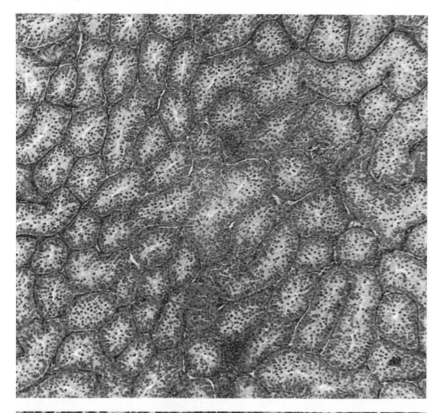

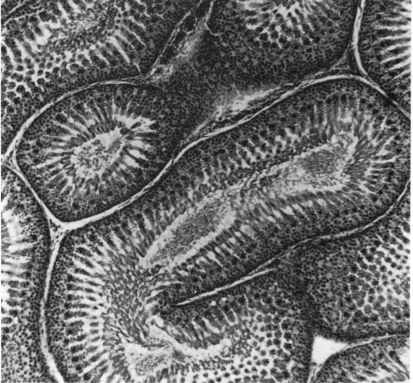

QUIESCENT AND ENLARGED TESTES of sparrows, shown in section in these micrographs, are proof that a seasonal readiness to mate, although stimulated by longer hours of daylight, does not depend on the birds' eyesight; the donors of these specimens were blinded before the experiment began. Each bird was exposed for two months to a "day" of predetermined length in the laboratory. A bird illuminated for only six out of every 24 hours produced the testis tissue at top; the many small tubules are no more developed than those in the testes of blinded birds kept in continuous darkness for the same period. The tissue at bottom, seen at the same magnification, contains very large tubules. The donor's "days" were 16 hours long, and the testis development equals that of normal wild sparrows when they react to the longer hours of daylight that prepare them to mate.

individually housed in a lightproof box equipped with overhead lights operated by a timer. When the bird is active, it jumps on and off the perches in its cage a good deal of the time. The perches are connected to microswitches that automatically relay the bird's movements to a strip-chart recorder [see top illustration on preceding page].

Circadian rhythms are so widespread among animals that we were not surprised to find them in the house sparrow. Its locomotor rhythm is readily entrained by artificial light cycles. If the phase of the entraining cycle is shifted, there are three to six transient, or intermediate, cycles before the bird reorients its activity to the new regime. The phase angle, or temporal relation, between the entraining light cycle and the locomotor rhythm depends on several factors, chiefly the period at which the light cycle is presented and on the ratio of light to darkness.

If a bird that has been entrained to a particular light cycle is suddenly placed in constant darkness, the rhythm persists indefinitely with a period that is no longer exactly 24 hours long and that reflects the free-running rate of its internal clock. If a bird that is free-running in constant darkness is then exposed to light for a single interval of a few hours' duration, the bird responds with several transient cycles that lead to a shift in the phase of its free-running locomotor rhythm [see bottom illustration on preceding page]. If a free-running bird is placed in dim constant light, the length of the free-running period is found to depend on the light intensity. In moderately bright constant light free-running birds become continuously active and therefore arhythmic.

Other investigators have reported similar responses to artificial light cycles in the circadian rhythms of many other animals and plants. The observations raise fundamental questions about the nature of the responding biological clock or clocks. Here it is sufficient to note two facts that emerged early in our own work. The first is that house sparrows live perfectly well in constant darkness, untended except for a monthly change of food and water. The second fact is that their free-running period in constant darkness is seldom if ever exactly 24 hours. It is therefore possible to use entrainment to test for the existence of photoreception. The difference between an entrained bird and a free-running one is immediately obvious from inspection of the strip-chart record of locomotor activity. A bird will clearly not be entrained to a light cycle it cannot perceive.

The observation that the house sparrow lives well in constant darkness suggested to us that it would also tolerate being blinded. In fact, maintaining blinded sparrows turned out to be no more difficult than maintaining blinded rats or blinded mice. With characteristic adaptability our blinded sparrows learned the location not only of their food and water jars but also of their perches. They stayed healthy indefinitely and continued to produce activity records.

Knowing of Benoit's work with ducks, we placed a sparrow that had been blinded by bilateral optic enucleation in one of our experimental chambers and set the light timers, as we had done so often with birds that could see. Almost immediately the blind sparrow became entrained to the artificial light cycle. Further experiments showed that blinded birds followed the imposed light cycles no matter how the cycles were phased with respect to the real day [*see illustration on next page*].

It was always possible, of course, that the blinded birds were responding not to the light cycle but to secondary cues. We noted, for example, that the fluorescent lamps used in the experimental chambers produced a slight hum and raised the temperature in the chamber one or two degrees Celsius. In an early control experiment we found that if we wrapped the lamps with black tape, the birds no longer became entrained to the light-dark cycle. When we unwrapped the lamps, entrainment promptly followed. The wrapping eliminates both visible and ultraviolet radiation but does not affect the sound or the temperature rise produced by the lamp. Although the wrapping distorts infrared emission, it does not eliminate it. The results of the experiment were consistent with the hypothesis that the sparrows, although blind, were able to perceive visible light.

We had at this point in our study no idea about the sensitivity of whatever sensory system was involved. We therefore decided to try a much dimmer light source that in addition had a less complex emission spectrum. For other reasons entirely we had already built into our light-controlled boxes exactly the kind of light source we needed: small electroluminescent panels made by Sylvania, widely sold as "Nite-Lites." These panels produce a rather narrow band of radiation that peaks in the green part of the spectrum; they produce no sound,

do not heat the chamber and emit negligible amounts of ultraviolet or infrared radiation. Furthermore, they produce only a thousandth as much visible light as the fluorescent lamps.

The amount of electroluminescent light received by our birds was roughly equivalent in intensity, although not in color, to bright moonlight. When we exposed blind sparrows to 12 hours of this faint light alternating with 12 hours of darkness, we found that about half of the birds became entrained and that the other half ignored the cycle and remained free-running as if they were in constant darkness. With this series of experiments we not only had strengthened the case for our hypothesis that sparrows possess a nonvisual light detector, which by this time we had begun to call the extraretinal receptor for entrainment, but also we had accidentally determined a crude operational threshold for the level at which the receptor begins to function.

We were now compelled to take seriously a suggestion by one of our more skeptical colleagues that the entire phenomenon was being caused by the sparrow's numerous ectoparasites, which were somehow transmitting information about the light cycle to their host. It was certainly conceivable that the ectoparasites might be roused even by dim light and that their activity would in turn rouse the sparrows. No matter what measures we took, we could never be certain that our sparrows were completely free of parasites. On the other hand, removing as many of them as we could did nothing to alter the entrainment behavior in the slightest. We were finally able to convince ourselves we

were dealing with a genuine extraretinal receptor on the basis of another series of experiments.

The new experiments were undertaken by Henry Keatts and me with the primary purpose of anatomically localizing the assumed photoreceptor. Again using electroluminescent light panels to provide the light cycle, we reduced the light intensity by adding pieces of black tape to the panel until, by becoming free-running, each blind bird demonstrated that it was not perceiving the light. Since we suspected that the light receptor was in the bird's brain, we looked for ways to manipulate the amount of light penetrating the skull.

When we plucked feathers from the top of the birds' heads, birds that had previously been free-running became entrained to the light cycle. Feathers plucked from other parts of the body had no effect. Later we measured the amount of light shielding normally provided by the head feathers and were surprised to find that between 100 and 1,000 times more light reached the top surface of the brain when the birds' heads were plucked.

The next step was to restore the opacity of the birds' heads and see if we could reverse the effect of plucking. We did this by injecting small amounts of India ink under the skin of the bald birds and massaging the skin to produce a fairly uniform layer of ink between the skin and the skull. Birds so treated lost their sensitivity to light and again became free-running. Finally we removed a flap of skin and the ink under it; the birds again became entrained to the cycle of very dim light that had been present throughout the experiments.

We were now fairly confident that

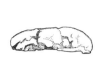
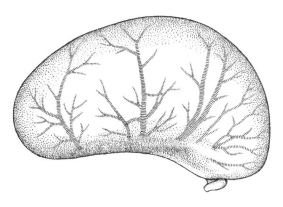

EFFECT OF LIGHT in stimulating testis growth through some kind of nonvisual channel was demonstrated in the 1930's by the French biologist Jacques Benoit, who used ducks as experimental animals. The two testes reproduced here are seen one-third larger than actual size; the smaller is from a normal duck that had its head and eyes shielded from light during 28 nights of artificial illumination. The larger is from a blinded duck that was left bareheaded during 27 nights of illumination. Its testes became as big as a breeding duck's.

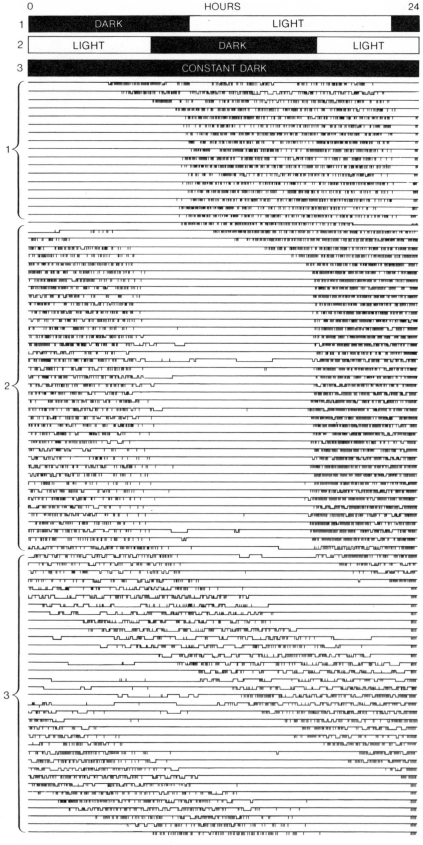

1   DARK   LIGHT

2   LIGHT   DARK   LIGHT

3   CONSTANT DARK

TWO ENTRAINMENTS appear in this consecutive record of a blinded sparrow's activity over a three-month period. At the start the daily period of cage illumination lasted from late morning to late evening (*Bar 1*) and the bird's circadian rhythm of activity soon came to match this period. After 18 days the pattern was shifted so that nights were illuminated and days were dark (*Bar 2*); prompt entrainment to the new pattern followed. When, 39 days later, the cage was darkened permanently (*Bar 3*), the rhythm became free-running.

light sensitivity was mediated by a photoreceptor in the brain similar to the one reported by Benoit in Pekin ducks but coupled to a different physiological system. In an attempt to further localize the receptor in sparrows we removed the pineal organ, a structure about the size of a mustard seed, from some of our blind sparrows to see if their light perception would be abolished. Entrainment persisted, ruling out the pineal as the sole site of photoreception in the brain. The interpretation of the result of these experiments, however, is complicated by the fact that removal of the pineal organ interferes with the circadian rhythm of locomotor activity itself. We cannot yet rule out the possibility that the pineal organ of sparrows, like the pineal of lower vertebrates, is photoreceptive and may constitute a part of a complex extraretinal photoreceptor for entrainment.

The eyes as well as the extraretinal photoreceptor appear to be involved in the light perception that affects the locomotor rhythm. Although the threshold for entrainment of blind birds is surprisingly low, the threshold of sighted birds is lower still: all sighted birds will entrain to the light from a single electroluminescent panel (about .1 lux, or .01 foot-candle), whereas only about half of blind birds will do so. Moreover, whereas sighted birds become continuously active in constant light of 50 to 500 lux, the activity of blind birds is still rhythmic at 2,000 lux or more. The relative contribution of the eyes and the extraretinal receptor, as well as the location of the extraretinal receptor in the brain and its physiology, remain subjects for continuing research.

Early in the course of our work with sparrows we naturally asked ourselves if brain photoreception was involved in the reproductive response to day length, as it is in ducks. Like most birds of the Temperate Zones, the house sparrow shows a dramatic seasonal cycle in the size and functional state of its gonads. In nature the timing of this cycle is largely regulated by the photoperiod; it can be readily manipulated in the laboratory merely by changing the length of the artificial days presented to the birds. Photoperiodism is least complex in male birds, and the most convenient indicator of the changes produced by light is the size or the weight of the testes.

Although many other organisms have annual reproductive cycles, birds in their seasonal changes in gonad weight surpass by orders of magnitude comparable changes found in other vertebrates. This is easy to understand: natural selection operates with particular stringency in flying animals to reduce total body weight and expenditure of energy. The gonads are an obvious target for such selection because they are active only during a short annual period. For eight months of the year the testes of wild sparrows represent a negligible fraction of the birds' total body weight of about 24 grams. During the breeding season the testes grow rapidly until they average close to a gram.

The annual regression of the gonads may enable the sparrow to survive with between 1 and 2 percent less food than it would otherwise need. If this does not seem like a very large saving, think of the commercial advantage that would accrue to a manufacturer who could reduce his budget for raw materials 2 percent below the budget of a competitor. Moreover, much of the effective reduction in energy requirement comes in winter, when food is scarce.

In order to learn whether or not the sparrow required a functioning retina to show testis growth in response to long days, we compared the response of a blind group and a sighted group to two months of artificial 16-hour days, beginning in the month of January. The testes of birds in both groups increased some 40 to 50 times in size. The testes of birds in two control groups, one normal and one blind, exposed to six-hour days for the same length of time showed no significant growth. In these initial experiments the number of birds used was too small to allow a quantitative comparison of the testis growth in blind and normal birds.

Herbert Underwood and I then conducted a series of experiments in which more than 500 birds were exposed to various lengths of day and intensities of light. The results demonstrated that the testes of blind and normal birds grew by the same amount and at the same rate when the birds were exposed equally to long days in winter. We concluded that sparrows, like ducks, have an extraretinal photoreceptor, presumably in the brain, that responds to seasonal changes in the number of daylight hours. We have called this receptor the extraretinal receptor for photoperiodism to emphasize that we reserve judgment about its relation to the extraretinal receptor for entrainment.

Our results led us to question whether the sparrow's eyes have anything at all to do with testis growth. In order to

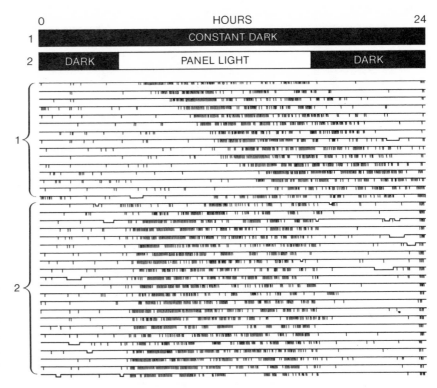

MUCH FAINTER LIGHT, which also caused neither noise nor a temperature change in the cages, was used to determine the minimum illumination threshold for response. The source was an electroluminescent panel, emitting light with about the intensity of bright moonlight. Of the 20 subjects of the experiment, roughly half responded as shown by this typical record: when a blinded sparrow, free-running for two weeks in the dark (Bar 1), was exposed to the faint panel light (Bar 2), its circadian rhythm was promptly entrained.

assess the role of the eyes one would like to remove the extraretinal receptor for photoperiodism. This we could not do, of course, because we did not know the receptor's precise location. Assuming that the receptor was somewhere in the brain, however, we could alter the amount of light reaching it without tampering with the amount of light reaching the eyes. Two experimental tricks were already open to us: we could pluck a bird's head feathers and thereby increase the amount of light passing through its skull, and by injecting India ink under the skin we could reduce the amount of light. We also knew from the work of George A. Bartholomew of the University of California at Los Angeles that in normal sparrows a light intensity of at least 10 lux is needed to stimulate slow but measurable growth of the testes.

Accordingly Richard Roberts, Jeffrey Elliot, Underwood and I set up an experiment in which two large groups of birds with normal sight and with gonads in the regressed condition were exposed to 16-hour days at a light intensity of 10 lux. We plucked the feathers from the heads of the birds in one group, effectively raising the light intensity above

10 lux, and injected ink under the skin of the fully feathered heads of the birds in the other group, effectively lowering the light intensity below the 10-lux threshold. Because the eyes of both groups were exposed to the 10-lux intensity, we reasoned that if birds' eyes were involved in photoperiodic photoreception, we should observe some testis growth in both groups. If, on the other hand, the eyes were not involved, we should see testis growth in the plucked birds and none in the India-ink group. This was exactly the result we obtained [see bottom illustration on page 21]. Furthermore, it indicates that the eyes are not involved in the photoperiodic response to light, although they are involved in entrainment.

At about the time we finished this study we learned of some ingenious experiments that had just been carried out at the University of Tokyo by Kazutaka Homma. He had made tiny beads incorporating a radioluminescent paint of the kind used to paint numerals on watch dials; he then implanted the beads in various regions of the brain and also directly in the eye of Japanese quail. Homma subjected his birds to short days,

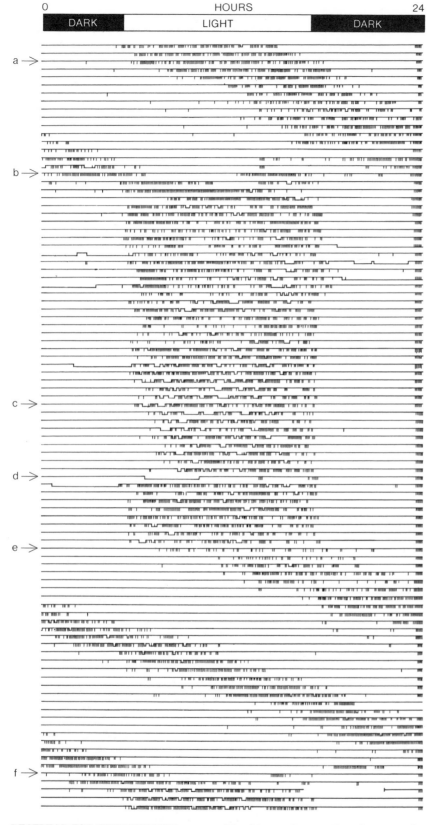

DARK   LIGHT   DARK

RECEPTOR FOR ENTRAINMENT was proved by this experiment and similar ones to lie somewhere within the sparrow's skull. Light far weaker than the previously determined threshold value illuminated the cages throughout the experiment. When feathers were plucked from the birds' backs (*a*), their free-running rhythm stayed unchanged, but when the head feathers were plucked (*b*), entrainment followed. After 30 days (*c*) regrowth of the feathers started to affect entrainment, but a second plucking (*d*) restored it. When injections of ink made the birds' skulls opaque to light (*e*), the sparrows' rhythm became free-running again. When the ink was removed (*f*), however, entrainment was reestablished.

which would not normally cause their gonads to grow. He could thereby determine if the continuous light emanating from the luminous beads had any growth-stimulating effect. The experiments disclosed two general regions of the quail brain whose stimulation by light induced growth of the gonads. Homma also found that placing the luminous beads in the birds' eyes had no effect.

Our results with sparrows and Homma's with quail both argue very strongly that photoperiodic photoreception is mediated exclusively by brain receptors without any participation by the retina. Benoit, however, has maintained for some time that in ducks both the eyes and a brain photoreceptor are involved. He has come to this conclusion on the basis of experiments in which ducks with severed optic nerves showed slower testis growth in response to light than intact animals did. Do these conflicting results merely reflect differences among the species of bird used in the experiments?

Perhaps, but it also seems possible that the experiments can be reconciled. In a recent extension of their earlier work Benoit, Ivan Assenmacher and their colleagues have come to the conclusion that the retinal response in ducks is much less sensitive to light than the response of the brain photoreceptor and that, unlike the brain receptor, the retina is sensitive only in the orange-red region of the spectrum. If this is true, then neither our results nor Homma's have adequately ruled out retinal participation. Homma's radioluminous beads emit only a very dim light. Our own experiments were based on threshold values that Bartholomew obtained with "daylight" fluorescent sources, whereas our experiments were performed with "cool white" fluorescent lights. Because the "daylight" bulbs emit more strongly in the red than "cool white" sources, it seems possible that there was not enough red light present in our experimental conditions to stimulate the red-sensitive retinal photoreceptors, but that enough light of other wavelengths was present to stimulate the brain receptor, with its greater sensitivity and range of response. If Benoit's proposed red-sensitive retinal receptors do exist generally among birds, their adaptive significance, when it is discovered, ought to be of great interest. Considering the degree of skepticism with which Benoit's findings were first greeted by biologists in 1935, it seems ironic that today it is the role of the eyes and not the existence of brain photoreception that still remains unresolved.

Extraretinal photoreception is not limited to birds. It is common in the invertebrates and may be a very general phenomenon among vertebrates. Underwood and I have shown in experiments with three species of lizard that locomotor rhythms can be entrained by artificial light cycles even after one has removed the lizards' two eyes and also the parietal "eye" on top of the head and the associated pineal organ. Other workers have reported various effects of light on the behavior of blinded fish and amphibians.

Working with sensitive photocells, William F. Ganong of the University of California School of Medicine in San Francisco has measured the penetration of visible light into the brain of the sheep, but in spite of a few tantalizing studies no one has yet demonstrated a clear-cut physiological response to extraretinally perceived light in any mammal. There are, in fact, several studies indicating that the circadian rhythms of blind mammals do not entrain to light cycles even when the light level is very high. Although it is too early to be certain, it seems possible that mammals are exceptional in not utilizing brain photoreceptors to mediate entrainment.

Many people, even when they are faced with the kind of evidence presented here, have difficulty accepting the fact that visible light does penetrate through structures they have always thought of as being opaque. The simplest way to remove any lingering doubts one may have on this score is to perform an experiment that most of us have done as children but have forgotten because the results appear to conflict with our everyday experience. In a completely dark room place an ordinary flashlight against your palm, switch it on and look at the back of your hand. This should convince you that light does penetrate living tissue, and furthermore that it is the long wavelengths that penetrate best. In effect the human hand, although it is almost an inch thick, is a moderately transparent red filter. The experiments described here, in addition to raising many specific questions concerning the ways in which environmental light cycles control rhythmic and reproductive events, underline the fact, of more general concern to biologists, that energy in the visible portion of the spectrum may well have effects on the activities of cells once thought to be completely shielded from it.

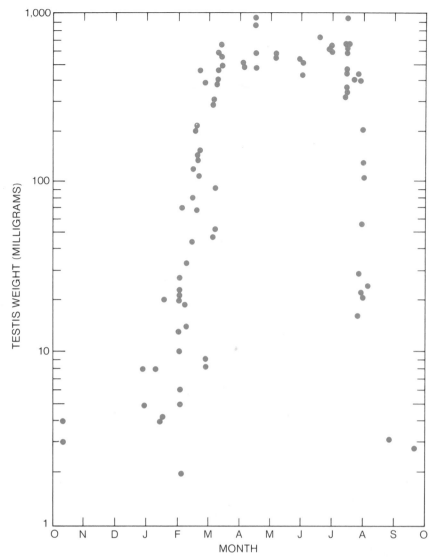

SEASONAL TESTIS GROWTH in a population of wild house sparrows in Texas begins in January and February and peaks in March and April. Regression, a return to nonmating dimensions, starts in July and early August. Each dot on the graph records the combined weight of the testes of one bird captured at the time indicated; the scale is logarithmic.

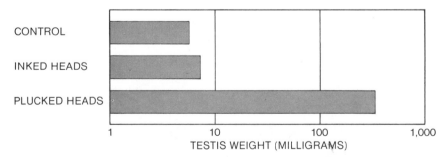

FINAL DEMONSTRATION proved that, like the receptor governing entrainment, the one governing testis growth must be located somewhere within the sparrow's skull. The subjects whose testis weight scarcely exceeded five milligrams (top bar) were a control group; these birds were sacrificed before the start of the experiment. The subjects whose testis weight remained below 10 milligrams (center bar) retained normal vision but, like the blinded birds in the preceding entrainment experiment, they were given ink injections to render their skulls opaque. The third group also had normal vision (bottom bar), but like the blinded birds in the preceding experiment their head feathers were plucked. Their testes enlarged greatly. Because both the inked and the plucked birds' vision was normal the experiment proves that eyesight is not involved in the birds' photoperiodic response.

3

The Reproductive Behavior of Ring Doves

by Daniel S. Lehrman
November 1964

An account of experiments showing that the changes in activity that constitute the behavior cycle are governed by interactions of outside stimuli, the hormones and the behavior of each mate

In recent years the study of animal behavior has proceeded along two different lines, with two groups of investigators formulating problems in different ways and indeed approaching the problems from different points of view. The comparative psychologist traditionally tends first to ask a question and then to attack it by way of animal experimentation. The ethologist, on the other hand, usually begins by observing the normal activity of an animal and then seeks to identify and analyze specific behavior patterns characteristic of the species.

The two attitudes can be combined. The psychologist can begin, like the ethologist, by watching an animal do what it does naturally, and only then ask questions that flow from his observations. He can go on to manipulate experimental conditions in an effort to discover the psychological and biological events that give rise to the behavior under study and perhaps to that of other animals as well. At the Institute of Animal Behavior at Rutgers University we have taken this approach to study in detail the reproductive-behavior cycle of the ring dove (*Streptopelia risoria*). The highly specific changes in behavior that occur in the course of the cycle, we find, are governed by complex psycho-

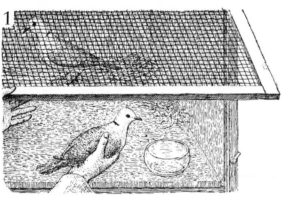 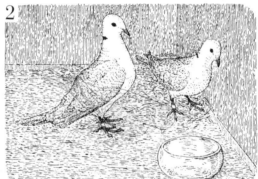 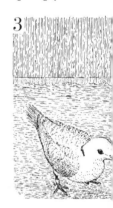

REPRODUCTIVE-BEHAVIOR CYCLE begins soon after a male and a female ring dove are introduced into a cage containing nest-ing material (hay in this case) and an empty glass nest bowl (*1*). Courtship activity, on the first day, is characterized by the "bowing

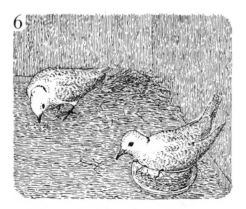 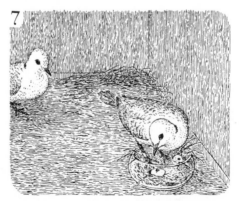 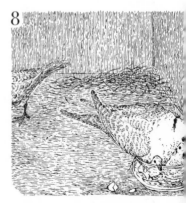

CYCLE CONTINUES as the adult birds take turns incubating the eggs (*6*), which hatch after about 14 days (*7*). The newly hatched squabs are fed "crop-milk," a liquid secreted in the gullets of the adults (*8*). The parents continue to feed them, albeit reluctantly,

biological interactions of the birds' inner and outer environments.

The ring dove, a small relative of the domestic pigeon, has a light gray back, creamy underparts and a black semicircle (the "ring") around the back of its neck. The male and female look alike and can only be distinguished by surgical exploration. If we place a male and a female ring dove with previous breeding experience in a cage containing an empty glass bowl and a supply of nesting material, the birds invariably enter on their normal behavioral cycle, which follows a predictable course and a fairly regular time schedule. During the first day the principal activity is courtship: the male struts around, bowing and cooing at the female. After several hours the birds announce their selection of a nest site (which in nature would be a concave place and in our cages is the glass bowl) by crouching in it and uttering a distinctive coo. Both birds participate in building the nest, the male usually gathering material and carrying it to the female, who stands in the bowl and constructs the nest. After a week or more of nest-building, in the course of which the birds copulate, the female becomes noticeably more attached to the nest and difficult to dislodge; if one attempts to lift her off the nest, she may grasp it with her claws and take it along. This behavior usually indicates that the female is about to lay her eggs. Between seven and 11 days after the beginning of the courtship she produces her first egg, usually at about five o'clock in the afternoon. The female dove sits on the egg and then lays a second one, usually at about nine o'clock in the morning two days later. Sometime that day the male takes a turn sitting; thereafter the two birds alternate, the male sitting for about six hours in the middle of each day, the female for the remaining 18 hours a day.

In about 14 days the eggs hatch and the parents begin to feed their young "crop-milk," a liquid secreted at this stage of the cycle by the lining of the adult dove's crop, a pouch in the bird's gullet. When they are 10 or 12 days old, the squabs leave the cage, but they continue to beg for and to receive food from the parents. This continues until the squabs are about two weeks old, when the parents become less and less willing to feed them as the young birds gradually develop the ability to peck for grain on the floor of the cage. When the young are about 15 to 25 days old, the adult male begins once again to bow and coo; nest-building is resumed, a new clutch of eggs is laid and the cycle is repeated. The entire cycle lasts about six or seven weeks and—at least in our laboratory, where it is always spring because of controlled light and temperature conditions—it can continue throughout the year.

The variations in behavior that constitute the cycle are not merely casual or superficial changes in the birds' preoccupations; they represent striking changes in the overall pattern of activity and in the atmosphere of the breeding cage. At its appropriate stage each of the kinds of behavior I have described represents the predominant activity of the animals at the time. Furthermore, these changes in behavior are not just responses to changes in the external situation. The birds do not build the nest merely because the nesting material is available; even if nesting material is in the cage throughout the cycle, nest-building behavior is concentrated,

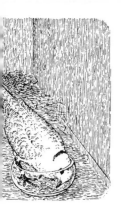
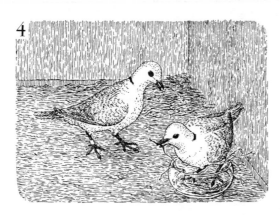
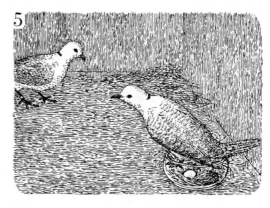

coo" of the male (2). The male and then the female utter a distinctive "nest call" to indicate their selection of a nesting site (3).

There follows a week or more of cooperation in nest-building (4), culminating in the laying of two eggs at precise times of day (5).

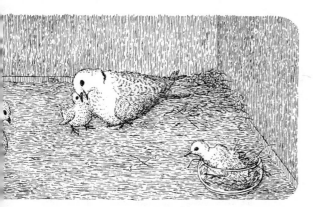
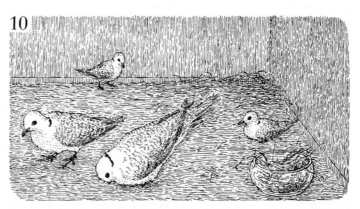

as the young birds learn to peck for grain themselves (9). When the squabs are between two and three weeks old, the adults ignore

them and start to court once again, and a new cycle begins (10). Physical changes during the cycle are shown on the next page.

as described, at one stage. Similarly, the birds react to the eggs and to the young only at appropriate stages in the cycle.

These cyclic changes in behavior therefore represent, at least in part, changes in the internal condition of the animals rather than merely changes in their external situation. Furthermore, the changes in behavior are associated with equally striking and equally pervasive changes in the anatomy and the physiological state of the birds. For example, when the female dove is first introduced into the cage, her oviduct weighs some 800 milligrams. Eight or nine days later, when she lays her first egg, the oviduct may weigh 4,000 milligrams. The crops of both the male and the female weigh some 900 milligrams when the birds are placed in the cage, and when they start to sit on the eggs some 10 days later they still weigh about the same. But two weeks afterward, when the eggs hatch, the parents' crops may weigh as much as 3,000 milligrams. Equally striking changes in the condition of the ovary, the weight of the testes, the length of the gut, the weight of the liver, the microscopic structure of the pituitary gland and other physiological indices are correlated with the behavioral cycle.

Now, if a male or a female dove is placed alone in a cage with nesting material, no such cycle of behavioral or anatomical changes takes place. Far from producing two eggs every six or seven weeks, a female alone in a cage lays no eggs at all. A male alone shows no interest when we offer it nesting material, eggs or young. The cycle of psychobiological changes I have described is, then, one that occurs more or less synchronously in each member of a pair of doves living together but that will not occur independently in either of the pair living alone.

In a normal breeding cycle both the male and the female sit on the eggs almost immediately after they are laid. The first question we asked ourselves was whether this is because the birds are always ready to sit on eggs or because they come into some special condition of readiness to incubate at about the time the eggs are produced.

We kept male and female doves in isolation for several weeks and then placed male-female pairs in test cages, each supplied with a nest bowl containing a normal dove nest with two eggs. The birds did not sit; they acted almost as if the eggs were not there. They courted, then built their own nest (usually on top of the planted nest and its eggs, which we had to keep fishing out to keep the stimulus situation constant!), then finally sat on the eggs—five to seven days after they had first encountered each other.

This clearly indicated that the doves are not always ready to sit on eggs; under the experimental conditions they changed from birds that did not want to incubate to birds that did want to incubate in five to seven days. What had induced this change? It could not have been merely the passage of time since their last breeding experience, because this had varied from four to six or more weeks in different pairs, whereas the variation in time spent in the test cage before sitting was only a couple of days.

Could the delay of five to seven days represent the time required for the birds to get over the stress of being handled and become accustomed to the strange cage? To test this possibility we placed pairs of doves in cages without any nest bowls or nesting material and separated each male and female by an opaque partition. After seven days we removed the partition and introduced nesting material and a formed nest with eggs. If the birds had merely needed time to recover from being handled and become acclimated to the cage, they should now have sat on the eggs immediately. They did not do so; they sat only after five to seven days, just as if they had been introduced into the cage only when the opaque partition was removed.

The next possibility we considered was that in this artificial situation stimulation from the eggs might induce the change from a nonsitting to a sitting "mood" but that this effect required five to seven days to reach a threshold value at which the behavior would change.

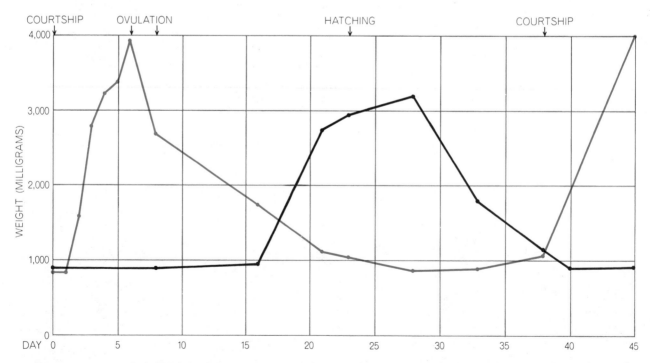

ANATOMICAL AND PHYSIOLOGICAL changes are associated with the behavioral changes of the cycle. The chart gives average weights of the crop (*black curve*) and the female oviduct (*color*) at various stages measured in days after the beginning of courtship.

We therefore placed pairs of birds in test cages with empty nest bowls and a supply of nesting material but no eggs. The birds courted and built nests. After seven days we removed the nest bowl and its nest and replaced it with a fresh bowl containing a nest and eggs. All these birds sat within two hours.

It was now apparent that some combination of influences arising from the presence of the mate and the availability of the nest bowl and nesting material induced the change from nonreadiness to incubate to readiness. In order to distinguish between these influences we put a new group of pairs of doves in test cages without any nest bowl or nesting material. When, seven days later, we offered these birds nesting material and nests with eggs, most of them did not sit immediately. Nor did they wait the full five to seven days to do so; they sat after one day, during which they engaged in intensive nest-building. A final group, placed singly in cages with nests and eggs, failed to incubate at all, even after weeks in the cages.

In summary, the doves do not build nests as soon as they are introduced into a cage containing nesting material, but they will do so immediately if the nesting material is introduced for the first time after they have spent a while together; they will not sit immediately on eggs offered after the birds have been in a bare cage together for some days, but they will do so if they were able to do some nest-building during the end of their period together. From these experiments it is apparent that there are two kinds of change induced in these birds: first, they are changed from birds primarily interested in courtship to birds primarily interested in nest-building, and this change is brought about by stimulation arising from association with a mate; second, under these conditions they are further changed from birds primarily interested in nest-building to birds interested in sitting on eggs, and this change is encouraged by participation in nest-building.

The course of development of readiness to incubate is shown graphically by the results of another experiment, which Philip N. Brody, Rochelle Wortis and I undertook shortly after the ones just described. We placed pairs of birds in test cages for varying numbers of days, in some cases with and in others without a nest bowl and nesting material. Then we introduced a nest and eggs into the cage. If neither bird sat within three hours, the test was scored as nega-

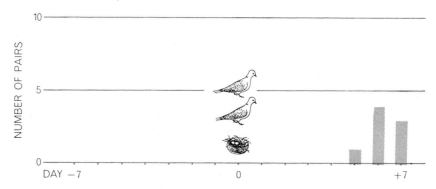

READINESS TO INCUBATE was tested with four groups of eight pairs of doves. Birds of the first group were placed in a cage containing a nest and eggs. They went through courtship and nest-building behavior before finally sitting after between five and seven days.

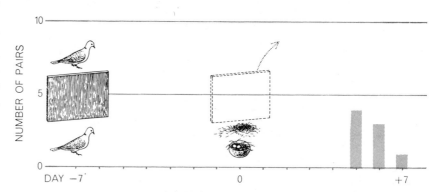

EFFECT OF HABITUATION was tested by keeping two birds separated for seven days in the cage before introducing nest and eggs. They still sat only after five to seven days.

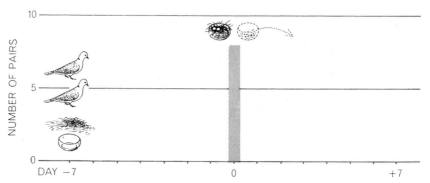

MATE AND NESTING MATERIAL had a dramatic effect on incubation-readiness. Pairs that had spent seven days in courtship and nest-building sat as soon as eggs were offered.

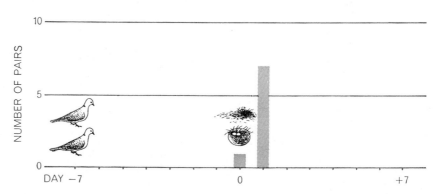

PRESENCE OF MATE without nesting activity had less effect. Birds that spent a week in cages with no nest bowls or hay took a day to sit after nests with eggs were introduced.

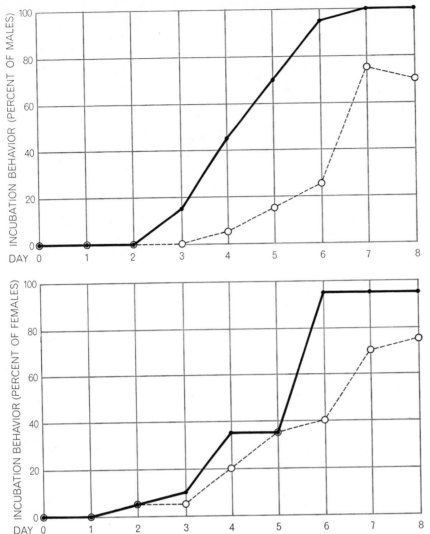

DURATION OF ASSOCIATION with mate and nesting material affects incubation behavior. The abscissas give the length of the association for different groups of birds. The plotted points show what percentage of each group sat within three hours of being offered eggs. The percentage increases for males (*top*) and females (*bottom*) as a function of time previously spent with mate (*open circles*) or with mate and nesting material (*solid dots*).

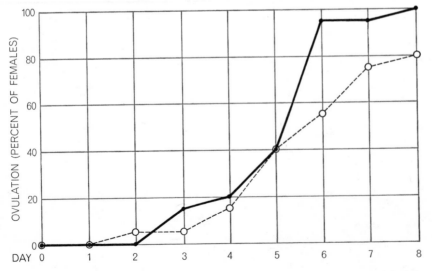

OVULATION is similarly affected. These curves, coinciding closely with those of the bottom chart above, show the occurrence of ovulation in the same birds represented there.

tive and both birds were removed for autopsy. If either bird sat within three hours, that bird was removed and the other bird was given an additional three hours to sit. The experiment therefore tested—independently for the male and the female—the development of readiness to incubate as a function of the number of days spent with the mate, with or without the opportunity to build a nest.

It is apparent [*see top illustration at left*] that association with the mate gradually brings the birds into a condition of readiness to incubate and that this effect is greatly enhanced by the presence of nesting material. Exposure to the nesting situation does not stimulate the onset of readiness to incubate in an all-or-nothing way; rather, its effect is additive with the effect of stimulation provided by the mate. Other experiments show, moreover, that the stimulation from the mate and nesting material is sustained. If either is removed, the incidence of incubation behavior decreases.

The experiments described so far made it clear that external stimuli normally associated with the breeding situation play an important role in inducing a state of readiness to incubate. We next asked what this state consists of physiologically. As a first approach to this problem we attempted to induce incubation behavior by injecting hormones into the birds instead of by manipulating the external stimulation. We treated birds just as we had in the first experiment but injected some of the birds with hormones while they were in isolation, starting one week before they were due to be placed in pairs in the test cages. When both members of the pair had been injected with the ovarian hormone progesterone, more than 90 percent of the eggs were covered by one of the birds within three hours after their introduction into the cage instead of five to seven days later. When the injected substance was another ovarian hormone—estrogen—the effect on most birds was to make them incubate after a latent period of one to three days, during which they engaged in nest-building behavior. The male hormone testosterone had no effect on incubation behavior.

During the 14 days when the doves are sitting on the eggs, their crops increase enormously in weight. Crop growth is a reliable indicator of the secretion of the hormone prolactin by the birds' pituitary glands. Since this growth coincides with the development of incubation behavior and culminates in the secretion of the crop-milk the birds feed to their young after the eggs hatch, Brody and I have recently examined the effect of injected prolactin on incubation behavior. We find that prolactin is not so effective as progesterone in inducing incubation behavior, even at dosage levels that induce full development of the crop. For example, a total prolactin dose of 400 international units induced only 40 percent of the birds to sit on eggs early, even though their average crop weight was about 3,000 milligrams, or more than three times the normal weight. Injection of 10 units of the hormone induced significant increases in crop weight (to 1,200 milligrams) but no increase in the frequency of incubation behavior. These results, together with the fact that in a normal breeding cycle the crop begins to increase in weight only after incubation begins, make it unlikely that prolactin plays an important role in the initiation of normal incubation behavior in this species. It does, however, seem to help to maintain such behavior until the eggs hatch.

Prolactin is much more effective in inducing ring doves to show regurgitation-feeding responses to squabs. When 12 adult doves with previous breeding experience were each injected with 450 units of prolactin over a seven-day period and placed, one bird at a time, in cages with squabs, 10 of the 12 fed the squabs from their engorged crops, whereas none of 12 uninjected controls did so or even made any parental approaches to the squabs.

This experiment showed that prolactin, which is normally present in considerable quantities in the parents when the eggs hatch, does contribute to the doves' ability to show parental feeding behavior. I originally interpreted it to mean that the prolactin-induced engorgement of the crop was necessary in order for any regurgitation feeding to take place, but E. Klinghammer and E. H. Hess of the University of Chicago have correctly pointed out that this was an error, that ring doves are capable of feeding young if presented with them rather early in the incubation period. They do so even though they have no crop-milk, feeding a mixture of regurgitated seeds and a liquid. We are now studying the question of how early the birds can do this and how this ability is related to the onset of prolactin secretion.

The work with gonad-stimulating hormones and prolactin demonstrates that the various hormones successively produced by the birds' glands during their reproductive cycle are capable of inducing the successive behavioral changes that characterize the cycle.

Up to this point I have described two main groups of experiments. One group demonstrates that external stimuli induce changes in behavioral status of a kind normally associated with the progress of the reproductive cycle; the second shows that these behavioral changes can also be induced by hormone administration, provided that the choice of hormones is guided by knowledge of the succession of hormone secretions during a normal reproductive cycle. An obvious—and challenging—implication of these results is that external stimuli may induce changes in hormone secretion, and that environment-induced hormone secretion may constitute an integral part of the mechanism of the reproductive behavior cycle. We have attacked the problem of the environmental stimulation of hormone secretion in a series of experiments in which, in addition to examining the effects of external stimuli on the birds' behavioral status, we have examined their effects on well-established anatomical indicators of the presence of various hormones.

Background for this work was provided by two classic experiments with the domestic pigeon, published during the 1930's, which we have verified in the ring dove. At the London Zoo, L. H. Matthews found that a female pigeon would lay eggs as a result of being placed in a cage with a male from whom she was separated by a glass plate. This was an unequivocal demonstration that visual and/or auditory stimulation provided by the male induces ovarian development in the female. (Birds are quite insensitive to olfactory stimulation.) And M. D. Patel of the University of Wisconsin found that the crops of breeding pigeons, which develop strikingly during the incubation period, would regress to their resting state if the incubating birds were removed from their nests and would fail to develop at all if the birds were removed before crop growth had begun. If, however, a male pigeon, after being removed from his nest, was placed in an adjacent cage from which he could see his mate still sitting on the eggs, his crop would develop just as if he were himself incubating! Clearly stimuli arising from participation in incubation, including visual stimuli, cause the doves' pituitary glands to secrete prolactin.

Our autopsies showed that the incidence of ovulation in females that had associated with males for various periods coincided closely with the incidence of incubation behavior [see bottom illustration on opposite page]; statistical analysis reveals a very high degree of association. The process by which the dove's ovary develops to the point of ovulation includes a period of estrogen secretion followed by one of progesterone secretion, both induced by appropriate ovary-stimulating hormones from the pituitary gland. We therefore conclude that stimuli provided by the male, augmented by the presence of the nest bowl and nesting material, induce the secretion of gonad-stimulating hormones by the female's pituitary, and that the onset of readiness to incubate is a result of this process.

As I have indicated, ovarian development, culminating in ovulation and egg-laying, can be induced in a female dove merely as a result of her seeing a male through a glass plate. Is this the result of the mere presence of another bird or of something the male does because he is a male? Carl Erickson and I have begun to deal with this question. We placed 40 female doves in separate cages, each separated from a male by a glass plate. Twenty of the stimulus animals were normal, intact males, whereas the remaining 20 had been castrated several weeks before. The intact males all exhibited vigorous bow-cooing immediately on being placed in the cage, whereas none of the castrates did so. Thirteen of the 20 females with intact males ovulated during the next seven days, whereas only two of those with the castrates did so. Clearly ovarian development in the female is not induced merely by seeing another bird but by seeing or hearing it act like a male as the result of the effects of its own male hormone on its nervous system.

Although crop growth, which begins early in the incubation period, is apparently stimulated by participation in incubation, the crop continues to be large and actively secreting for quite some time after the hatching of the eggs. This suggests that stimuli provided by the squabs may also stimulate prolactin secretion. In our laboratory Ernst Hansen substituted three-day-old squabs for eggs in various stages of incubation and after four days compared the adults' crop weights with those of birds that had continued to sit on their eggs dur-

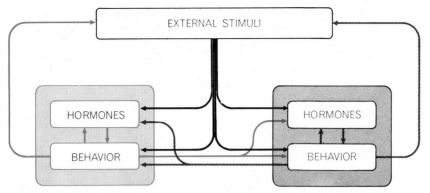

INTERACTIONS that appear to govern the reproductive-behavior cycle are suggested here. Hormones regulate behavior and are themselves affected by behavioral and other stimuli. And the behavior of each bird affects the hormones and the behavior of its mate.

ing the four days. He found that the crops grow even faster when squabs are in the nest than when the adults are under the influence of the eggs; the presence of squabs can stimulate a dove's pituitary glands to secrete more prolactin even before the stage in the cycle when the squabs normally appear.

This does not mean, however, that any of the stimuli we have used can induce hormone secretion at *any* time, regardless of the bird's physiological condition. If we place a pair of ring doves in a cage and allow them to go through the normal cycle until they have been sitting on eggs for, say, six days and we then place a glass partition in the cage to separate the male from the female and the nest, the female will continue to sit on the eggs and the male's crop will continue to develop just as if he were himself incubating. This is a simple replication of one of Patel's experiments. Miriam Friedman and I have found, however, that if the male and female are separated from the beginning, so that the female must build the nest by herself and sit alone from the beginning, the crop of the male does

not grow. By inserting the glass plate at various times during the cycle in different groups of birds, we have found that the crop of the male develops fully only if he is not separated from the female until 72 hours or more after the second egg is laid. This means that the sight of the female incubating induces prolactin secretion in the male only if he is in the physiological condition to which participation in nest-building brings him. External stimuli associated with the breeding situation do indeed induce changes in hormone secretion.

The experiments summarized here point to the conclusion that changes in the activity of the endocrine system are induced or facilitated by stimuli coming from various aspects of the environment at different stages of the breeding cycle, and that these changes in hormone secretion induce changes in behavior that may themselves be a source of further stimulation.

The regulation of the reproductive cycle of the ring dove appears to depend, at least in part, on a double set of reciprocal interrelations. First, there

is an interaction of the effects of hormones on behavior and the effects of external stimuli—including those that arise from the behavior of the animal and its mate—on the secretion of hormones. Second, there is a complicated reciprocal relation between the effects of the presence and behavior of one mate on the endocrine system of the other and the effects of the presence and behavior of the second bird (including those aspects of its behavior induced by these endocrine effects) back on the endocrine system of the first. The occurrence in each member of the pair of a cycle found in neither bird in isolation, and the synchronization of the cycles in the two mates, can now readily be understood as consequences of this interaction of the inner and outer environments.

The physiological explanation of these phenomena lies partly in the fact that the activity of the pituitary gland, which secretes prolactin and the gonad-stimulating hormones, is largely controlled by the nervous system through the hypothalamus. The precise neural mechanisms for any complex response are still deeply mysterious, but physiological knowledge of the brain-pituitary link is sufficiently detailed and definite so that the occurrence of a specific hormonal response to a specific external stimulus is at least no more mysterious than any other stimulus-response relation. We are currently exploring these responses in more detail, seeking to learn, among other things, the precise sites at which the various hormones act. And we have begun to investigate another aspect of the problem: the effect of previous experience on a bird's reproductive behavior and the interactions between these experiential influences and the hormonal effects.

The Social Order of Japanese Macaques

by G. Gray Eaton
October 1976

*Long-term observation of a troop of these monkeys
confined in an Oregon corral indicates that the
biological component of their behavior is much
modified by the social component*

Japanese macaques are perhaps best known in the form of the three wise-looking wooden monkeys that mime the Buddhist proverb "See no evil, hear no evil, speak no evil" on the world's souvenir stands. The choice of models is apt, because in real life macaques are among the most intelligent of primates. Relatives of the rhesus monkey and the Barbary ape, they live in cohesive troops of 50 to 150 individuals. They have a complex social order that like all other social orders has been created by the interaction of biological and social forces. What is particularly interesting about the social order of macaques is that the social forces play a larger role than one might expect.

In their natural forest habitat Japanese macaques are shy and difficult to observe, and ethologists interested in their social behavior have been obliged either to provision wild troops or to study them in captivity. Over the past six years my colleagues and I have spent more than 8,000 hours observing a typical macaque troop in a grassy two-acre corral at the Oregon Regional Primate Research Center. Our troop had originally roamed free near Mihara City in the Hiroshima prefecture of Japan, until complaints from local farmers prompted the Japan Monkey Center to capture nearly all the 49 troop members in 1964. The following year they were transplanted to our corral in Oregon, and since then they have thrived.

The macaques in our troop were not studied before their capture, so that it is difficult to assess the effect confinement has had on them. We assume, however, that provisioning and confinement tend to increase the frequency of all types of social interaction, since the restriction of movement and the freedom from having to spend hours foraging for food have increased the animals' unoccupied time. When on occasion we have fed our macaques by scattering grain throughout the corral instead of doling out their usual ration of monkey chow, we have

noticed how quiet they become when they are foraging for food.

The most striking feature of social behavior in the troop is the fact that a few males dominate all the other animals. Next one notices several old females that attack other females without retali-

ation, and many adult females that threaten and chase males. It soon becomes apparent that there is a rigid dominance hierarchy, analogous to a pecking order. The top position, that of the "leader," or "alpha" monkey, is almost always occupied by a mature adult

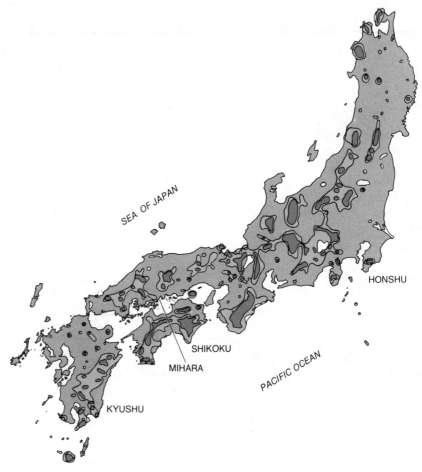

SHRINKING RANGE of Japanese macaques is shown in this superposition of distribution maps made by K. Hasebe in 1932 (*light color*) and by K. Kishida in 1953 (*dark color*). The most northerly-living of nonhuman primates, their distribution extremes have remained unchanged during the past half-century, but deforestation has caused decreases in every area. Today macaques are considered a national treasure, and the Japanese government bans their export.

male that sometimes does not attain this rank until he is 18 or 19 years old. (Males normally reach puberty at four and full body growth at eight to 10.) Immediately below the alpha male are typically five or six "subleader" males, followed by most of the adult females, which reach puberty at three years and full body size at six to eight and together with their infant and juvenile offspring form the middle of the hierarchy. The remainder of the adult males are at the bottom of the hierarchy, and in the wild they live on the periphery of the troop.

Rank is not highly correlated with aggressiveness, so that we cannot determine the order of the hierarchy simply by counting the number of attacks. Instead the troop is organized in such a way that the highest-ranking animal is attacked by the smallest number of other animals, with the progressively lower-ranking animals being attacked by an increasingly large number of others. Dominance rank is basically linear, but there are occasional reversals, that is, animal X chases animal Y, Y chases Z and Z chases X.

By the same token, high rank does not necessarily entail a high frequency of aggressive behavior. Our second- and third-ranking males, named Greater Than and Perfect, are both more aggressive than the alpha male, Arrowhead, because, among other reasons, Arrow-

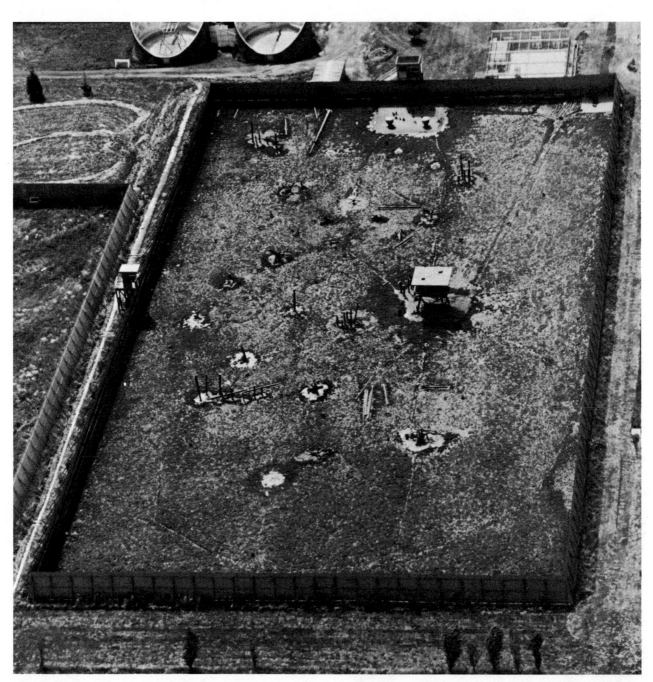

GRASSY TWO-ACRE CORRAL at the Oregon Regional Primate Research Center confines the author's 230-member troop of Japanese macaques. (The monkeys appear as black dots scattered throughout the enclosure.) The walls are of corrugated steel, 3.5 meters high, and slant inward about 15 degrees. Poles and tree stumps provide climbing surfaces for this largely ground-dwelling but occasionally arboreal species; the trails in the grass were made by the monkeys as they wandered between preferred areas. Three observation towers are visible, and at left is part of a newly built corral identical with the first that will be used in the near future for a population experiment.

head receives more "respect" from the other troop members and therefore does not need to maintain his position by constantly attacking other animals or even threatening them. For example, when the monkeys are fed, Arrowhead is given more personal space than Greater Than, and when a prized food such as a peanut is thrown near either of them, Arrowhead's mere presence is enough to keep the other animals away, whereas Greater Than often has to chase them away.

Paradoxically the dominant males are not at the top of the hierarchy because of fighting ability or physical characteristics such as size. Arrowhead is one of the smallest of the adult males, and he has no canine teeth and only one eye, but we have never observed any challenge to his authority as the alpha male. Moreover, when he attacks other males, they do not fight back but merely struggle to get free. Of the subleader males, Bruno and Perfect also lack canine teeth, and Greater Than achieved his rank before his canine teeth had fully erupted. If size and canine teeth play no role in attaining or maintaining a high dominance rank, what is the basis of the macaque "pecking order"?

After observing wild troops Japanese ethologists concluded that the dominance rank of an animal is closely correlated with the rank of its mother. The role of the mothers in determining the rank of their offspring can be observed during juvenile fights, most of which begin when play gets too rough. One juvenile screams, inciting its mother to run over and bite the other juvenile, which is in turn aided by its mother. The two mothers then fight, and the dominant female and her offspring chase the lower-ranking female, whose son or daughter flees with her. Once this has happened several times, the offspring of the lower-ranking female will run away from those of the higher-ranking female even when she is not nearby. Occasionally a young macaque will be unusually aggressive and will rise above its mother's rank, but that is exceptional.

We have several adult males in our troop that are still defended by their mothers. When the current second-ranked male, Greater Than, was third in the male hierarchy, he was occasionally attacked by the second-ranked male, One-Eye, and the alpha male, Arrowhead. At those times Greater Than's mother, Red Witch, would distract the dominant monkeys by leaping on their back, enabling her son to escape.

In the wild only the sons of very high-ranking females are allowed to stay in the center of the troop; the other males are driven to the periphery when they are about five years old, about a year after they have reached puberty. At that age they probably have to fight for a

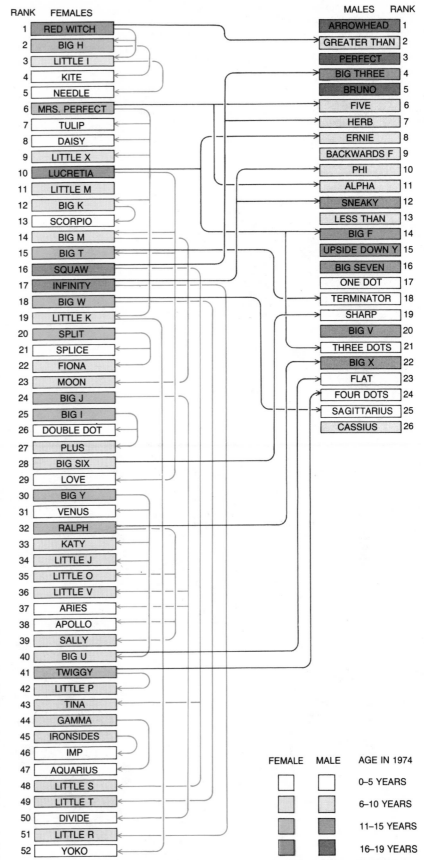

ADULT DOMINANCE HIERARCHIES for the Oregon troop are shown as they stood in 1974. Female hierarchy (*color*) and male hierarchy (*gray*) are listed separately because dominance relationships change during the mating season, when low-ranking males attack females. Arrows indicate maternal relationships to show how rank is influenced by maternal status.

place in the peripheral male hierarchy without the physical assistance of their mothers. The mothers' influence may still carry over, because many macaque fights are bluffing matches, and the sons of high-ranking females would presumably be more self-confident than those of low-ranking females.

Superimposed on the maternally determined dominance hierarchy is a sec-ond system of organization we have found to be even more important in determining the overall social order: each monkey has a specific function or role to perform within the troop that is dependent on its age, sex and dominance rank. These roles can be as simple and interchangeable as watching for predators or as complex and fixed as rearing an infant, but together they constitute the es-sence of a society as opposed to a simple aggregation of individuals.

The role of the alpha male appears to be one of directing the movement of the troop and defending it. Since movements of our troop are restricted by a fence, Arrowhead no longer leads, but he still defends. Once a year, when we round up the entire troop for general

1

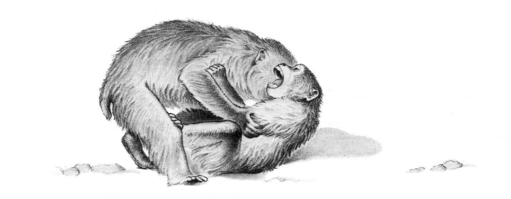

2

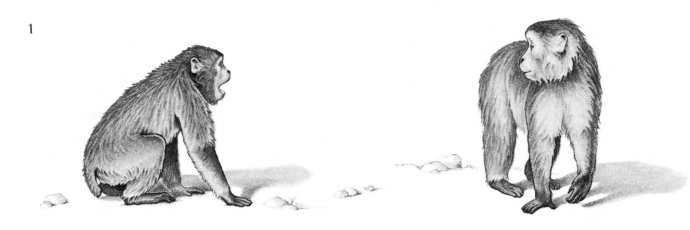

3

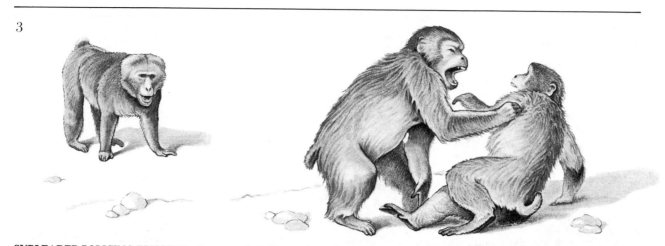

SUBLEADER POLICING EPISODE lasting one and a half seconds was drawn from a series of photographs taken with a motor-drive camera by Kurt B. Modahl. The sequence begins when Tulip, a juvenile female, threatens Infinity, an adult female (*1*). Infinity responds by fiercely attacking and punishing Tulip (*2 and 3*). Tulip's screams prompt Greater Than, the second-ranking subleader male, to rush in from the rear left (*4*) and break up the fight by pursuing Tulip a short distance (*5*) and then threatening her with a stare (*6*). The subleaders

housekeeping purposes, he is conspicuous in his disregard for his own safety in defending the troop. Because of the limited size of the catching pen at the west end of the corral we try to detach small, manageable groups of animals from the main troop and drive them along the corral's north wall. As we do so Arrowhead leaves the main troop and joins the group being herded into the catching pen. Instead of facing away from us and toward the pen as the other animals do he faces toward us and makes threats as he moves backward with the others. Once the other monkeys have been driven into the pen, Arrowhead breaks through the line of animal handlers, returns to the main troop and repeats the performance with the next small group.

Occasionally we have to remove a sick or wounded animal from the corral. As we attempt to do so Arrowhead leads many of the low-ranking males, one or two of the subleader males and some of the adult females in threatening us, while the rest of the subleader males move away and stay close to the mothers and infants in the main troop. The cry of an infant makes Arrowhead and the other adult males appear to be par-

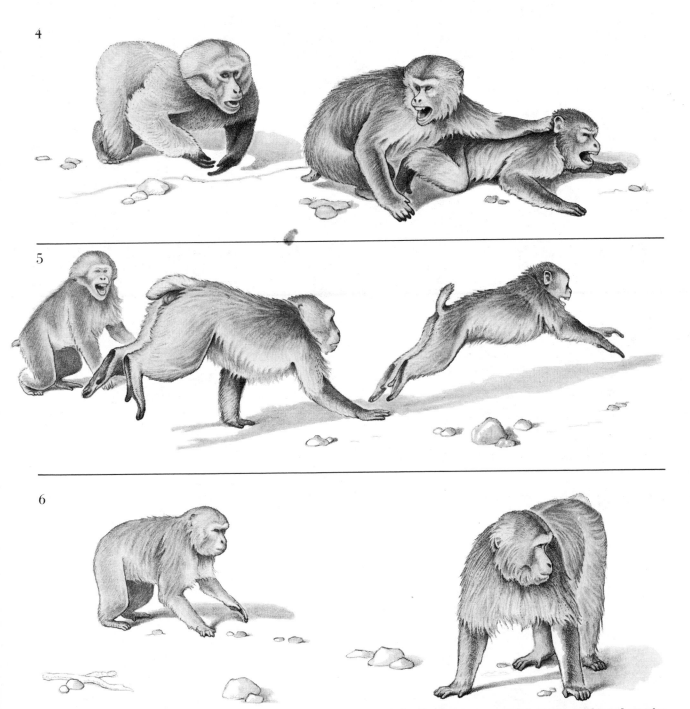

4

5

6

usually attack the dominant combatant; in this case, however, Greater Than chased the losing Tulip. He did so apparently because she may have inadvertently threatened him when she started the fight, and because he seems to like Infinity, although this interpretation is speculative. In any case macaque behavior is variable and complex and cannot be reduced to formulas. The presence of the alpha male, male-female alliances and the personal likes and dislikes of the individual subleaders are all factors that may influence policing behavior.

ticularly enraged, and they advance shoulder to shoulder, growling, bobbing their heads and slapping the ground with their hands.

The principal role of the subleader males is to stop fights. This they usually do by chasing away the more aggressive of the combatants. Such behavior favors the underdog, but it cannot be regarded as "ethical" because it seems to be an automatic response to the dynamics of the fight situation. The screams, grimaces and cringing posture of the losing monkey are signs of submission that tend to inhibit aggression by the subleader males, whereas the growls, gapes and ear-flattening display of the attacking monkey are threatening gestures that are likely to incite the subleader males to attack.

The alpha male occasionally plays a secondary role in this policing behavior. In his presence the subleader males appear uncertain and alternately threaten the combatants and turn with exaggerated motions to look at him. If the alpha male turns away as though ignoring the entire affair, the subleader males may or may not attack the aggressor in the fight; if he threatens the subleaders themselves, they will leave the area; if he joins them in threatening the combatants, they will attack and end the fight.

Role-specialization in a troop of Japanese macaques is largely determined by class membership. Some learning nonetheless seems to be necessary. When Big Three rose from the peripheral class to the subleader class after defeating the subleader Bruno, he appeared to assume the subleader role of policing, but his behavior differed from that of the more experienced subleader males. When a fight started, he would become overly excited and attack animals that were not involved. Over a period of several months, however, he gradually became more proficient, and he is now one of the most effective subleaders in checking aggression.

In the wild the primary role of the peripheral males is apparently to give warning of predators and to help the alpha male defend the troop. They also play with and discipline juvenile males and are groomed by them; the juveniles undoubtedly learn a great deal about social behavior through this interaction. In addition the peripheral males move from one troop to another and thus provide a mechanism of genetic exchange that prevents continuous inbreeding. In our corral the peripheral males are not really on the periphery because the corral is not large enough. They are generally accepted by the rest of the troop and are only occasionally harassed.

The role of the adult females is to raise their offspring and protect them. A newborn macaque is relatively helpless, able only to cling to its mother's breast, and for the first few days the mother supports the infant with one hand as she moves about. The infant develops rapidly and soon attempts to crawl away from its mother. It rarely gets far; the mother is adept at controlling the infant with her foot while she uses both hands to eat or groom. When the infant is about two weeks old, the mother appears to teach it to walk by placing it on the ground and then backing away, encouraging it by smacking her lips. During these developmental stages wide individual differences are apparent. Some females prefer having their infant ride jockey style on their back. Others seem not to care; we have occasionally observed a mother dragging her one- or two-year-old offspring along the ground as it clung to her abdomen.

Infants are a great source of interest to other females, particularly to older sisters and females that do not have offspring of their own. The mothers are extremely protective, however, and do not allow another female to pick up the infant until it is several weeks old. Some females use a rather deceptive stratagem to circumvent this protectiveness: they patiently groom the mother until she is sufficiently distracted and then surreptitiously touch the infant while it is still at its mother's breast.

Sex differences in behavior develop as the infants begin to venture away from their mothers. Juvenile males tend to spend more of their time roughhousing in play groups consisting of their peers and an occasional adult male than juvenile females do; the females are mostly occupied in grooming activities with their mothers and sisters. Occasionally a female joins a male play group, but she usually does not stay long before she returns to less strenuous activities. Juvenile males seldom groom other monkeys, but they groom themselves more frequently than females do. When juvenile males and females groom others, they both tend to groom adults of their own sex.

Siblings defend one another and their mother; after puberty, however, the males no longer defend the mother. The bond between mother and daughter remains strong throughout their lives. They spend much time grooming each other; it is not uncommon to see two or three fully grown sisters deftly picking through their mother's fur as their own offspring play beside them.

Adult females also form alliances with one another, a kind of behavior that is rarely observed in unrelated males. These alliances may be the reason many males are driven from wild troops or are low-ranking in our troop. If a male fights with a female, other females will usually come to her aid, whereas adult males rarely assist one another. Groups of females occasionally fight, and in the wild the social disruption caused by continued fighting may result in the fission of the troop, that is, the departure of several families to form a new troop. Female alliances therefore appear to be more important in regulating the cohesiveness of the macaque social order than sexual attraction between males and females, which in this species is seasonal and transitory.

A male may, however, form an alliance with a female and defend her against attack. In our troop the female Gamma is treated in this way by two of the subleader males. One of them, the old male Bruno, "adopted" Gamma when her mother died. Bruno groomed, cuddled and defended her; even now, eight years later, Gamma still runs to him for support. The fact that Bruno has never mated with Gamma leads us to believe that in Japanese macaques the "incest taboo," as a result of which male macaques do not mate with their mothers or sisters, is not genetically determined but has its source in a developmental process. Gamma's other protector, Big Three, does mate with her, but he also defends her during the nonbreeding season.

The seasonality of the macaques' behavior is striking. Their mating is confined to fall and winter; October and November are the months of peak activ-

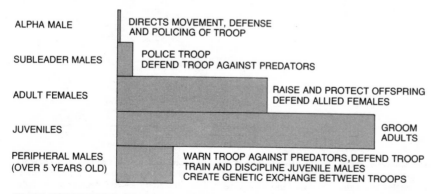

ALPHA MALE	DIRECTS MOVEMENT, DEFENSE AND POLICING OF TROOP
SUBLEADER MALES	POLICE TROOP DEFEND TROOP AGAINST PREDATORS
ADULT FEMALES	RAISE AND PROTECT OFFSPRING DEFEND ALLIED FEMALES
JUVENILES	GROOM ADULTS
PERIPHERAL MALES (OVER 5 YEARS OLD)	WARN TROOP AGAINST PREDATORS, DEFEND TROOP TRAIN AND DISCIPLINE JUVENILE MALES CREATE GENETIC EXCHANGE BETWEEN TROOPS

CLASS STRUCTURE of the macaque social order is determined by age, sex and dominance rank. Each class has specific social roles to perform. Bars show relative proportions in 1974.

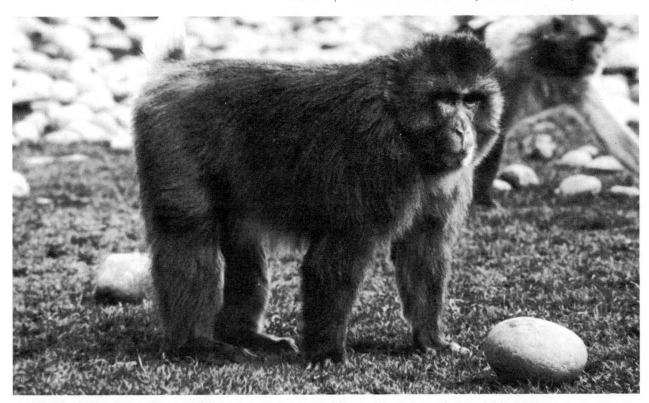

"ALPHA," OR DOMINANT, MALE of a troop of Japanese macaques kept under seminatural conditions in a two-acre corral at the Oregon Regional Primate Research Center is named Arrowhead. The alpha male is responsible for directing the movement, defense and policing of the troop. Arrowhead is about 25 years old, and he was probably the alpha male when the troop roamed wild in Japan. Although he is one of the smallest males, has no canine teeth and is missing an eye, a challenge to his leadership has never been observed.

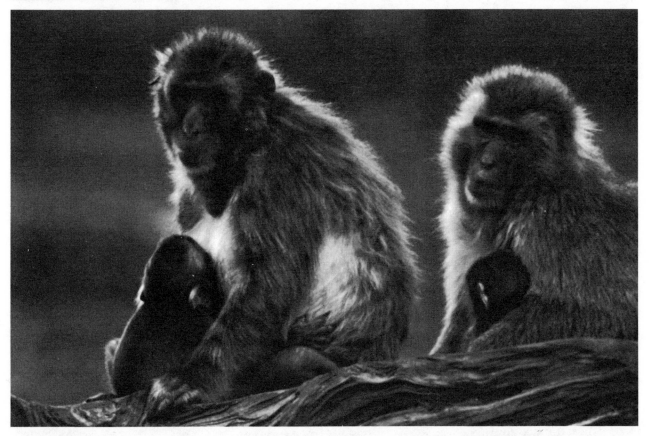

ADULT FEMALE MACAQUES huddle with their infants atop a dead tree stump in the Oregon corral. The single offspring are born in April and May and are nursed throughout the summer. After the infant is about two weeks old, the mother teaches it to walk and which foods to eat. The female macaques are very protective and do not allow other females to touch the infant until it is several weeks old.

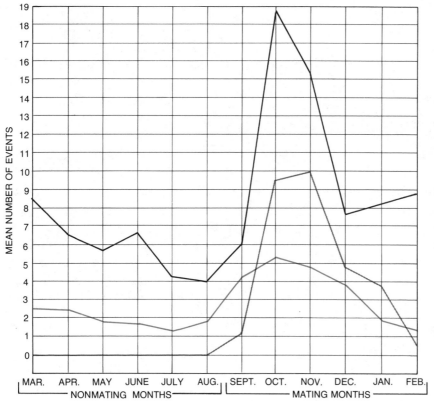

SEASONALITY of certain kinds of macaque behavior is striking: male aggressive attacks (*color*), mating (*gray*) and male courtship displays (*black*) are largely confined to fall and winter.

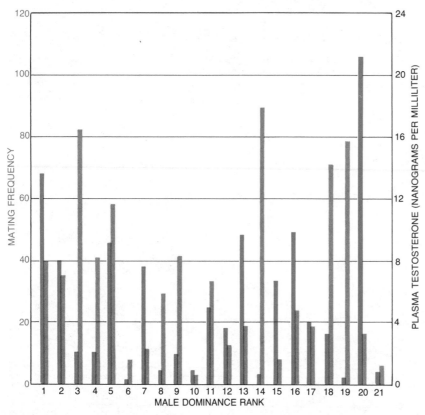

LEVELS OF MALE SEX HORMONE (testosterone) in the blood of male macaques (*gray bars*) are not correlated with dominance rank or mating frequency (*colored bars*). Although high hormone levels may lower the threshold for aggressive behavior, social and developmental factors are more important than biological factors in determining the macaque social order.

ity. The majority of the young are born about six months later, in April and May. Summer is a quiet season, with the females nursing their infants and grooming one another while the males lie about in the sun. As fall approaches there is a change in behavior, first in the males. Holding their stubby tails erect, they begin to strut around the corral. From the rear the view is striking: the bright white fur on the underside of the male's tail contrasts with the deep scarlet of the skin of the scrotum and perineum. This display of color is a form of courtship behavior, resembling the behavior of a peacock fanning his tail in front of the peahen. The males also shake objects such as the uprooted tree stumps scattered around the corral, and they leap rhythmically up and down and drum their feet. The shaking, leaping and drumming seem to serve a courtship function, since the males that do them most frequently mate most frequently.

As time passes, the males begin to groom the females more often than they do during the nonmating season, and they often fight among themselves and threaten or attack the females. Far from being repelled by this behavior, the females become increasingly attracted to the males until mating pairs form. Not all the animals pair, however, and among those that do the relationship is somewhat casual. The male and female may stay together for a few hours, seldom longer than a few days, and then the pair breaks up; one partner or both may enter into a new pairing. Most of the animals mate with several different partners in the course of the breeding season.

Dominance rank is not correlated with mating either in the males or in the females. Arrowhead, the alpha male, is one of the more active males, but Big V, one of the lowest-ranking males, has mated much more frequently in the years we have observed the two. High-ranking females also mate with low-ranking males in an apparently similar random fashion. The male takes the active role in courting, but the ultimate choice of partner appears to be made by the female. Over the years we have seen a number of females refuse Arrowhead simply by not standing still when he indicated (by pushing lightly on the female's back) that he was ready to mount. In each of these cases Arrowhead followed the female for a few days to a week before turning his attention to a more willing partner. Meanwhile the original female might have mated with several other males she apparently preferred to Arrowhead. Because we do not have a reliable paternity test we do not know which males are making the greatest contribution to the gene pool, but a preliminary data analysis indicates that the dominant males were not involved in a disproportionately large number of matings about the time of conception.

The changes in male aggressive behavior during the mating season are presumably caused by an increase in the male sex hormone testosterone. The relation between testosterone and aggression is complex, however, and is subject to modification by social factors. Although we have not measured the hormone throughout the year, we sampled every adult male at the beginning of two separate mating seasons and compared the measurement with the dominance rank of the animal. To our surprise there was no correlation between a male's dominance rank and his testosterone levels. We concluded that although testosterone may help to lower the thresholds of aggressive reactions during the mating season, it is less important than social stimuli in eliciting masculine patterns of aggressive behavior.

The end of the mating season is signaled by the cessation of pairing and by play activity among the adult males. The same monkeys that viciously attacked one another during the mating season now spend much time wrestling and tumbling with one another and with juvenile males. It is amusing to see one of the large males lying on his back waving his legs in the air while a juvenile jumps up and down on his belly and then executes a mock diving attack on his throat. The adult males also show considerable parental concern at this time and not only play with the juveniles but also groom them, defend them, huddle with them and carry them around on their backs. According to Junichiro Itani of Kyoto University, this paternal care, which is unrelated to dominance rank in our troop, is displayed only by high-ranking males in the wild Takasakiyama troop in Japan.

The difference is not necessarily related to the confinement of our troop but may simply reflect protocultural differences. Shunzo Kawamura of Osaka City University, who has studied protocultural behavior in free-ranging troops in Japan, has found that different troops have different diets. The Shodoshima-O troop, for example, normally feeds on rice being grown by farmers, whereas the Takagoyama troops never pillage rice paddies even though they pass through them in the course of their wanderings. Kawamura also observed a young female of the Koshima Island troop washing sand off sweet potatoes in a stream that runs through the island beach. The habit then spread to other members of the troop, until all the monkeys began to wash the sweet potatoes in the sea, apparently to season them.

Protocultural differences in macaque courtship have been recorded by Gordon R. Stephenson of the University of Wisconsin, who found significant dif-

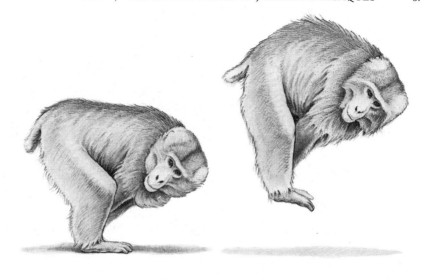

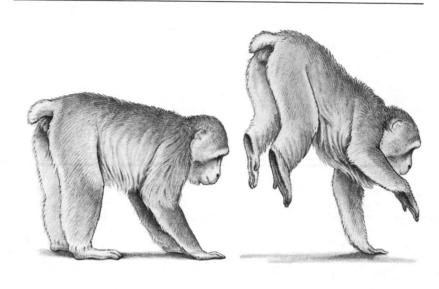

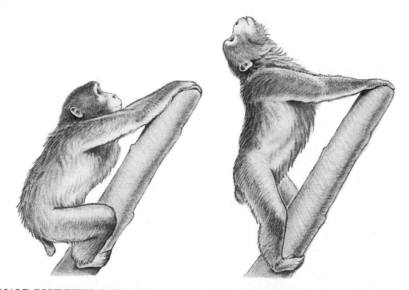

MALE COURTSHIP DISPLAYS occur primarily during the fall and winter mating season. Individual males tend to prefer one type of display and perform it repetitively on a stump, a log or the ground. The most common display is leaping (*top*), followed in frequency by kicking (*middle*) and tossing (*bottom*). Some macaques combine kicking and tossing in a single motion.

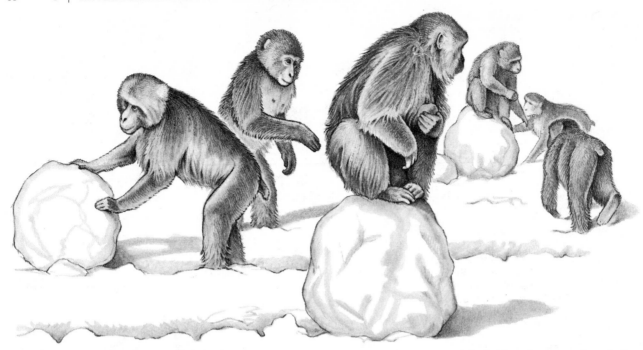

SNOWBALL-MAKING is a protocultural behavior observed in the Oregon troop. It first appeared on January 13, 1971, when Big X, a low-ranking male, made a small snowball while eating snow and proceeded to roll it until it had reached a diameter of about one and a half feet. Every winter since then he and other macaques have con- **structed several large snowballs that have become centers of attention for the troop. Although unconnected with aggressive or feeding behavior (unlike most tool use in animals), the improvisation of snowballs and other objects may serve an adaptive function by preparing the macaques to adapt to new situations and a variety of habitats.**

ferences in courtship behavior among the Miyajima, Arashiyama and Koshima troops. Female macaques are known to court males by mounting them, yet the three troops differed in this behavior: only low-ranking females mounted males in the Miyajima troop, all females did so in the Arashiyama troop and no female was ever observed to mount a male in the Koshima troop. In our troop only a few females mount males, and they do so without relation to their rank or the male's.

We have observed an unusual form of protocultural behavior in our troop. In the winter of 1970–1971 one of the peripheral males, Big X, rolled a snowball along the ground until it was about a foot and a half in diameter. Every winter since then other macaques have made similar snowballs; they have been centers of attention for infants and juveniles, who play on them, and for adults, who simply sit on them. The snowballs do not seem to have any functional significance for the macaques but appear to be the product of their manipulative skill, intelligence and leisure time.

Since the fence around our corral prevents a monkey's escape from an aggressor that is chasing it, the frequency of aggression is undoubtedly higher than it would be in the wild. We have tried to provide a form of escape by placing small steel drums on their side in the

corners of the corral, bolting them to the ground and fitting them with a handle on the inside to which the aggressee can cling if the aggressor tries to pull him out. These barrels are often used as hiding places by the low-ranking males and seem to effectively stop group attacks.

Occasionally many members of the troop attack one animal. Why they do it is a mystery. The mobbing does not seem to be caused by crowding. Bruce Alexander, who is now at Simon Fraser University, looked into the matter by crowding our troop into a pen 50 feet square adjacent to the corral. He recorded the type and frequency of aggressive interactions during three crowding periods in the pen and three control periods in the corral. Surprisingly the crowding did not result in a breakdown of the social structure of the troop; indeed, the dominance hierarchy was stabler in the pen than it was in the corral. Mobbing and severe aggression increased during the crowding periods, but their frequency decreased over the span of the three crowding periods. This suggested that the increased frequency of mobbing observed under crowded conditions was due more to the removal of the animals from a familiar habitat than to increased density. Alexander's hypothesis is supported by the fact that our troop's initial move from an 1,100-square-foot holding pen into the two-acre corral was

immediately followed by an increase in severe aggression that lasted for three weeks and left one low-ranking male dead and three others badly wounded.

My own research on the troop is concerned with the effects of increasing population density on both reproduction and aggression. I am following a procedure similar to the classic one of John B. Calhoun of the National Institute of Mental Health, who allowed populations of laboratory rodents to reproduce in a confined space until they developed abnormal patterns of behavior that invariably led to a disastrous decline in population [see "Population Density and Social Pathology," by John B. Calhoun; SCIENTIFIC AMERICAN Offprint 506]. We too have allowed the population of our macaques to grow without restriction within the confines of their corral.

Our troop gives no indication of developing abnormal patterns of behavior in spite of its rapid growth from the original 46 members captured in 1964 to 230 in 1976. In fact, we recorded a significant decrease in aggressive encounters among the adult males between the 1971 and 1972 mating seasons, when the population of the troop increased by 17 percent. (The number of adult males remained stable at 21.) A more detailed analysis showed that the higher frequency of aggression during the 1971 season was associated with a change in the hierarchy that involved the six highest-ranking males, whereas in 1972 the hierarchy had stabilized. It therefore appears that our macaques are unlike rodents in their response to increasing population density because their social structure is a critical factor in regulating their aggressive behavior.

On the other hand, even though the macaques are confined in a space more than 100 times smaller than their original home range, which was probably a minimum of 250 acres, the crowding may not yet have reached the pathological limit. Daniel S. Stokols of the University of North Carolina has distinguished between the physical condition of density, defined purely in terms of spatial parameters, and the experience of crowding, a motivational state aroused through the interaction of spatial, social and individual factors. With this distinction in mind I have observed the Arashiyama West troop of Japanese macaques, which is confined in a 107-acre enclosure near Laredo, Tex. There I found that although the 150 troop members move through a minimum of eight to 10 acres a day when they are feeding and cover the entire 107 acres every few days, at most times of the day or night the entire troop appears to be grouped in a space of less than two acres. It is therefore possible that our troop is not yet "crowded" but is only limited in range.

It seems unlikely, however, that the corral population can continue to increase at the present rate without eventual pathological changes in the animals. Deterioration in social structure has been reported to precede troop fission in the Gagusan troop in Japan, which has maintained its size between

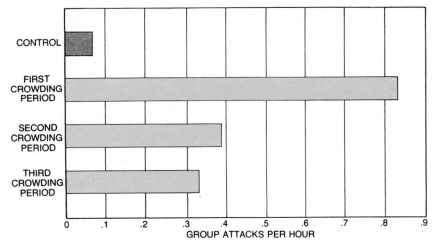

GROUP ATTACKS on a low-ranking monkey, involving up to 35 animals and often resulting in severe wounding or death, greatly increased in frequency when the Oregon troop was crowded into a 50-foot-square pen in an experiment conducted by Bruce Alexander. Over three sequential crowding periods, however, the frequency of mobbing decreased, suggesting that severe aggression was due largely to unfamiliar environment and not to crowding per se.

130 and 160 by frequently dividing. Such fission may be evidence that the sensitivity of the macaque social structure to increased numbers evolved as part of an intrinsic mechanism for population control. Alexander has speculated that once a threshold population level has been reached territorial interactions within the troop will lead to fission without a decrease in fertility.

We plan to test this hypothesis in the near future. We have just finished a new corral adjacent to the original one and shall soon connect the two by a runway in order to determine whether fission will occur when rising population density threatens the stability of the social order or whether the troop will simply expand its home range. If fission does take place without any indication of reduced fertility, it will suggest that Japanese macaques have evolved popula-

tion-control mechanisms fundamentally different from those of rodents.

The fission of our troop, if it occurs, will also provide us with a unique opportunity for studying the formation of a new social order. Which families will emigrate? Which males will be subleaders? Which will be the alpha male? What effect will the old dominance relationships have on the new social order? What will happen to the old social order if and when its key members leave?

Beyond the intrinsic interest of studies of primate societies, they may shed some light on the vastly more complex structure of human social behavior. To survive is to adapt, and man's understanding of the macaques' successful adaptation to many different environments may ultimately contribute to his own survival.

II

INTERNAL REGULATION
OF SEX HORMONES

II INTERNAL REGULATION OF SEX HORMONES

INTRODUCTION

Hormones are chemical substances that are released into the bloodstream from ductless (endocrine) glands. Most authors date the birth of endocrinology in 1849, when A. A. Berthold began his study of the endocrine actions of the testis. Since that time other endocrine organs have been identified and the chemical structure of their secretions elucidated. Sir Solly Zuckerman's article describes the basic concepts of endocrinology as they were understood in the mid-1950s.

Although the role of hormones as chemical messengers integrating life processes was appreciated at this juncture, Zuckerman's article demonstrates that the regulation of hormone secretion and the mechanisms by which hormones act on cells were far less clearly understood. Zuckerman summarizes data showing that the secretions of the anterior pituitary gland regulate the endocrine activity of the gonads and several other endocrine glands. In turn, the endocrine products of the gonads and other glands feed back onto the anterior pituitary and partially regulate the endocrine activity of this gland. However, this type of "feedback" loop between gonads and pituitary could not account for many aspects of reproductive function. For example, how could factors in the external environment alter secretion by the gonads?

To account for environmental effects, one would have to postulate a functional connection between the nervous system and the anterior pituitary–gonad loop. One clue came from the research of Ernst and Berta Scharrer, who showed that certain brain cells were capable of secreting hormones. In the 1950s, Sir Geoffrey Harris and others postulated that the hypothalamic area of the brain produces chemicals that travel in the bloodstream down a stalk connecting the hypothalamus to the pituitary gland. If neural pathways to the sense organs could be traced to the hypothalamus, a mechanism for the alteration of gonadal function by the external environment would be apparent (see Wurtman's and Menaker's chapters in Section I).

Harris's proposal was put to experimental test, and about 25 years later Roger Guillemin and A. Schally were awarded the Nobel Prize for discovering the structure of the polypeptide hormone of the hypothalamus that stimulates production of reproductive hormones by the anterior pituitary gland. This discovery is described in the article by Guillemin and Roger Burgus. All of this research, conducted in a variety of animal species, led to a better understanding of the physiology of reproduction in humans.

In Sheldon J. Segal's article we see how the interactions among brain, anterior pituitary gland, and gonads become integrated in the adult human. With this information it is possible for us to intervene at points of vulnerability and manipulate the reproductive process in order to enhance or diminish fertility.

The final article of the section, by Seymour Levine, describes the differences in the brain–pituitary–gonad loops of females and males. Why do females have a cyclic pattern of hormone secretion and males an acyclic pattern of hormone secretion in adulthood? The work of C. Pfeiffer and G. Harris suggests that this differentiation between females and males is attributable to an action of a testicular hormone on the brain early in life (prenatally in some species) (see the article by Bruce S. McEwen in Section III for a description of the biochemistry of this effect). Although this concept may be valid for some species, there is still doubt about its applicability to humans. The same may be said of the amazing finding, first established by W. C. Young's laboratory, that testis hormone produced prenatally affects sex differences in adult behavior (see the article by Jean Lipman-Blumen in Section V for a discussion of the social determinants in sexual differentiation of behavior in humans).

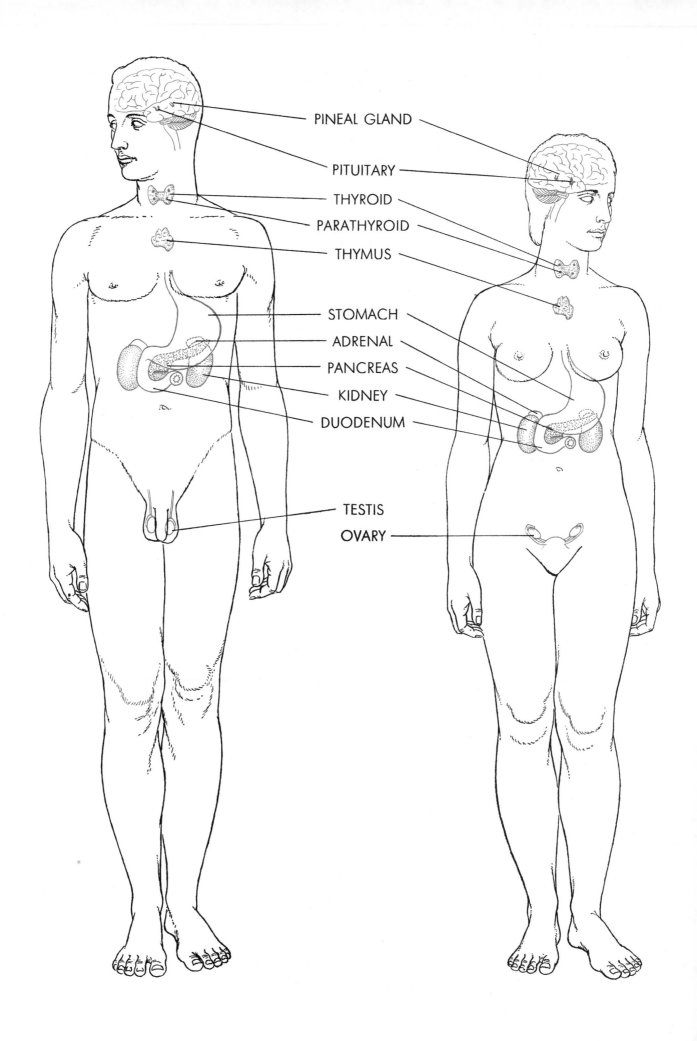

PINEAL GLAND

PITUITARY

THYROID

PARATHYROID

THYMUS

STOMACH

ADRENAL

PANCREAS

KIDNEY

DUODENUM

TESTIS

OVARY

Hormones

5

by Sir Solly Zuckerman
March 1957

*These potent biological substances are called
the chemical messengers of the body. They may also
be viewed as members of a larger system which
integrates the phenomena of life*

When a cockerel is castrated, it fails to develop into a rooster. Normal development of the secondary sexual characters that mark a male fowl depends upon a chemical substance which is secreted by the testes and transported by the bloodstream to all parts of the body, including the germ buds of the feathers and the region of the comb and wattles. The maleness and femaleness of most animals is determined in this chemical way.

The idea that something of this kind happens in the body came early in man's speculation about his physiological workings. Aristotle made observations about the effects of castration, and so did many after him. John Hunter, the distinguished 18th-century English anatomist, went a step further and experimented on transplanting the testes. When they were regrafted to another part of the abdominal cavity, the animal developed normally. This implied that the mechanism of their effects must be chemical rather than nervous, for the original nerve connections of the testes to the body were cut by the operation. But it was not until 1849 that A. A. Berthold, a young German zoologist, made a detailed study of the effects of removal and replacement of testicular tissue and so discovered the principle of what is now called endocrine action. His short paper on the subject provides the essential foundation of the modern study of hormones.

Soon afterward the observation by Claude Bernard, the famous French

physiologist, that the liver "secretes" sugar into the blood led to the general understanding that there are special endocrine glands which pour their secretions directly into the bloodstream. The whole concept was given a specific meaning when, in 1904, the English physiologists Ernest Starling and William Bayliss conceived the endocrine system as a complex of chemical messengers which coordinate the functions of different tissues of the body. Starling observed that these "hormones," as he named them, "have to be carried from the organ where they are produced to the organ which they affect, by means of the bloodstream, and the continually recurring physiological needs of the organism must determine their repeated production and circulation through the body."

Modern endocrinology, in spite of all the attention it has received, remains essentially an empirical science, for we have only a vague understanding of the fundamental mechanisms of endocrine action. We observe the physiological effects of hormones, but we know little about how they act upon cells. We have nothing like a full list of the hormones themselves, or of the organs that produce them. The usual method of identifying a hormone is to remove the organ suspected of secreting a chemical messenger, analyze the effects of its removal and then try to extract the active agent. But obviously these methods are inapplicable to an organ such as the lungs, whose removal would mean immediate death. We have no present means of determining with certainty whether or not such organs secrete hormones, although they may well do so.

Of the established endocrine organs, the most important is the pituitary gland, attached to the base of the brain. It has two lobes. The posterior lobe secretes

hormones which stimulate the contractions of the uterus during childbirth and also the release of milk from the mammary gland. Posterior lobe secretions also control the amount of fluid filtered by the kidneys. Hormones of the pituitary's anterior lobe control the functioning of most of the other endocrine organs of the body. They include the thyrotrophic hormone (TSH), which acts upon the thyroid gland; the adrenocorticotrophic hormone (ACTH), which stimulates the cortex (outer part) of the adrenal glands, and the gonadotrophic hormones (FSH and LH), which control the secretion of sex hormones by the ovaries and the testes, respectively. In addition, the anterior lobe produces a growth hormone, somatotrophin (STH), which acts on the whole body.

Other endocrine organs are the pancreas, which secretes insulin; the parathyroids, four beads of tissue embedded in the back of the thyroid; the adrenal medulla, the core of the adrenal glands; certain cells lining the first part of the gut; the pineal gland, attached to the brain, and the thymus gland, behind the breastplate.

Effects on Growth

We know that hormones are concerned in almost every living process, including every phase of the growth of the body. If an immature animal is deprived of the anterior lobe of its pituitary gland, it ceases to grow or mature. To grow it must be supplied with the growth hormone (STH), and for sexual maturation it requires the gonad-stimulating hormones (FSH and LH). The growth of the body as a whole is also influenced by the male sex hormones produced by the testes. This is shown by the fact that about the time of puberty

5

HORMONE-SECRETING ORGANS of man are outlined in color in the figures on the opposite page. Except for the gonads, the organs are the same in the male and female.

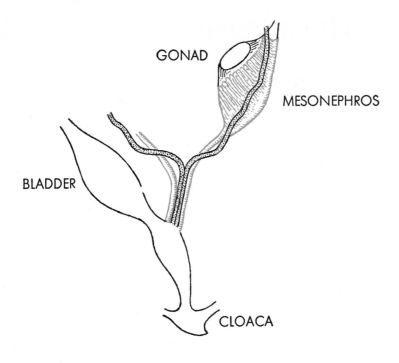

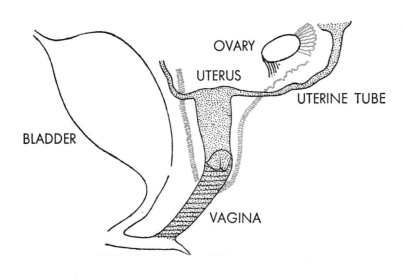

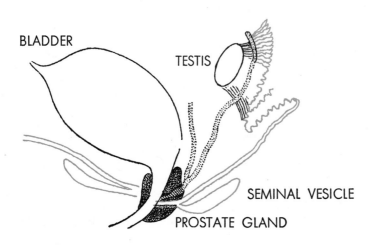

the male begins to grow bigger than the female. Indeed, it is through hormones that the animal's sex itself is determined. In the early stages the embryo is sexually neutral, possessing tissues out of which either female or male reproductive organs can be formed. If the embryo is a genetic male, its embryonic gonad produces hormone which promotes the development of masculine organs and suppresses the feminine.

The development of the body is also profoundly affected by the hormones of the thyroid gland (thyroxine and triiodothyronine). Removal of this gland from a young animal will inhibit growth, delay bone formation and prevent proper development of the reproductive system. These disturbances of growth combine to produce cretinism. The physical basis of the retardation of mental development in cretins has recently been clarified by experiments on rats. In an animal deprived of thyroid hormone there is a reduction in development of the network of dendrites, the tendril-like processes which act as contacts between nerve cells, and also in growth of the nerve axon, down which impulses are fired from one nerve cell to the next. As a result the animal's reflex responses are considerably slower than normal. The nerve cells of such an animal can be stimulated to resume normal growth by giving it thyroxine, if the hormone is supplied before it is too late. The treatment restores some, but not all, of its adaptive behavior.

The parathyroid glands also influence growth, by their control over calcium and phosphorus metabolism, and of course so too does the adrenal cortex; when it ceases to pour its secretions in normal fashion into the bloodstream, not only growth but life itself must stop.

Effects on Metabolism

Hormones regulate metabolism in the body in intricate and far-reaching ways. Consider the metabolism of sugar. For good health the supply or level of sugar

GONADAL SYSTEM of vertebrates is sexually neutral in the early embryo (*schematic drawing at top*). The mesonephros, an excretory organ, retains its function even after birth. If the embryo develops into a female (*center*), the outer tubes (*color*) regress while the uterine tube, uterus and vagina form from the inner ones. In the male (*bottom*), the inner tubes practically disappear while the outer ones (*color*) form the seminal vesicles and ducts from testes.

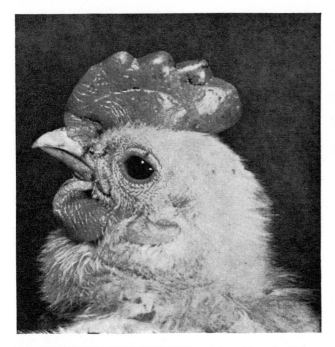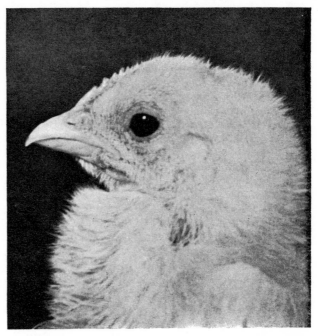

MALE HORMONE TESTOSTERONE was injected into the 18-day-old chick at left by Hans Selye of the University of Montreal. The injection resulted in male characteristics. The normal chick at right, which is the same age, lacks precocious comb and wattles.

in the blood must be held fairly constant. Four factors enter here: (1) the rate of use of sugar for energy by the tissues; (2) the rate of absorption of sugar by the blood from the intestines and of reabsorption from the fluid filtered by the kidneys; (3) the release of sugar from the carbohydrate-storing tissues (*e.g.*, the liver and muscle), and (4) the formation of sugar from fats and proteins. In all these processes hormones play a part. Insulin, produced in the pancreas, speeds up the rate at which the tissues use sugar. If the body is deprived of this hormone, by removal or poor functioning of the pancreas (as in the disease diabetes mellitus), the level of sugar in the blood rises considerably. This can lead to death, unless insulin is given to depress the blood-sugar level. On the other hand, if the anterior lobe of the pituitary gland, as well as the pancreas, is removed from an animal, it may survive for months, in spite of the lack of insulin. Evidently the anterior pituitary normally has something to do with supplying sugar to the blood, and its removal therefore reduces the sugar level.

The pituitary apparently acts indirectly to promote both the formation of sugar and its release into the bloodstream. For example, the pituitary hormone ACTH stimulates the adrenal cortex to secrete hormones which in turn stimulate the tissues to synthesize glycogen (animal starch) from proteins. Again, the anterior pituitary causes the thyroid to release a hormone which speeds up the oxidation of sugar by the tissues and also affects the rate at which sugar is absorbed into the bloodstream through the gut.

The metabolism of proteins likewise is considerably influenced by hormonal reactions. So too is the retention or shift of water between and within cells, which is determined mainly by the movement of sodium and potassium ions across cell membranes. One of the hormones involved in water metabolism is aldosterone, produced by the adrenal cortex: it promotes the retention of sodium and chloride in the tissues and stimulates the excretion of potassium. Other hormones that affect the body's retention of water are the hormone serotonin (found in brain tissue and in certain cells of the gut) and an antidiuretic hormone of the posterior pituitary. The sex hormones also influence water metabolism to some extent.

Controls

These examples illustrate that hormones play a vital part in the orderly development and functioning of the body, in general metabolic processes and in specific bodily adaptations such as the cyclic changes in the female reproductive organs. How are all these mechanisms organized into an orderly pattern of operation?

The pattern of control seems to be made up of sets of reciprocal interactions between the endocrine organs. For example, the anterior pituitary and the adrenal cortex are parts of a feedback system. The pituitary hormone ACTH stimulates the adrenal cortex to secrete its steroid hormones. If one adrenal gland is removed, the ACTH stimulation causes the cortex of the remaining adrenal to increase in size. If, on the other hand, the anterior pituitary lobe is removed, the resultant lack of ACTH leads to a considerable atrophy of the cortex of both adrenal glands. If ACTH is then injected, the adrenals return to their usual size. It appears that under normal conditions the concentration of adrenal cortex hormones in the bloodstream controls the secretion of stimulating ACTH by the pituitary: when this concentration is high, less ACTH is released; when it is low, the release of ACTH increases. The same sort of "push-and-pull" mechanism is believed to operate in other cases of hormones stimulating a specific target organ. The secretion of sex hormones by the ovaries and testes is subject to a similar feedback control, and the various sex hormones in turn interact with each other. Thus the effects of estrogen, one of the two hormones produced by the ovaries, may be neutralized by an extra output of progesterone, the other ovarian hormone.

There is considerable ignorance about how all these sets of interactions are organized into a pattern. One possibility is that a chain reaction involving several endocrine organs may be called forth by a general metabolic condition or need of the body. For example, during exercise the muscles require more sugar. This single need may call a number of hormonal processes into play. Insulin stimulates the transformation of glycogen in the liver and muscle into glucose. The release and conversion of this glycogen is also promoted by adrenalin from the adrenal medulla, which is activated by nerve impulses during exercise or stress. In addition, the secretion of adrenalin apparently stimulates the anterior pituitary to secrete ACTH, which in turn causes the adrenal cortex to release hormones that promote the synthesis of glycogen from protein. Adrenalin may also stimulate the anterior pituitary to produce ACTH indirectly by way of its effects on the hypothalamus, to which the posterior part of the pituitary is connected. Finally, it has been suggested that a low level of sugar in the blood itself directly stimulates the secretion of ACTH. These various possibilities indicate the complex interplay of events that must be involved even in a single metabolic process.

The problems become still more complex in responses in which the nervous system plays a part. An example is the seasonal reproductive behavior of animals whose breeding is conditioned by the length of the day, or exposure to light. A female ferret, which is sexually dormant during the autumn and winter, can be brought into heat at that time by keeping it in artificial light for a few hours after sunset each day. But it will not respond if it is blind or if its pituitary gland or its ovaries are removed. The chain of reactions clearly follows the sequence: stimulation of the retina by light, transmission of impulses along the optic nerves to the brain, stimulation of the anterior pituitary to secrete the gonadotrophic hormone, which stimulates the ovaries to secrete estrogen which in turn produces sexual heat, marked by swelling of the genital organs. The main gap in our knowledge here is: How do the nervous impulses reaching the brain via the optic nerves trigger the secretion of gonadotrophic hormone by the anterior pituitary?

The hypothalamus, at the base of the brain, is connected to the pituitary by a stalk of nerve fibers. These are known to pass to the posterior lobe, but whether any reach the anterior lobe of the pituitary, which produces the gonadotrophic hormone, is still unsettled, in spite of considerable study. If they do, one might suppose that nerve impulses directly activate the anterior pituitary to release the hormone; if not, we might assume that the hypothalamus sends a chemical messenger to the anterior pituitary by way of the bloodstream. But unfortunately the whole problem is made completely mysterious by the experimental finding that the anterior pituitary can secrete the gonadotrophic hormone even when its nerve and blood-vessel connections to the hypothalamus are completely severed!

Hormones from Nerve Cells

There is considerable evidence, however, that the hypothalamus itself does produce hormones—hormones previously supposed to be secreted by the posterior pituitary. The hormones in question include oxytocin, which triggers labor contractions of the uterus and the release of milk by the mammary glands, and vasopressin, which raises blood pressure and reduces the excretion of urine.

Some years ago the anatomist Ernst A. Scharrer (now at the Albert Einstein College of Medicine) drew attention to the fact that certain nerve cells in the hypothalamus contained what looked like secretory granules. He therefore argued that the hypothalamus, in addition to being a primitive motor center of the brain, was also in effect a secretory organ. Similar granules were later found also within the nerve fibers of the pituitary stalk. When the stalk was tied or cut, secretory material collected in the fibers immediately above the knot, and the part of the posterior pituitary below the ligature rapidly became depleted of such material. Other experiments showed that extracts of the hypothalamus have the properties of the hormones that had been thought to be produced by the posterior pituitary. It is now believed that the hypothalamus is the source of the hormones and the posterior lobe of the pituitary is essentially a storehouse for them, although very likely it also modifies them chemically.

Action in the Cell

The concept of nerve cells secreting hormones immediately raises some provocative questions. For example, can the same cell generate a nerve impulse and secrete a hormone? However, the whole subject of the way hormonal mechanisms operate at the cell level is clouded by ignorance. It is tempting to suppose that hormones act in the cell by regulating enzyme reactions, which are involved in all metabolic transformations (*e.g.*, the

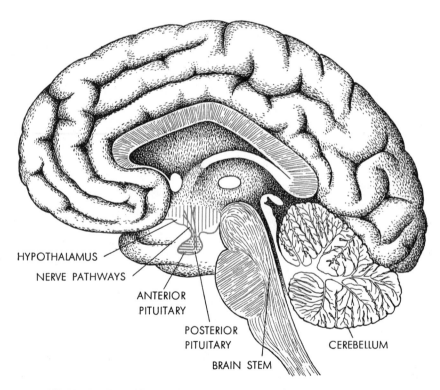

HYPOTHALAMUS

NERVE PATHWAYS

ANTERIOR PITUITARY

POSTERIOR PITUITARY

BRAIN STEM

CEREBELLUM

SECTION OF THE HUMAN BRAIN indicates the close relationship between the pituitary and the hypothalamus. The two structures are connected by a stalk of nerve fibers. It is not clear, however, whether the hypothalamus stimulates the secretions of the pituitary.

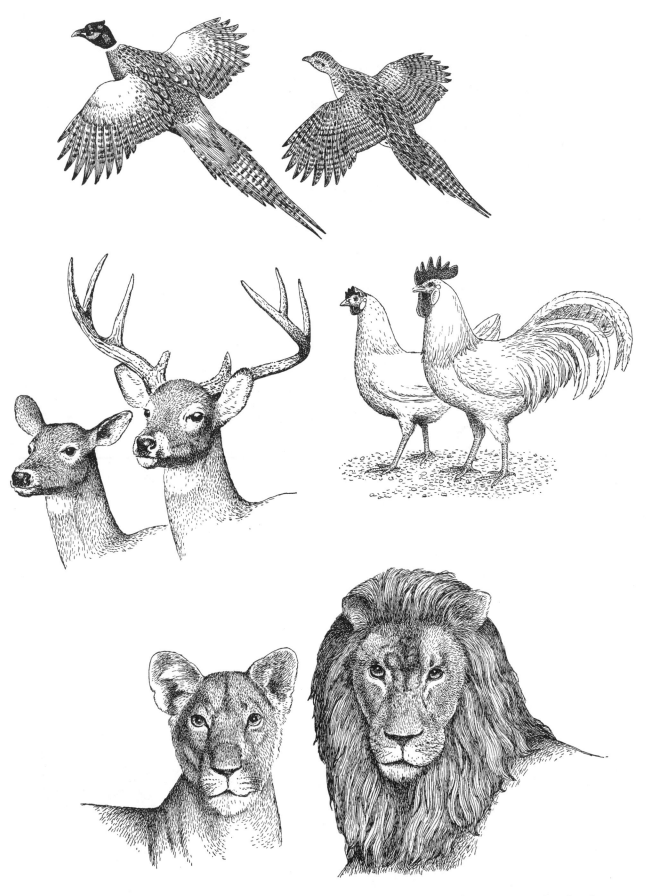

SECONDARY CHARACTERISTICS of male and female animals are brought out by hormones acting in concert with hereditary factors. Estrogen produces the plumage of the female pheasant (*top right*). Testosterone causes the development of comb and spurs in the white leghorn rooster (*right center*), the antlers of the white-tailed deer (*left center*) and probably the mane of the lion (*bottom*).

1 TESTOSTERONE

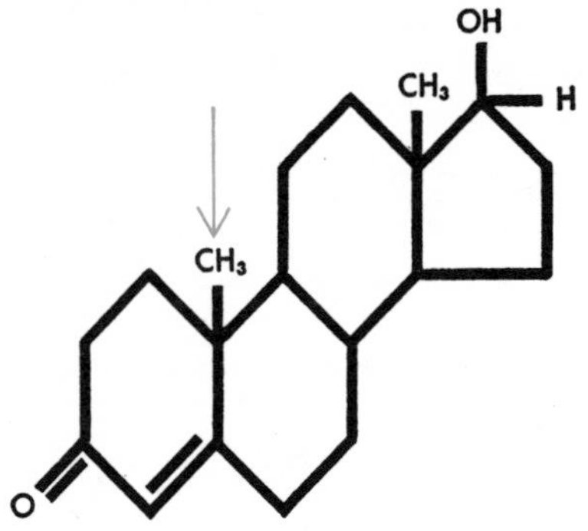

2 19-NOR-TESTOSTERONE

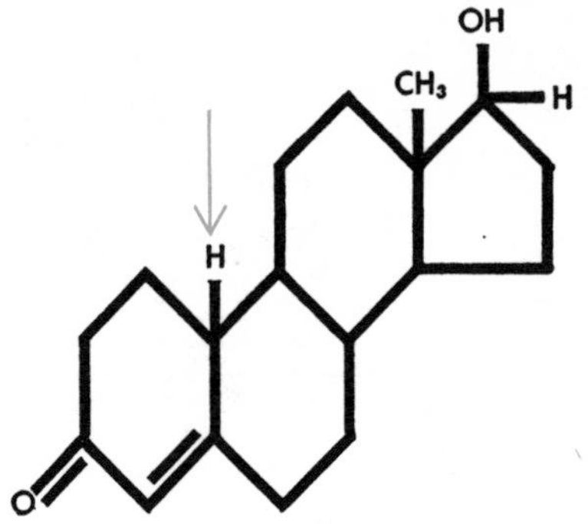

3 PROGESTERONE

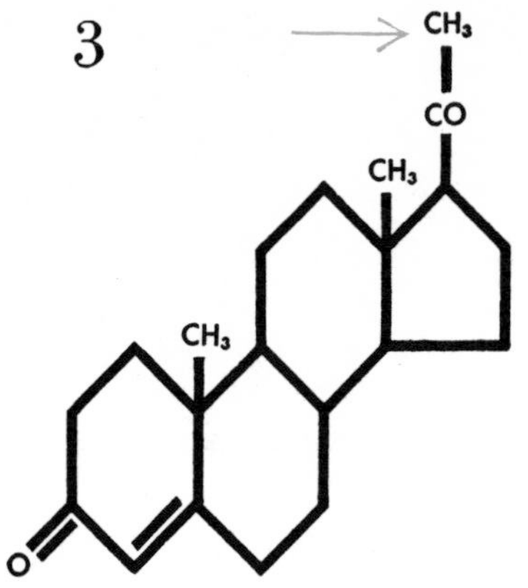

ANDROGENS and related compounds have the molecular structures depicted in these diagrams, in which carbon rings are abbreviated. The arrows in the diagrams emphasize significant differences in structure. Male characteristics are induced by compounds 1

1 DESOXYCORTICOSTERONE

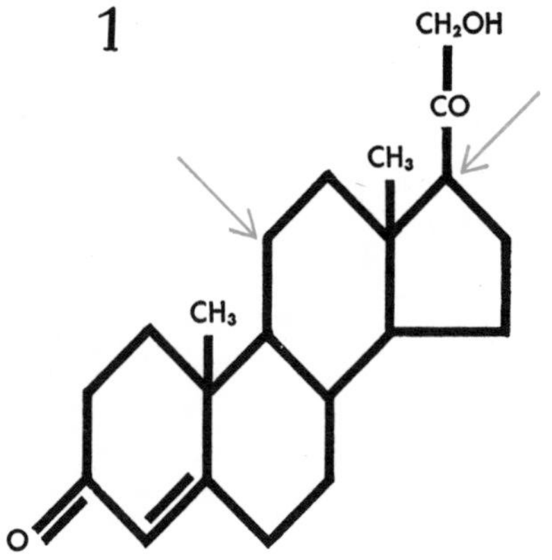

2 HYDROCORTISONE

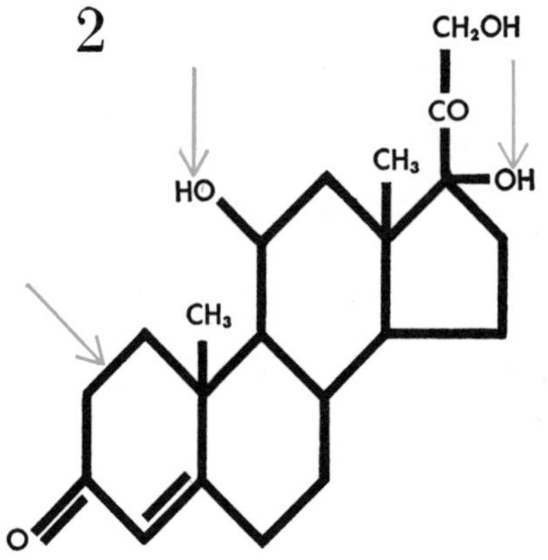

3 PREDNISOLONE

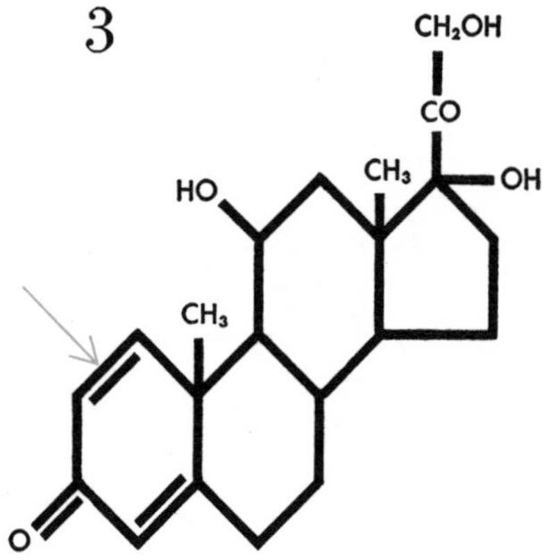

ADRENOCORTICAL STEROIDS and related compounds are important in the treatment of certain diseases. Compounds 1 and 4 are associated with retention of sodium and water, while 2 is associated with excretion of sodium and water and with carbohydrate-

1 ESTRADIOL

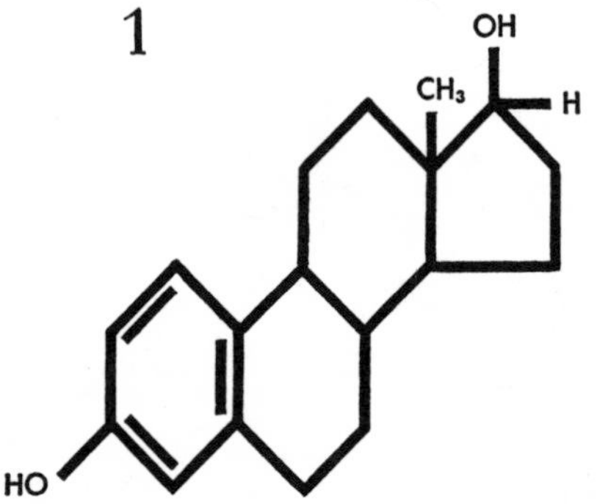

2 DIETHYLSTILBESTROL

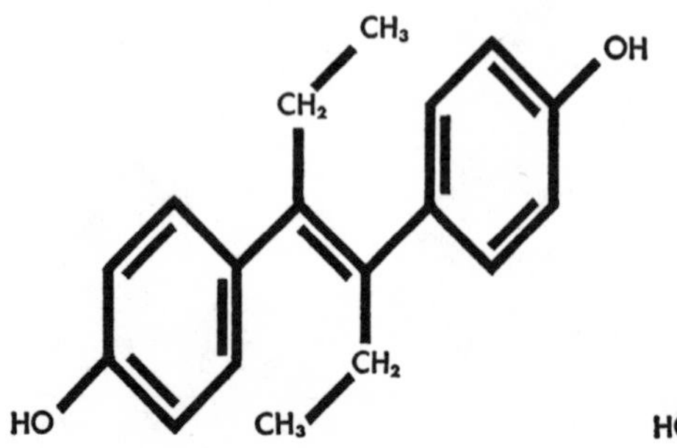

3 DIMETHYLSTILBESTROL

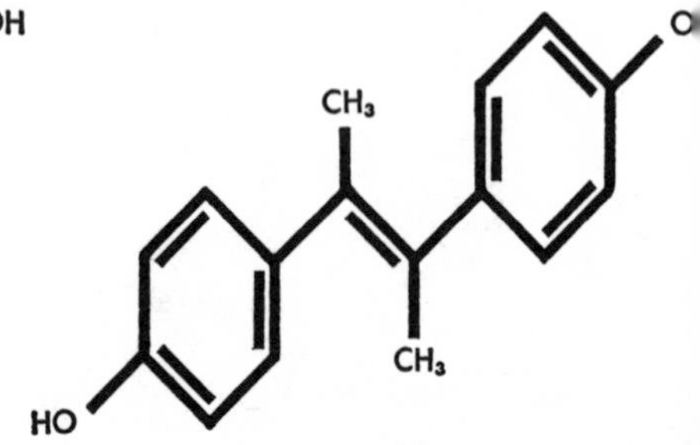

ESTROGENS and related compounds do not all have the configuration of four joined rings characteristic of the steroid hormones. Estradiol (1) is the natural female hormone. Synthetic compounds 2 and 3 are closely related but only 2 has estrogenic properties.

4

CH₂F

21-FLUORO-PROGESTERONE

5

AMPHENONE-B

and 2, but 1 is considerably more potent. Progesterone (3) is produced by the ovary. Compounds 4 and 5 have properties similar to 3, even though the structure of 5 is unrelated.

4

ALDOSTERONE

forming properties. Both 2 and 3 may be made synthetically; 3 is the more potent.

4

GENISTEIN

Genistein is extracted from subterranean clover, a spreading species of clover genus.

conversion of liver glycogen to glucose). If so, they must act in a great variety of ways, because the hormones are chemically very diverse: those secreted by the adrenal cortex and the gonads are steroids; insulin is a protein; the gonadotrophins are glycoproteins; the posterior pituitary hormones are polypeptides; thyroxine is an amino acid combined with iodine; adrenalin is an amine derivative. A further indication of the hormones' chemical versatility is the fact that a single hormone may act upon various enzymes: estrogen is apparently able to influence at least six enzyme reactions.

Yet all the enzyme systems with which we are acquainted appear to be able to function without the intervention of any hormone, and it has not yet been possible to trace the physiological action of hormones to their chemical action. According to some authorities, it is even possible that hormones exercise their effects not by modulating the action of particular enzymes but by influencing energy transfers. For example, it has been suggested that estrogens increase the availability of energy to the cell by altering the physical state of a part of the cell where glucose is formed. By so doing they provide energy for the synthetic processes which underlie cellular division. In addition, estrogens possibly regulate the permeability of tissues to water, partly by altering the ground substance in which the cells of the body are embedded.

Hormones which apparently differ

only slightly in molecular structure sometimes have vastly different effects. In some cases, on the other hand, compounds of very different structure produce the same effect [*see formulas in bottom row at the left*]. There is no obvious explanation for such facts, but in the case of the natural estrogen estradiol and the synthetic estrogen stilbestrol, the similarity of their biological effects may be due to a correspondence of interatomic distance between the two hydroxylic groups of the molecule.

Among the difficulties which prevent any real understanding of the relation of chemical structure to hormonal action is the fact that the experimentalist can rarely be certain that an isolated hormone is chemically identical with its form in the body. There is always a danger that the extracted, "chemically pure" hormone has lost some of the activities which it normally exercises in the body. It frequently turns out, too, that several pure substances are isolated from extracts of an endocrine organ and it is difficult to decide which of them is the natural hormone. For example, several clearly defined estrogens have been isolated from the ovaries. Are they all normal secretions, or are some laboratory artifacts? And in view of the chemical transformations that natural estrogens undergo in the body, can we be certain which of its natural forms is the one that acts on estrogen-sensitive tissues? Again, of some 30 different steroids isolated from the adrenal cortex, only a few are biologically active. Which of them is the important hormone? We still do not know how many active steroids the adrenal cortex produces under normal conditions, and what their respective effects are on the metabolism of carbohydrates, proteins and minerals. Studies with radioactive tracers may soon answer some of these questions, however. Such studies have already helped greatly in elucidating stages in the chemical breakdown of hormones before their excretion from the body.

One of the remarkable features of the endocrine glands is the capacity of the same cell to produce a number of different hormones. We have just seen that the cells of the adrenal cortex make several different biologically active steroids. From just a few types of cells in the anterior pituitary come diverse secretions which stimulate the thyroid, the gonads, the adrenal cortex, the mammary glands and other organs, not to speak of body growth in general. In the testes the same cells can produce male and female hormones. In fact a stallion gives forth more

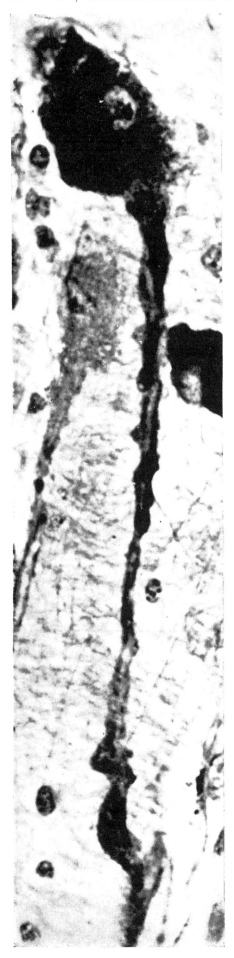

NERVE CELL of the hypothalamus secretes the dark-staining material which fills the cell body (*top*) and most of its long, thin axon. The material exudes from the end of the axon. This preparation was made from a dog's hypothalamus by Walther Hild of the University of Texas School of Medicine in Galveston. It is magnified 1,100 diameters.

estrogen than a mare does, except during a brief period of the mare's gestation!

Most hormones are produced only by a specific organ and effect a specific reaction. In some cases the target is a reaction that takes place throughout the body: for instance, the adrenal hormone aldosterone affects the water balance of all tissues. In others the target is a specific organ: the pituitary gonadotrophin acts basically on the testes or ovaries. Yet, to add to the complexity of the hormonal system, there are deviations even from this fundamental concept of specificity. The adrenal cortex can produce sex hormones; the gonads, conversely, can secrete substances with the properties of adrenocortical hormones. Some specialized reactions may be triggered by several types of stimulation: for example, menstrual bleeding, normally brought on by cessation of stimulation by ovarian hormone, can also be induced experimentally by certain adrenocortical steroids.

Hormones and Disease

In view of the complex, interlocking character of the endocrine system, it is not surprising that a derangement of the functioning of an endocrine gland produces far-reaching effects. A marked deficiency of secretion by the adrenal cortex results in Addison's disease, which manifests a variety of symptoms—extreme weakness, wasting, gastro-intestinal disturbances, a pronounced darkening of the skin—and was almost invariably fatal until the recent development of hormonal treatment. On the other hand, overactivity of the adrenal cortex may lead to various disorders: among other things, it may cause women to develop masculine characteristics, because it produces steroids with the properties of the male sex hormone. When the anterior pituitary gland functions poorly, growth of the body is impaired and puberty is delayed; development of the reproductive organs may even fail altogether. Conversely, overactivity of the pituitary leads to gigantism or, in an adult, to overgrowth of the head, hands and feet—the condition known as acromegaly. In the case of the thyroid gland, under-

functioning in childhood produces cretinism, and in adulthood it leads to a strange thickening of the skin, loss of hair, great lethargy and mental slowness. Overactivity of the thyroid (called Graves' disease) results in the familiar symptoms of a high rate of metabolism, great excitability and protruding eyes. And of course everyone knows that a deficiency of secretion of insulin by the pancreas is responsible for diabetes.

The results of derangement of the endocrine system are so pervasive that it is natural to suspect it of complicity in various systemic diseases. The estrogenic hormones are chemically related to some of the hydrocarbons that induce cancer when applied to the skin of rats and mice. These hormones stimulate the growth of cells in the reproductive organs of women, including the breast. Could they initiate malignant growth in those organs? So far all that has been proved is that estrogenic stimulation does play a part in the triggering of cancer in strains of mice genetically susceptible to the disease. Paradoxically, estrogen can be used as a treatment for certain forms of cancer—for example, cancer of the prostate.

Hans Selye of Montreal has grouped together arthritis, hypertension and kidney disease as a set of disorders resulting from derangement of the pituitary-adrenal system. The basic idea is that when the body is subjected to some general stress (such as extreme cold or shock), the adrenal cortex immediately releases and becomes temporarily depleted of its steroid hormones. If the stress continues, the anterior pituitary secretes so much ACTH as to overstimulate the adrenal cortex. This leads to pathological results, including rheumatoid arthritis. Popular interest in the idea was excited when it was found that ACTH and cortisone had an almost miraculous effect in relieving the symptoms of rheumatoid arthritis. However, the relief lasts only so long as the hormones are being administered, and if administered too long, they frequently have dangerous side effects.

The "adaptation syndrome" has been hailed as a "unified concept of disease." This seems too sweeping and overambitious a view. Nevertheless it is difficult to exaggerate the importance of the study of endocrinology. The past 10 years have seen the development of the concept of secretions by nerve cells, the synthesis of the hormones of the pituitary posterior lobe, the discovery of such potent adrenal hormones as aldosterone and hydrocortisone and the complete working out of the structure of the insulin molecule. They have also brought to light the

possible roles of hormones in immunological reactions, in the genesis of cancer
and in the control of fertility—a subject
which may have enormous importance
for the future welfare of the world. Other
vast fields of endocrine action have been
found in invertebrate animals and in
plants. Hormones are no longer regarded
merely as chemical messengers in the
bloodstream. They play a part in almost
every, if not every, living process.

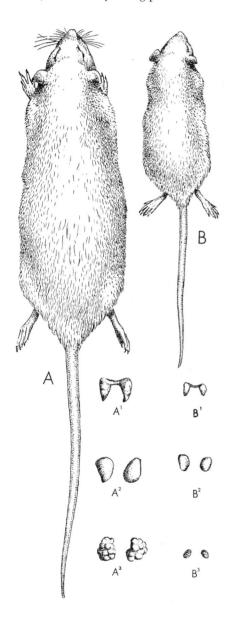

EFFECT OF PITUITARY HORMONE on
growth may be demonstrated in the rat. The
pituitary was removed from one of two lit-
termates 36 days after birth, at which time
both rats had the same weight. After several
months the normal animal (*left*) had
tripled its weight and had matured while
the other (*right*) had gained little weight
and was maturing much more slowly. At left
are the thyroids (A1), adrenals (A2), and
ovaries (A3) of the normal rat, and at right
are glands (B1, B2, B3) of operated rat.

6

The Hormones
of the Hypothalamus

by Roger Guillemin and Roger Burgus
November 1972

*The anterior pituitary gland, which controls the
peripheral endocrine glands, is itself regulated by
"releasing factors" originating in the brain. Two of these
hormones have now been isolated and synthesized*

The pituitary gland is attached by a stalk to the region in the base of the brain known as the hypothalamus. Within the past year or so, after nearly 20 years of effort in many laboratories throughout the world, two substances have been isolated from animal brain tissue that represent the first of the long sought hypothalamic hormones. Because the molecular structure of the new hormones is fairly simple the substances can readily be synthesized in large quantities. Their availability and their high activity in humans has led physiologists and clinicians to consider that the hypothalamic hormones will open a new chapter in medicine.

It has long been known that the pituitary secretes several complex hormones that travel through the bloodstream to target organs, notably the thyroid gland, the gonads and the cortex of the adrenal glands. There the pituitary hormones stimulate the secretion into the bloodstream of the thyroid hormones, of the sex hormones by the gonads and of several steroid hormones such as hydrocortisone by the adrenal cortex. The secretion of the thyroid, sex and adrenocortical hormones thus has two stages beginning with the release of pituitary hormones. Studies going back some 50 years culminated in the demonstration that the process actually has three stages: the release of the pituitary hormones requires the prior release of another class of hormones manufactured in the hypothalamus. It is two of these hypothalamic hormones that have now been isolated, chemically identified and synthesized.

One of the hypothalamic hormones acts as the factor that triggers the release of the pituitary hormone thyrotropin, sometimes called the thyroid-stimulating hormone, or TSH. Thus the hypothalamic hormone associated with TSH is called the TSH-releasing factor, or TRF. The other hormone is LRF. Here again "RF" stands for "releasing factor"; the "L" signifies that the substance releases the gonadotropic pituitary hormone LH, the luteinizing hormone. A third gonadotropic hormone, FSH (follicle-stimulating hormone), may have its own hypothalamic releasing factor, FRF, but that has not been demonstrated. It is known, however, that the hypothalamic hormone LRF stimulates the release of FSH as well as LH.

Studies are continuing aimed at characterizing several other hypothalamic hormones that are known to exist on the basis of physiological evidence but that have not yet been isolated. One of them regulates the secretion of adrenocorticotropin (ACTH), the pituitary hormone whose target is the adrenal cortex. Another hormone (possibly two hormones with opposing actions) regulates the release of prolactin, the pituitary hormone involved in pregnancy and lactation. Still another hormone (again possibly two hormones with opposing actions) regulates the release of the pituitary hormone involved in growth and structural development (growth hormone).

That the hypothalamus and the pituitary act in concert can be suspected not only from their physical proximity at the base of the brain but also from their development in the embryo. During the early embryological development of all mammals a small pouch forms in the upper part of the developing pharynx and migrates upward toward the developing brain. There it meets a similar formation, resembling the finger of a glove, that springs from the base of the primordial brain. Several months later the first pouch, now detached from the upper oral cavity, has filled into a solid mass of cells differentiated into glandular types. At this point the second pouch, still connected to the base of the brain, is rich with hundreds of thousands of nerve fibers associated with a modified type of glial cell, not too unlike the glial cells found throughout the brain. The two organs are now enclosed in a single receptacle that has formed as an open spherical cavity within the sphenoid bone, on which the brain rests.

This double organ, now ensconced in the sphenoidal bone, is the pituitary gland, or hypophysis. The part that migrated from the brain is the posterior lobe, or neurohypophysis; the part that migrated from the pharynx is the anterior lobe, or adenohypophysis. Both parts of the gland remain connected to the brain by a common stalk that goes through the covering flap of the sphenoidal cavity. For many years after the double embryological origin of the pituitary gland was recognized the role of the gland was no more clearly understood than it had been in the old days. Indeed, the name "pituitary" had been given to it in the 16th century by Vesalius, who thought that the little organ had to do with secretion of *pituita:* the nasal fluid.

We know now that the anterior lobe of the pituitary gland controls the secretion and function of all the "periph-

HYPOTHALAMIC FRAGMENTS of sheep brains were the source from which the authors' laboratory extracted one milligram of TRF, the first hypothalamic hormone to be characterized and synthesized. The photograph is of about 30 frozen hypothalamic fragments; some five million such fragments, dissected from 500 tons of sheep brain tissue, were processed over a period of four years.

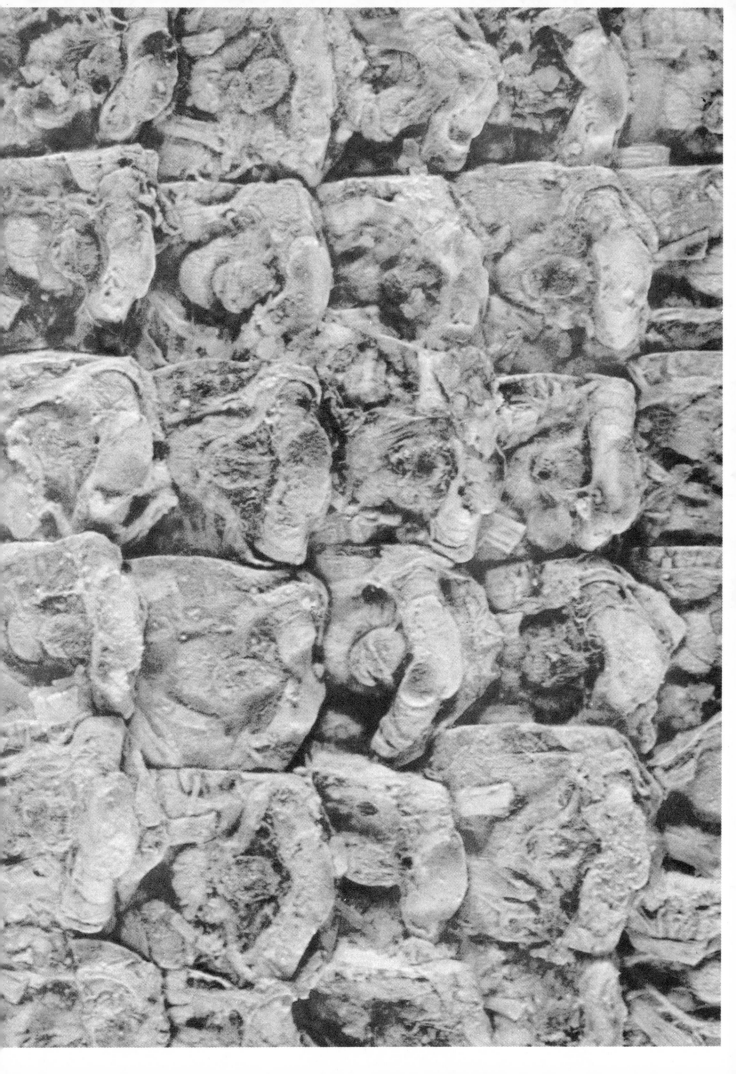

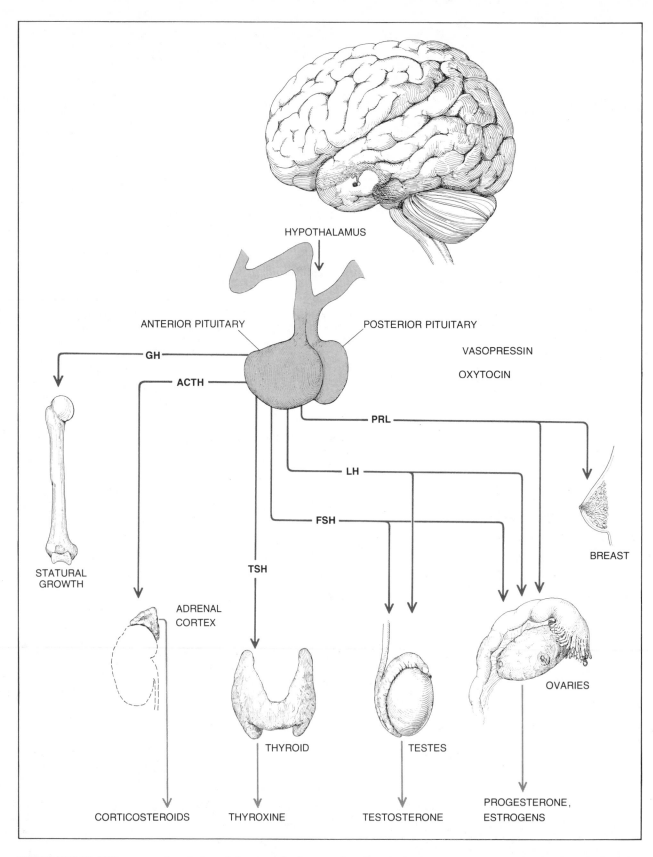

HYPOTHALAMUS

ANTERIOR PITUITARY   POSTERIOR PITUITARY

VASOPRESSIN

OXYTOCIN

GH

ACTH

PRL

LH

FSH

TSH

BREAST

STATURAL
GROWTH

ADRENAL
CORTEX

OVARIES

THYROID   TESTES

CORTICOSTEROIDS   THYROXINE   TESTOSTERONE   PROGESTERONE,
                                                       ESTROGENS

PITUITARY GLAND, connected to the hypothalamus at the base of the brain, has two lobes and two functions. The posterior lobe of the pituitary stores and passes on to the general circulation two hormones manufactured in the hypothalamus: vasopressin and oxytocin. The anterior lobe secretes a number of other hormones: growth hormone (GH), which promotes statural growth; adreno-corticotropic hormone (ACTH), which stimulates the cortex of the adrenal gland to secrete corticosteroids; thyroid-stimulating hormone (TSH), which stimulates secretions by the thyroid gland, and follicle-stimulating hormone (FSH), luteinizing hormone (LH) and prolactin (PRL), which in various combinations regulate lactation and the functioning of the gonads. Several of these anterior pituitary hormones are known to be controlled by releasing factors from the hypothalamus, two of which have now been synthesized.

eral" endocrine glands (the thyroid, the gonads and the adrenal cortex). It also controls the mammary glands and regulates the harmonious growth of the individual. It accomplishes all this by the secretion of a series of complex protein and glycoprotein hormones. All the pituitary hormones are manufactured and secreted by the anterior lobe. Why should this master endocrine gland have migrated so far in the course of evolution (a journey recapitulated in the embryo) to make contact with the brain? As we shall see, recent observations have answered the question.

The posterior lobe of the pituitary has been known for the past 50 years to secrete substances that affect the reabsorption of water from the kidney into the bloodstream. These secretions also stimulate the contraction of the uterus during childbirth and the release of milk during lactation. In the early 1950's Vincent Du Vigneaud and his co-workers at the Cornell University Medical College resolved a controversy of many years' standing by showing that the biological activities of the posterior lobe are attributable to two different molecules: vasopressin (or antidiuretic hormone) and oxytocin. The two molecules are octapeptides: structures made up of eight amino acids. Du Vigneaud's group showed that six of the eight amino acids in the two molecules are identical, which explains their closely related physicochemical properties and similar biological activity. Both hormones exhibit (in different ratios) all the major biological effects mentioned above: the reabsorption of water, the stimulation of uterine contractions and the release of milk.

As early as 1924 it was realized that the hormones secreted by the posterior lobe of the pituitary are also found in the hypothalamus: that part of the brain with which the lobe is connected by nerve fibers through the pituitary stalk. Later it was shown that the two hormones of the posterior pituitary are actually manufactured in some specialized nerve cells in the hypothalamus. They flow slowly down the pituitary stalk to the posterior pituitary through the axons, or long fibers, of the hypothalamic nerve cells [see top illustration on page 59]. They are stored in the posterior pituitary, which is now reduced to a storage organ rather than a manufacturing one. From it they are secreted into the bloodstream on the proper physiological stimulus.

These observations had led several

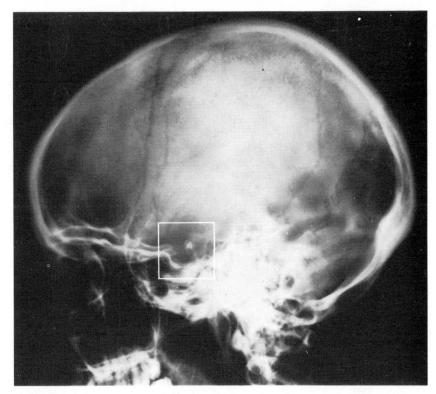

BONY RECEPTACLE in which the pituitary gland is enclosed is a cavity in the sphenoid bone, on which the base of the brain rests. White rectangle shows area diagrammed below.

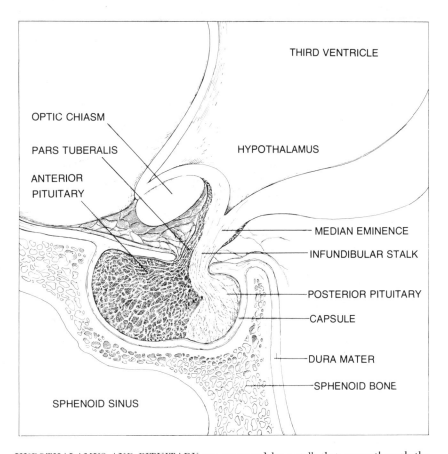

HYPOTHALAMUS AND PITUITARY are connected by a stalk that passes through the membranous lid of the receptacle in the sphenoid bone in which the pituitary rests. The double embryological origin of the two lobes of the pituitary is reflected in their differing tissues and functions and in the different ways that each is connected to the hypothalamus.

biologists, notably Ernst and Berta Scharrer, to the striking new concept of neurosecretion (the secretion of hormones by nerve cells). They suggested that specialized nerve cells might be able to manufacture and secrete true hormones, which would then be carried by the blood and would exert their effects in some target organ or tissue remote from their point of origin. The ability to manufacture hormones had traditionally been assigned to the endocrine glands: the thyroid, the gonads, the adrenals and so on. The suggestion that nerve cells could secrete hormones would endow them with a capacity far beyond their ability to liberate neurotransmitters such as epinephrine and acetylcholine at the submicroscopic regions (synapses) where they make contact with other nerve cells.

Even as these studies were in progress and these new concepts were being formulated other laboratories were reporting evidence that functions of the anterior lobe of the pituitary were somehow dependent on the structural integrity of the hypothalamic area and on a normal relation between the hypothalamus and the pituitary gland. For example, minute lesions of the hypothalamus, such as can be created by introducing small electrodes into the base of the brain in an experimental animal and producing localized electrocoagulation, were found to abolish the secretion of anterior pituitary hormones. On the other hand, the electrical stimulation of nerve cells in the same regions dramatically increased the secretion of the hormones [see illustration below].

Thus the question was presented: Precisely how does the hypothalamus regulate the secretory activity of the anterior pituitary? The results produced by electrocoagulation and electrical stimulation of the hypothalamus suggested some kind of neural mechanism. One objection to this theory was rather hard to overcome. Careful anatomical studies over many years had clearly established that there were no nerve fibers extending from the hypothalamus to the anterior pituitary. The only nerve fibers found in the pituitary stalk were those that terminate in the posterior lobe.

A way out of the dilemma was provided by an entirely different working hypothesis, suggested by the discovery in 1936 of blood vessels of a peculiar type that were shown to extend from the floor of the hypothalamus through the pituitary stalk to the anterior pituitary [see bottom illustration on opposite page]. If these tiny blood vessels were cut, the secretions of the anterior pituitary would instantly decrease. If the capillary vessels regenerated across the surgical cut, the secretions resumed.

Accordingly a new hypothesis was put forward about 1945 with which the name of the late G. W. Harris of the University of Oxford will remain associated. The hypothesis proposed that hypothalamic control of the secretory activity of the anterior pituitary could be neurochemical: some substance manufactured by nerve cells in the hypothalamus could be released into the capillary vessels that run from the hypothalamus to the anterior pituitary, where it could be delivered to the endocrine cells of the gland. On reaching these endocrine cells the substance of hypothalamic origin would somehow stimulate the secretion of the various anterior pituitary hormones.

The hypothesis that pituitary function is controlled by neurohormones originating in the hypothalamus was soon well established on the basis of intensive physiological studies in several laboratories. The next problem was therefore to isolate and characterize the postulated hypothalamic hormones. It was logical to guess that the hormones might be polypeptides of small molecular weight, since it had been well established that the two known neurosecretory products of hypothalamic origin, oxytocin and vasopressin, are each composed of eight amino acids. Indeed, in 1955 it was reported that crude aqueous hypothalamic extracts designed to contain polypeptides were able specifically to stimulate the secretion of ACTH, the pituitary hormone that controls the secretion of the steroid hormones of the adrenal cortex.

It was quickly demonstrated that none of the substances known to originate in the central nervous system (such as epinephrine, acetylcholine, vasopressin and oxytocin) could account for the ACTH-releasing activity observed in the extract of hypothalamic tissue. It therefore seemed reasonable to postulate the existence and involvement in this phenomenon of a new substance designated (adreno)corticotropin-releasing factor, or CRF. Several laboratories then undertook the apparently simple task of purifying CRF from hypothalamic extracts, with the final goal of isolating it and establishing its chemical structure. Seventeen years later the task still remains to be accomplished. Technical difficulties involving the methods

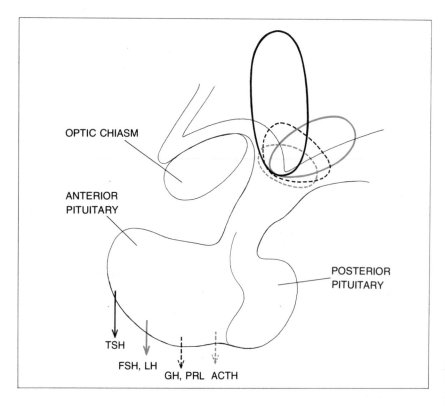

OPTIC CHIASM

ANTERIOR PITUITARY

POSTERIOR PITUITARY

TSH

FSH, LH

GH, PRL ACTH

RELATION between the hypothalamus and anterior pituitary was established experimentally. Lesions in specific regions of the hypothalamus interfere with secretion by the anterior lobe of specific hormones; electrical stimulation of those regions stimulates secretion of the hormones. The regions associated with each hormone are mapped schematically.

of assaying for CRF, together with certain peculiar characteristics of the molecule, have defied the enthusiasm, ingenuity and hard work of several groups of investigators.

More rewarding results were obtained in a closely related effort. About 1960 it was clearly established that the same crude extracts of hypothalamic tissue were able to stimulate the secretion of not only ACTH but also the three other pituitary hormones mentioned above: thyrotropin (TSH) and the two gonadotropins (LH and FSH). TSH is the pituitary hormone that controls the function of the thyroid gland, which in turn secretes the two hormones thyroxine and triiodothyronine. LH controls the secretion of the steroid hormones responsible for the male or female sexual characteristics; it also triggers ovulation. FSH controls the development and maturation of the germ cells: the spermatozoa and the ova. In reality the way in which LH and FSH work together is considerably more complicated than this somewhat simplistic description suggests.

Results obtained between 1960 and 1962 were best explained by proposing the existence of three separate hypothalamic releasing factors: TRF (the TSH-releasing factor), LRF (the LH-releasing factor) and FRF (the FSH-releasing factor). The effort began at once to isolate and characterize TRF, LRF and FRF. Whereas it was difficult to find a good assay for CRF, a simple and highly reliable biological assay was devised for TRF. At first, however, the assays for LRF and FRF still left much to be desired.

With a good method available for assaying TRF, progress was initially rapid. Within a few months after its discovery TRF had been prepared in a form many thousands of times purer. Preparations of TRF obtained from the brains of sheep showed biological activity in doses as small as one microgram. A great deal of physiological information was obtained with those early preparations. For example, the thyroid hormones somehow inhibit their own secretion when they reach a certain level in the blood. This fact had been known for 40 years and was the first evidence of a negative feedback in endocrine regulation. Studies with TRF showed that the feedback control takes place at the level of the pituitary gland as the result of some kind of competition between the number of available molecules of thyroid hormones and of TRF. Other significant observations were made on the gonadotropin-releasing factors when

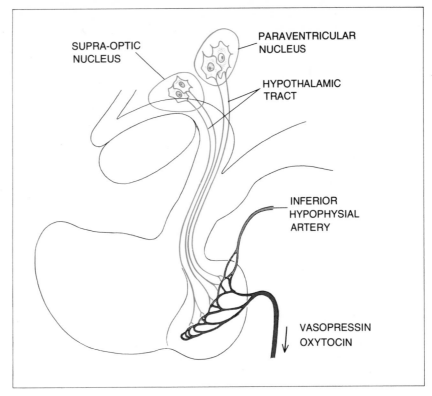

NEURAL CONNECTIONS could not explain the relation of the hypothalamus and the anterior lobe. The only significant nerve fibers connecting hypothalamus and pituitary run from two hypothalamic centers to the posterior lobe. They transmit oxytocin and vasopressin, two hormones manufactured in the hypothalamus and stored in the posterior lobe.

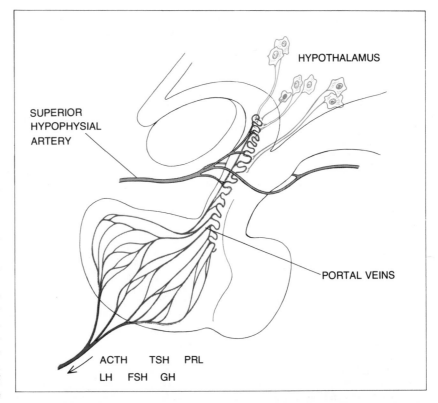

VASCULAR CONNECTIONS between hypothalamus and anterior lobe were eventually discovered: a network of capillaries reaching the base of the hypothalamus supplies portal veins that enter the anterior pituitary. Small hypothalamic nerve fibers apparently deliver to the capillaries releasing factors that stimulate secretion of the anterior-lobe hormones.

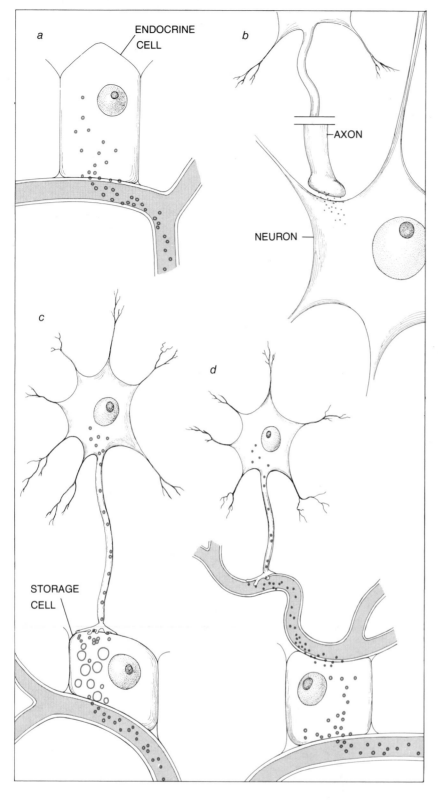

NEUROHUMORAL SECRETIONS involved in hypothalamic-pituitary interactions differ from classical hormone secretion and classical nerve-cell communication. A classical endocrine cell (such as those in the anterior pituitary or the adrenal cortex, for example) secretes its hormonal product directly into the bloodstream (a). At a classical synapse, the axon, or fiber, from one nerve cell releases locally a transmitter substance that activates the next cell (b). In neurosecretion of oxytocin or vasopressin the hormones are secreted by nerve cells and pass through their axons to storage cells in the posterior pituitary, eventually to be secreted into the bloodstream (c). Hypothalamic (releasing factor) hormones go from the neurons that secrete them into local capillaries, which carry them through portal veins to endocrine cells in the anterior lobe, whose secretions they in turn stimulate (d).

purified preparations, also active at microgram levels, were injected in experimental animals, for instance to produce ovulation.

It soon became apparent, however, that the isolation and chemical characterization of TRF, LRF and FRF would not be simple. The preparations active in microgram doses were chemically heterogeneous; they showed no clear-cut indication of a major component. It was also realized that each fragment of hypothalamus obtained from the brain of a sheep or another animal contained nearly infinitesimal quantities of the releasing factors. The isolation of enough of each factor to make its chemical characterization possible would therefore require the processing of an enormous number of hypothalamic fragments. Two groups of workers in the U.S. undertook this challenge: a group headed by A. V. Schally at the Tulane University School of Medicine and our own group, first at the Baylor University College of Medicine in Houston and then at the Salk Institute in La Jolla, Calif.

Over a period of four years the Tulane group worked with extracts from perhaps two million pig brains. Our laboratory collected, dissected and processed close to five million hypothalamic fragments from the brains of sheep. Since one sheep brain has a wet weight of about 100 grams, this meant handling 500 tons of brain tissue. From this amount we removed seven tons of hypothalamic tissue (about 1.5 grams per brain). Semi-industrial methods had to be developed in order to handle, extract and purify such large quantities of material. Finally in 1968 one milligram of a preparation of TRF was obtained that appeared to be homogeneous by all available criteria.

On careful measurement the entire milligram could be accounted for by the sole presence of three amino acids: histidine, glutamic acid and proline. Moreover, the three amino acids were present in equal amounts, which suggested that we were dealing with a relatively simple polypeptide perhaps as small as a tripeptide. In the determination of peptide sequences it is customary to subject the sample to attack by proteolytic enzymes, which cleave the peptide bonds holding the polypeptide chain together in well-established ways. Pure TRF, however, was shown to be resistant to all the proteolytic enzymes used. Since we could spare only a tiny amount of our precious one-milligram sample for studies of molecular weight, we could not obtain a

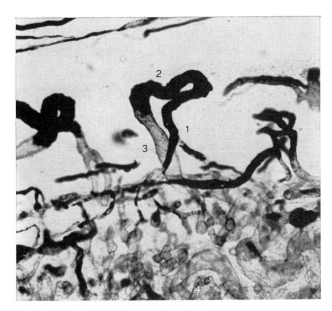

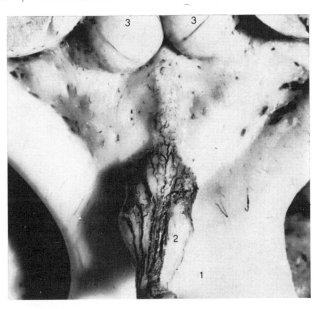

BLOOD VESSELS linking the hypothalamus and the anterior pituitary are seen in photographs made by Henri Duvernoy of the University of Besancon. The photomicrograph (*left*) shows some of the individual loops that characterize the capillary network at the base of the hypothalamus of a dog. The ascending branch of one loop is clearly seen (*1*); the loop comes close to the floor of the third ventricle (*2*) and then descends (*3*), carrying with it the releasing factors that are secreted by this region of the hypothalamus and entering the pars tuberalis of the anterior lobe (*4*). The photograph of the floor of the human hypothalamus (*right*) shows the optic chiasm (*1*), the posterior side of the pituitary stalk with its portal veins (*2*) and the mammillary bodies of the brain (*3*).

precise value for that important measurement. On the basis of inferential evidence, however, it seemed to be reasonable to assume that the molecular weight of TRF could not be more than 1,500.

With small molecules it is often possible to use methods based on the technique of mass spectrometry to obtain in a matter of hours the complete molecular structure of the compound under investigation. Because of the minute quantities of TRF available such efforts on our part were frustrated; the mass-spec-

trometric methods available to us in 1969 were not sensitive enough to indicate the structure of our unknown substance. Other approaches involve the use of infrared or nuclear magnetic-resonance spectrometry, which can provide direct insight into molecular structure. Here too the techniques then available were inadequate for providing clear-cut information about polypeptide samples that weighed only a few micrograms.

Confronted with nothing but dead ends, we decided on an entirely different

approach to finding the structure of TRF. That approach was first to synthesize each of six possible tripeptides composed of the three amino acids known to be present in TRF: histidine (abbreviated His), glutamic acid (Glu) and proline (Pro). The six tripeptides were then assayed for their biological activity. None showed any activity when they were injected at doses of up to a million times the level of the active natural TRF.

Was this another dead end? Not quite. Our synthetic polypeptides all had a

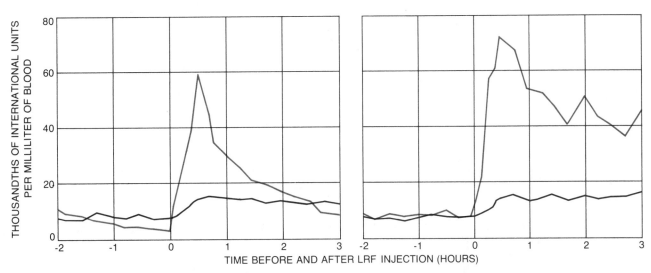

HYPOTHALAMIC HORMONES have clinical implications and applications. For example, women with no pituitary or ovarian defect respond to the administration of synthetic LRF by secreting normal amounts of the hormones LH and FSH. Curves show effect of LRF on secretion of LH (*color*) and FSH (*black*) in a normal woman on the third (*left*) and 11th (*right*) day of menstrual cycle.

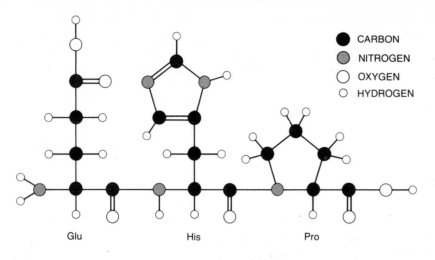

Glu　　　　His　　　　Pro

AMINO ACID CONTENT of TRF, the releasing factor for thyroid-stimulating hormone (TSH), was established: glutamic acid, histidine and proline in equal proportions. Each of six possible tripeptides was synthesized; one is diagrammed. None was active biologically.

free amino group (NH_2) at the end of the molecule designated the *N* terminus. We knew that in several well-characterized hormones the *N*-terminus end was not free; it was blocked by a small substitute group of some kind. Indeed, we had evidence from the small quantity of natural TRF that its *N* terminus was also blocked. To block the *N* terminus of our six candidate polypeptides was not difficult: we heated them in the presence of acetic anhydride, which typically couples an acetyl group (CH_3CO) to the *N* terminus. When these "protected" tripeptides were tested, the results were unequivocal. The biological activity of the sequence Glu-His-Pro, and that sequence alone, was qualitatively indistinguishable from the activity of natural TRF. Quantitatively, how-

ever, there was still a considerable difference between the synthetic product and natural TRF. Next it was shown that the protective effect of heating Glu-His-Pro with the acetic anhydride had been to convert the glutamic acid at the *N* terminus into a ring-shaped form known as pyroglutamic acid (pGlu).

We now had available gram quantities of the synthetic tripeptide pGlu-His-Pro-OH. (The OH is a hydroxyl group at the end of the molecule opposite the *N* terminus.) Accordingly we could bring into play all the methods that had yielded no information with the microgram quantities of natural TRF. Several of the techniques were modified, particularly with the aim of obtaining mass spectra of the synthetic

peptide at levels of only a few micrograms.

Meanwhile, armed with knowledge about the structure of other hormones, we modified the synthetic pGlu-His-Pro-OH to pGlu-His-Pro-NH_2 by replacing the hydroxyl group with an amino group (NH_2) to produce the primary amide [*see top illustration on opposite page*]. This substance proved to have the same biological activity as the natural TRF. At length the complete structure of the natural TRF was obtained by high-resolution mass spectrometry. It turned out to be the structure pGlu-His-Pro-NH_2. The time was late 1969. Thus TRF not only was the first of the hypothalamic hormones to be fully characterized but also was immediately available by synthesis in amounts many millions of times greater than the hormone present in one sheep hypothalamus. TRF from pig brains was subsequently shown to have the same molecular structure as TRF from sheep brains.

Characterization of the hypothalamic releasing factor LRF, which controls the secretion of the gonadotropin LH, followed rapidly. Isolated from the side fractions of the programs for the isolation of TRF, LRF was shown in 1971 to be a polypeptide composed of 10 amino acids. Six of the amino acids are not found in TRF: tryptophan (Trp), serine (Ser), tyrosine (Tyr), glycine (Gly), leucine (Leu) and arginine (Arg). The full sequence of LRF is pGlu-His-Trp-Ser-Tyr-Gly-Leu-Arg-Pro-Gly-NH_2 [*see bottom illustration on these two pages*]. Although this structure is more compli-

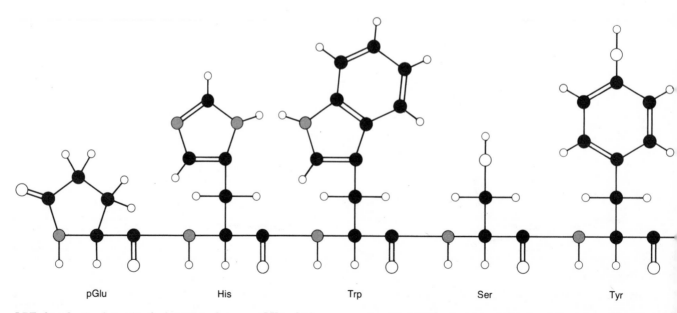

pGlu　　　　His　　　　Trp　　　　Ser　　　　Tyr

LRF, the releasing factor for the luteinizing hormone (LH), which affects the activity of the gonads, was characterized and synthesized

soon after. First the hormone was isolated and its amino acid content was determined. Then their intramolecular sequence was es-

cated than the structure of TRF, it begins with the same two amino acids (pGlu-His) and has the same group at the other terminus (NH₂).

It turns out that LRF also stimulates the secretion of the other gonadotropin, FSH, although not as powerfully as it stimulates the secretion of LH. It has been proposed that LRF may be the sole hypothalamic controller of the secretion of the two gonadotropins: LH and FSH.

There is good physiological evidence that the hypothalamus is also involved in the control of the secretion of the other two important pituitary hormones: prolactin and growth hormone. Curiously, prolactin is as plentiful in males as in females, but its role in male physiology is still a mystery. The hypothalamic mechanism involved in the control of the secretion of prolactin or growth hormone is not fully understood. It is quite possible that the secretion of these two pituitary hormones is controlled not by releasing factors alone but perhaps jointly by releasing factors and specific hypothalamic hormones that somehow act as inhibitors of the secretion of prolactin or growth hormone. If it should turn out that inhibitory hormones rather than stimulative ones are involved in the regulation of prolactin and growth hormone, one should not be too surprised. The brain provides many examples of inhibitory and stimulative systems working in parallel.

The hypothalamic hormones TRF and LRF are both now available by synthesis in unlimited quantities. Both are highly active in stimulating pituitary functions in humans. TRF is already a

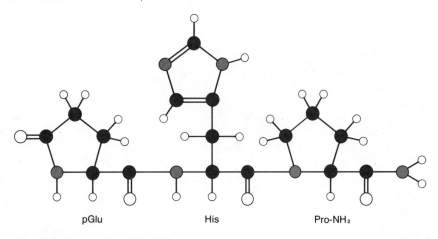

TRIPEPTIDES were modified in an effort to characterize the releasing factor. When the sequence glutamic acid–histidine-proline was modified by forming the glutamic acid into a ring and converting the proline end (*right*) to an amide, it was found to be TRF.

powerful tool for exploring pituitary functions in several diseases characterized by the abnormality of one or several of the pituitary secretions. There is increasing evidence that most patients with such abnormalities (primarily children) actually have normally functioning glands, since they respond promptly to the administration of synthetic hypothalamic hormones. Evidently their abnormalities are due to hypothalamic rather than pituitary deficiencies. These deficiencies can now be successfully treated by the administration of the hypothalamic polypeptide TRF.

Similarly, an increasing number of women who have no ovulatory menstrual cycle and who show no pituitary or ovarian defect begin to secrete normal amounts of the gonadotropins

LH and FSH after the administration of LRF. The administration of synthetic LRF should therefore be the method of choice for the treatment of those cases of infertility where the functional defect resides in the hypothalamus-pituitary system. Indeed, ovulation can be induced in women by the administration of synthetic LRF. On the other hand, knowledge of the structure of the LRF molecule may open up an entirely novel approach to fertility control. Synthetic compounds closely related to LRF in structure may act as inhibitors of the native LRF. Two such analogues of LRF, made by modifying the histidine in the hormone, have been reported as antagonists of LRF. It is therefore possible that LRF antagonists will be used as contraceptives.

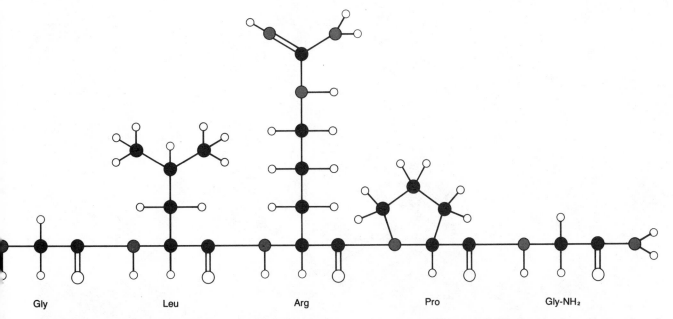

tablished and reproduced by synthesis; the synthetic replicate shown here was found to have full biological activity. In addition to stimulating LH activity, LRF also stimulates the secretion of another gonadotropic hormone, FSH, although not so powerfully.

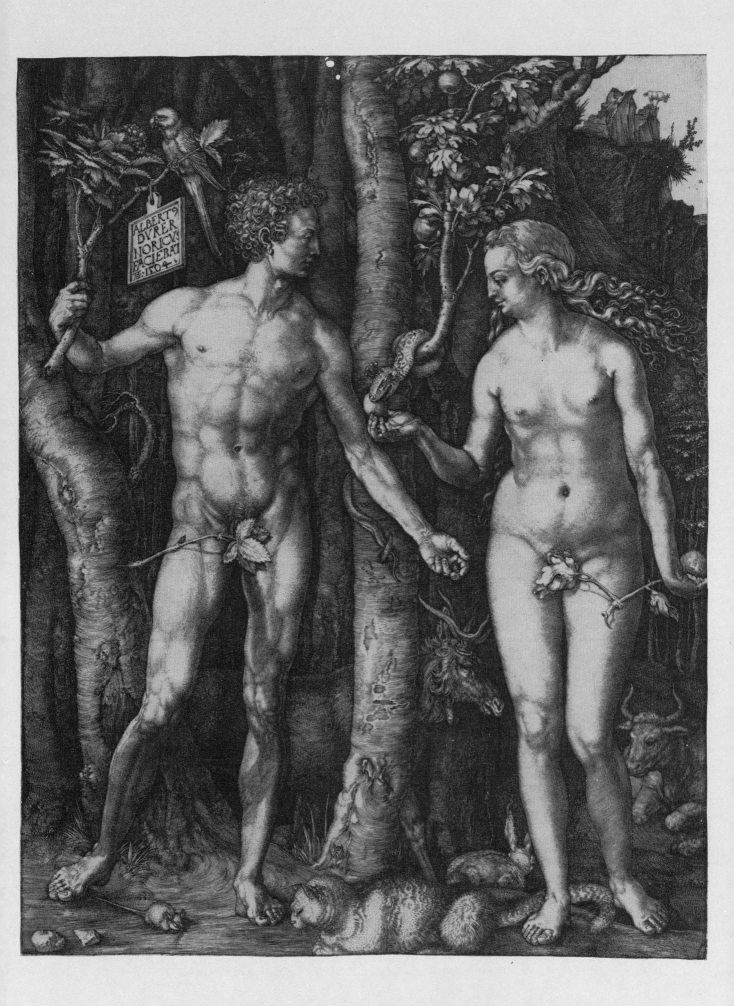

7

The Physiology of Human Reproduction

by Sheldon J. Segal
September 1974

Its complex series of events is organized by molecular messengers. Advancing knowledge of the system provides humane methods that enable couples to have the number of children they choose to have

The human reproductive process, on which the size and structure of individual families and of the populations of communities, nations and the world ultimately depend, is an orchestration of interrelated behavioral and physiological events and anatomical changes that proceed in perfect sequence and synchrony. At the center of the process are the gonads: the ovaries in the female and the testes in the male. These sex glands have two functions. They produce gametes (eggs and spermatozoa) and they produce the sex hormones. The role of the male ends with fertilization; the female goes on to harbor the fertilized egg in a protective and nutritive setting. The entire process is regulated by a series of chemical substances that issue from the brain and the pituitary gland to influence the gonads and then from the sex glands to order the successive events of egg or sperm development and transport, fertilization, implantation and gestation.

In both the female and the male this remarkable relay of molecular messages [*see illustrations on pages 68 and 69*] begins in specialized nerve cells in the brain. Sensory stimuli from the external environment and/or humoral stimuli from the bloodstream activate these neurons (whose location and pathways are as yet uncharted) and cause them to release small neurotransmitter molecules that reach neurosecretory cells in the hypothalamus at the base of the brain. On receiving the appropriate molecular message (which might signal, for example, a lowered blood level of an ovarian hormone) the hypothalamic cells discharge their stored supply of a gonadotropin-releasing factor, a small polypeptide hormone composed of 10 amino acid subunits. Aggregates of releasing-factor molecules move from the hypothalamic cells into a short local system of small capillaries and veins that carry them only a few centimeters, to the anterior lobe of the pituitary [see the article "The Hormones of the Hypothalamus," by Roger Guillemin and Roger Burgus, beginning on page 75]. The releasing factor causes the pituitary to discharge its stored supply of two gonadotropins, or gonad-influencing hormones: large glycoproteins called luteinizing hormone (LH) and follicle-stimulating hormone (FSH), which enter the bloodstream and are carried to the sex glands.

In the female the two gonadotropins participate in unison in stimulating ovarian function, but each has a specialized role. FSH is responsible chiefly for causing the maturation of the ovary's Graafian follicles, which contain the oöcytes, or immature eggs, in a multilayered sheath of granulosa cells. In the process the hormone-secreting cells of the follicle are stimulated to produce increasing amounts of estrogens, one of the two kinds of female steroid sex hormone, and the immature egg enclosed in the stimulated follicle is brought to the state of maturation necessary for ovulation. The other gonadotropin, LH, triggers the ovulation process, in which the mature egg leaves the follicle. The empty follicle is transformed into the corpus luteum, a structure that is in effect a temporary secretory organ. LH thereupon stimulates the new luteal cells to produce large amounts of progesterone, the second female sex steroid. (There is probably a role for a third gonadotropic hormone of the pituitary, prolactin, in maintaining the steroid-producing function of the corpus luteum for its usual 14-day life span, but there is some doubt whether this is true in humans.) Because of estrogen's and progesterone's extensive effects on sex behavior and secondary sex characteristics they are usually referred to as the sex steroids, but they also affect other organs, including bone, muscle, blood and the liver, and processes such as carbohydrate and calcium metabolism and water retention.

In the next steps of the molecular relay the steroid hormones act on individual cells of the reproductive organs. The cells that are targets for the sex hormones have unique large molecules in their cytoplasm that bind particular sex steroids. These receptors are highly specific: they are not found in other organs and in the target organs they do not bind other steroids. After binding, the complex of receptor and, say, an estrogen molecule is moved to the nucleus of the cell, where it interacts with the genetic material and changes the pattern of the cell's production of messenger RNA, thus altering the program of protein synthesis. In this manner a nonstimulated cell of the uterus, for example, is converted to the stimulated state.

ADAM AND EVE, the legendary initiators of human reproduction, were depicted by Albrecht Dürer in the illustration on the opposite page, a copper engraving made in 1504. The engraving is celebrated, according to the critic Erwin Panofsky, for the "splendor of a technique that does equal justice to the warm glow of human skin, to the chilly slipperiness of a snake, to the metallic undulations of locks and tresses, to the smooth, shaggy, downy or bristly quality of animals' coats...." Panofsky commented that the engraving is "intentionally a model of human beauty...two classic specimens of the nude human body, as perfect as possible both in proportions and in pose." Although Genesis relates that Adam was formed "of the dust of the ground" and Eve of "one of his ribs," Dürer drew them both with an umbilicus, the mark of placental gestation that characterizes their descendants. The print from which this reproduction is made is in the Museum of Fine Arts in Boston.

Identical molecules play analogous roles in the human male. As in females, integrated processes control both gamete and hormone production by the testis. Although the structures responsible for these two functions (respectively the seminiferous tubules and the Leydig cells) are more independent in the testis than they are in the ovary, they do respond to stimulation by the gonadotropins in a coordinated manner. And so the production, maturation and transport of the sperm and the stimulation of secondary sex characteristics, including the formation of the seminal fluid's normal chemistry, proceed under required hormonal conditions, much as egg production in the female is coordinated with the proper hormonal milieu for the subsequent steps of egg transport and nidation: the implantation of the egg in the uterine lining. The patterns of production of the hypothalamic releasing factor, the pituitary's gonadotropic hormones and the gonadal steroids are noncyclic in the male whereas they are cyclic in the female, but the hypothalamic and pituitary messengers are the same in both sexes. The main gonadal steroid in the male is testosterone.

So much for the general pattern of hormone interactions that serve to integrate the sequence of reproductive events in both sexes. Let me now describe those events in more detail, first in the female and then in the male.

Every month, from the time of sexual maturation, the human female prepares for a possible pregnancy. An egg is produced, the uterine cervix becomes receptive to the passage of spermatozoa, the muscular and secretory capacities of the uterus and the fallopian tubes become conducive to the transport of sperm and egg, and the endometrial lining of the uterus prepares to harbor a fertilized egg. All of this is accomplished by two distinct but cross-linked sequences of events, the ovulatory and the uterine, or menstrual, cycles.

The key event is the monthly development of an egg. As early as about the sixth week of embryonic age some 2,000 amoebalike oögonia, or germ cells, migrate into the human ovary from a specialized region of the yolk sac. In the course of embryonic and fetal development their number increases tremendously through cell division. At birth the two ovaries of the female infant contain nearly 500,000 primary follicles: individual oöcytes, the precursors of eggs, surrounded by a layer of follicle cells. Most of the follicles, however, are destined for spontaneous degeneration, a process that continues during childhood and adolescence and throughout the reproductive years. It is only the occasional egg that actually ovulates and has an opportunity to participate in fertilization—perhaps fewer than 400 in a woman's reproductive years.

From among the scores of thousands of primary follicles, a few start to develop as the circulating FSH levels rise each month a few days before a menstrual period. After about 10 days usually only one follicle continues to flourish and become fully mature, ready to release its egg. At mid-cycle, on approximately the 14th day, ovulation occurs, with the oöcyte bursting from the rupture point in a cascade of follicular cells and fluid. The released egg is swept from the surface of the ovary by the undulating open end of the fallopian tube. At this point the egg still has 46 chromosomes, the normal human complement; the process of reduction division whereby the complement is reduced to 23, to be matched by the 23 chromosomes of the fertilizing spermatozoon, begins during fetal life but is suspended for many years. Now the process is resumed with the expulsion of the first polar body carrying 23 of the chromosomes. The remaining 23 replicate once more, and it is only after a sperm makes contact with the surface of the egg that a second polar body is expelled, again reducing the genetic material by half, so that the union of egg and sperm will produce the normal complement of hereditary material.

Fertilization, once thought to be a simple matter of sperm-egg interaction, is an intricate series of steps that begins when a spermatozoon makes contact with the zona pellucida, a viscous en-

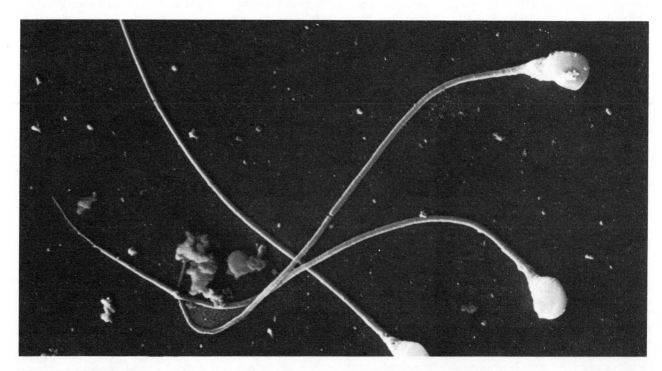

HUMAN SPERMATOZOA are enlarged some 4,000 diameters in this scanning electron micrograph made by David M. Phillips of the Population Council. The sperm were removed from semen by centrifugation and shadowed with platinum. The sperm head consists of densely packed chromatin, the hereditary material, covered by the acrosomal cap containing the enzymes that accomplish the penetration of the egg. Behind the head is a short segment containing mitochondria that supply energy to power the long flagellum.

velope surrounding the egg. By enzymatic action the sperm slices through the zona and makes contact with the surface of the egg. This initiates a series of functional and structural responses. A key event is an immediate blockade against the entry of additional sperm. In fact, without the evolutionary development of a means of preventing polyspermy (the entry of additional sperm) sexual reproduction would not be a successful means of maintaining any species, since polyspermy is almost invariably nonviable. The barriers to polyspermy include changes in the zona pellucida that make it impenetrable and alterations in the egg's surface that preclude the attachment of additional sperm, but the precise nature of the blocks remains unknown. The fertilizing sperm passes through the outer membrane of the egg into the cytoplasm in several stages, in the process both activating the egg to complete its second reduction division and orienting the axis of future development. Even then it is not clear at all that the egg is "fertilized." For about 12 hours the formation within the cytoplasm of distinct egg and sperm pronuclei unfolds. The pronuclei, which are large organelles with a complex structure, move together gradually. Then, following further structural changes, the maternal and paternal hereditary contributions intermingle, and with this event the first cell division of the zygote begins. After 36 hours the single cell has become two. Two days later the fertilized egg may have divided twice more to form a microscopic ball of eight cells. In this condition the egg completes its passage through the fallopian tube and enters the uterus.

Four days after fertilization the egg is a cluster of 32 or 64 cells, which are beginning to divide more rapidly. This stage corresponds to about day 19 or 20 of the menstrual cycle. The cluster of cells remains unattached for one or two days and assumes the form of a signet ring: an inner mass of cells encircled by a single row of aligned trophoblastic, or nourishing, cells. This preembryo state is called the blastocyst. Under the proper conditions the outer ring of cells nestles into the endometrium and begins to form the placenta. The inner cell mass, after several more days of cell divisions and internal rearrangements, becomes a human embryo.

In an integrated manner a second sequence takes place concurrently to ensure the egg a protective and supportive nesting place in the uterus. Early in the four-week menstrual cycle, before

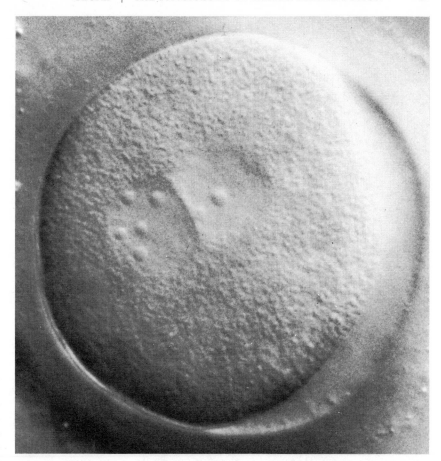

HUMAN EGG is enlarged 1,200 diameters in a photomicrograph made by Pierre Soupart and Larry L. Morgenstern of the Vanderbilt University School of Medicine. Here differential-interference micrography focuses sharply on the equatorial plane of the egg, revealing the female pronucleus and the male pronucleus, derived from the sperm head, in close apposition; nucleoli are visible in each pronucleus. The egg proper is surrounded by the viscous zona pellucida. At this stage, some 20 hours after the sperm's penetration, the hereditary material is replicating within the pronuclear membranes. The membranes will break down as the chromosomes condense and pair up for first division of fertilized egg.

ovulation, the ovary secretes in ever increasing amounts the estrogenic steroids, principally estradiol. These hormones stimulate the endometrium to proliferate and to become much richer in blood vessels. The final surge of estrogen production heralds (and also induces, by means of the hypothalamic recognition of blood estrogen levels) a mid-cycle peak in the LH level. Ovulation follows within 24 hours, and at about this time ovarian steroid production is switched over from a predominance of estrogen to a predominance of progesterone. In response the cells of the endometrium become still more numerous and more corpulent. The endometrial glands grow rapidly in length and thickness and begin to accumulate secretions. The entire endometrial surface, by the 20th day of the cycle, has become a highly vascular, spongy nest ready to accept, protect and nurture a fertilized and dividing egg if one should arrive from the fallopian tube. The tube itself has developed cilia and

increased its flow of glandular fluids for transporting an egg to the uterus.

The uterine lining is now under the remarkable influence of progesterone produced by the corpus luteum. In a nonfertile month the luteal cells begin to reduce their progesterone production about 10 days after ovulation; some four or five days later the level is low enough to result in a sloughing off of the endometrium and menstruation. If an egg is fertilized, the first crisis to be overcome is therefore the avoidance of menstruation. For the pregnancy to survive there must be a source of progesterone to continue the support of the endometrium; without it the blastocyst, or later the new embryo, would pass out with the sloughed-off endometrium and menstrual blood.

The maintenance of progesterone—and indeed the synchrony of maturation, release and fertilization of the egg on the one hand and preparation of the uterus as a proper environment for nida-

INTERRELATIONS OF ORGANS involved in the reproductive process are shown in this flow diagram. The central nervous system, prompted by external or internal stimuli, causes the hypothalamus to secrete a releasing factor that stimulates the anterior pituitary gland. The pituitary thereupon releases the gonadotropic hormones FSH and LH, which stimulate specific structures in the gonads to secrete the steroid hormones: either estrogen and progesterone or testosterone. The gonadal steroids affect reproductive organs and feed back to the hypothalamus and perhaps to other structures to stimulate and/or inhibit their activity.

To pass the first crisis, in other words, the embryo produces a gonadotropin that stimulates maternal hormonal production; to meet the second crisis the developing embryo itself assumes the required endocrine function, thus becoming self-sufficient in this respect. By five and a half weeks the pregnancy can continue even if the maternal ovaries cease to function or are removed [see illustration on page 72].

The noteworthy characteristics of the chain of reproductive events in the female are the restriction of the multiplication phase of oögenesis to the fetal ovary, the dramatic rate of depletion of the oöcytes and the cyclic patterns of pituitary-gonodal interaction. The male reproductive process differs in each of these respects in spite of the similarity of its molecular relay system.

A man produces many billions of spermatozoa in a lifetime, all of which derive from the 1,000 or 2,000 spermatogonia, or germ cells, that migrate into the embryonic testis before the end of the second month of intrauterine life. This process is made possible by the way in which the male germ cells multiply: when the spermatogonia divide, many of the daughter cells are kept in reserve while others undergo further cell divisions and then complete spermatogenesis in the seminiferous tubules. In contrast to the multiplication phase of oögenesis in the ovary, which is confined to a few weeks of fetal life, the multiplication phase of spermatogenesis in the testis begins in the fetal period and continues throughout life. Since there is no significant depletion of the germ-cell stores, there is no gradual loss of gamete-producing function as there is in the ovary; the testis goes on producing millions upon millions of spermatozoa and, in the normal gonad, there always remain additional germ cells to provide the capability of producing millions more. (It is not uncommon, however, for the vascular changes of aging to affect the testis or pituitary and indirectly cause a loss of testicular function.) In the course of spermatogenesis the two important objectives are reduction of the chromosome number from the diploid number (46) of the spermatogonium to the haploid number (23) of the spermatozoon and the preparation of the spermatozoon for its role in fertilization. A complex series of transformations involving both the cytoplasm and the nucleus changes the large, round spermatogonium into streamlined and motile spermatozoa in approximately 74 days.

The testis, like the ovary, must be

tion on the other—is achieved because the hormones involved in each process have such exquisitely integrated and interrelated functions. Consider the implications of the hormonal events of a nonfertile cycle. After ovulation the gonadal steroid hormones feed back at mid-cycle to suppress the pituitary secretion of FSH and LH, and the progressive decline in the concentration of the pituitary gonadotropins in the blood prevents any supplementary ovulations that might interfere with a possible pregnancy. In the absence of a pregnancy, however, a decline in blood steroid concentration in the late luteal phase causes a rise in LH and FSH. In other words, once it is clear that a cycle has been infertile there is an immediate signal to the brain to initiate the events that prepare an egg for release the next month; menstruation intervenes, but the new cycle has already begun. In response to the increase in secretion of FSH and LH follicular maturation proceeds, and with it egg development and increases in gonadal steroid-hormone production. Late in the follicular phase, approaching the period of the maximal rate of follicular enlargement and maximal steroid production, the patterns of FSH and LH di-

verge. FSH secretion declines but LH secretion increases gradually until rising estrogen levels signal the preovulatory surge of both LH and FSH, linking follicular maturation and steroid production to the ovulatory stimulus from the pituitary.

In the case of pregnancy, as I have indicated, avoiding the crisis of menstruation requires an uninterrupted supply of progesterone. The initial source is the corpus luteum, which receives a signal to continue making the steroid. The signal comes from the newly formed blastocyst. Even before nidation the outer cells of the early blastocyst copiously produce a gonadotropic molecule, usually called human chorionic gonadotropin (HCG), that is very similar in function and structure to pituitary LH. The blastocyst's gonadotropin stimulates the maternal corpus luteum to keep on producing progesterone beyond the time of the first expected menstrual period. A second critical point lies ahead, however. The corpus luteum, in spite of maximum stimulation, has a limited life span. Before this time limit is reached, at about the fifth week of gestation, the placenta itself begins to produce sufficient quantities of progesterone to maintain the pregnancy.

stimulated by pituitary gonadotropins to produce sex hormones and sperm, but there is still some uncertainty about the relative roles of FSH and LH. It appears that the role of LH is primarily to stimulate the Leydig cells, which lie between the seminiferous tubules, to produce their steroid hormones, mainly testosterone; the testosterone in turn has an important effect on the process of sperm production, since the tubules require a

high local concentration of the hormone to maintain spermatogenesis. FSH binds specifically to the Sertoli cells of the seminiferous tubules, which implies that its role is in the maintenance of spermatogenesis.

The sperm's voyage can be described even though many of its control mechanisms are poorly understood. A limited number of collecting ducts funnel the spermatozoa coming from the seminifer-

ous tubules to the epididymis, a long tube convoluted into a compact body adjacent to the testis. These immature sperm are not yet able to fertilize an egg or even to move under their own power. As they pass from the head of the epididymis through its slender body to its distended tail they achieve motility and a degree of maturity, but the final critical changes that enable them to penetrate and fertilize an egg are achieved

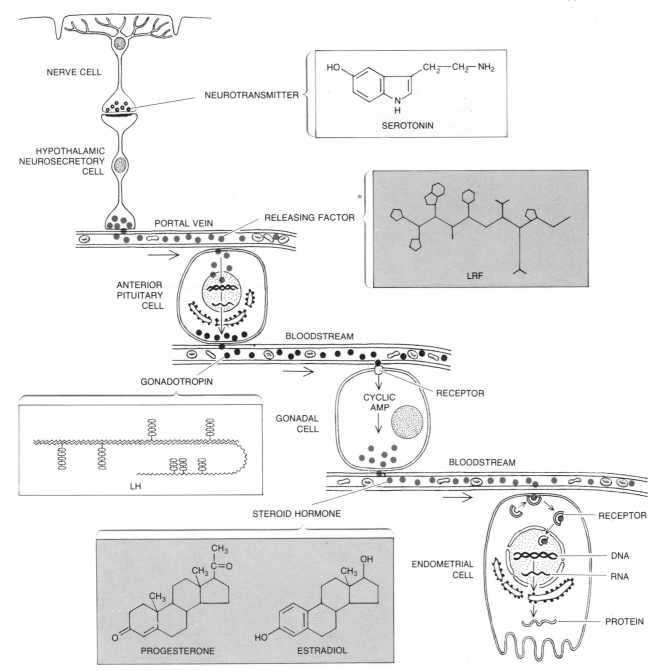

MOLECULAR RELAY that interrelates the reproductive organs is shown in more detail. A neurotransmitter (perhaps serotonin) is released from a specialized brain cell and excites a neurosecretory cell in the hypothalamus. The hypothalamic cell secretes a gonadotropin-releasing factor, the polypeptide LRF, into short portal veins that supply cells in the anterior pituitary and cause them to release their gonadotropins. These are large glycoproteins (whose structure is merely suggested here) that enter the general

circulation. On reaching a specialized gonadal cell each of the gonadotropins acts, by way of the cyclic adenosine monophosphate "second messenger" system, to stimulate the synthesis of a specific steroid hormone; the two major female hormones are diagrammed. The gonadal steroids move through the bloodstream to reproductive-organ target cells, where they bind to receptors that carry them into the nucleus. There they either activate or "derepress" genes to make new proteins and thus affect the organ's structure or function.

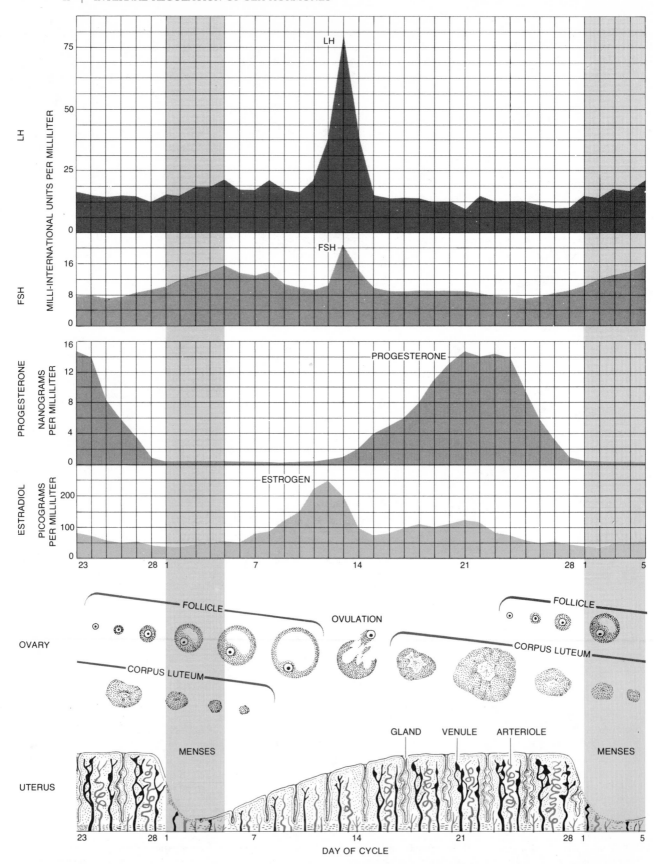

OVULATORY AND MENSTRUAL CYCLES are charted in terms of fluctuating blood levels of gonadotropins and gonadal steroids, development of a follicle and corpus luteum in the ovary and changes in the thickness and in the blood vessels and glands of the endometrial lining of the uterus. A rising FSH level stimulates follicular development, causing the ovaries to secrete estrogen (primarily estradiol), which, once menstruation is over, promotes anew the thickening and vascularization of the endometrium. Estradiol also signals a peak in LH release that brings on ovulation: an egg is released from the developed follicle, which is converted into a corpus luteum. The corpus luteum now secretes the steroid progesterone, which further prepares the endometrium for pregnancy. In the absence of fertilization, however, progesterone production falls and the endometrium is sloughed off with menstruation.

only in the female reproductive tract, and even there only if the tract is in the proper hormonal balance: precisely the estrogen-dominated status of about the time of ovulation. Thus, remarkably, the interrelations that link the ovary's hormone production and the physiology of the female gamete are extended to the male gamete once it is deposited in the female tract.

From the tail of the epididymis the sperm proceed into the continuation of the epididymal tube known as the vas deferens, which empties into the urethra below the bladder. Some of the sperm die and are disposed of by white blood cells; others enter the urethra in a steady stream and are carried away in the urine. The remainder leave the male tract at ejaculation, when sperm are forced rapidly into the urethra by muscular contractions. These sperm are mixed with the fluid secretions of several accessory glands, including the prostate, whose ducts lead into the terminal portion of the vas deferens or into the urethra. The contributions from these sources and the secretions from the testis, the epididymis and the vas deferens together constitute the semen, which serves primarily as a vehicle to carry the sperm to the vagina. Most of the spermatozoa go no farther. Of the hundreds of millions that are ejaculated only tens of thousands enter the cervix, where there is further attrition, so that only a few thousand reach the uterus proper. A few hundred spermatozoa ultimately complete the journey to the upper part of each fallopian tube, where one of them may penetrate and fertilize an egg.

In addition to providing more insight into human biology in general and improved diagnosis and treatment of various diseases and abnormal conditions, increased understanding of the reproductive process has deep significance for the human condition. Recent years have seen important advances in the physician's ability to help people have the children they want to have, notably through the hormonal induction of ovulation and prevention of spontaneous abortion; artificial insemination can also make a pregnancy possible for some subfertile couples. On the other hand, contraceptive technology has improved to the point where it can facilitate efforts to cope with the rapid increase in population that has come with better medical care, public health and nutrition, and the consequent reduction in mortality, first in the developed and now in the underdeveloped countries.

There is, however, a danger of think-

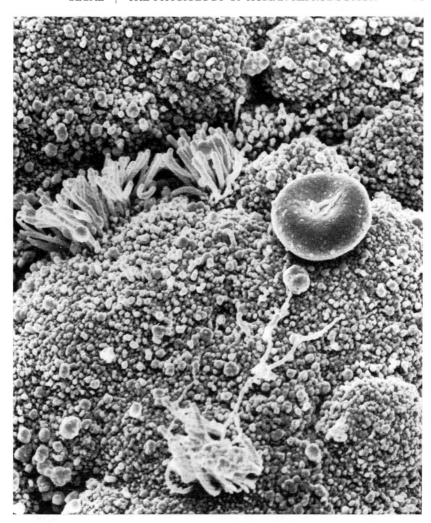

ENDOMETRIAL SURFACE is seen at the height of the secretory phase, at day 23 of the uterine cycle, in a scanning electron micrograph made by Alvaro Cuadros of the Population Council. The enlargement is some 4,500 diameters. A lone red blood cell sits on the surface (*middle right*). Individual endometrial cells, grown large and protuberant in this phase, are separated in some cases by intercellular ridges. Some of the cells have fingerlike cilia on their surfaces; all are covered by pebbly microvilli. A gland opening (*bottom left*) is discharging secretion granules, aggregates of molecules that constitute the uterine fluid.

ing that the regulation of fertility is a simple matter of the development and dissemination of contraceptive technology. The fact is that contraceptive technology is only part of the story along with social and economic conditions and the motivation of individuals. Yet the development of new technology can contribute in major ways. It can provide methods that encourage effective family planning at lower levels of motivation, and at any given level of motivation it can provide safer and more effective methods.

The age-old way to avoid a pregnancy has been for the male to withdraw prior to ejaculation. Blockage of sperm transport has been achieved with the condom, by the introduction of a variety of spermicides into the vagina, retroactively by postcoital douching and more

recently by the diaphragm. And permanent blockage has been achieved by surgical interruption of either the fallopian tubes or the vas deferens.

The rhythm method (periodic abstinence timed to avoid coitus near the day of ovulation) was the first method of fertility regulation that had as its basis scientific understanding of ovulation, since it was only in this century that even the identity of the human egg was established and the relation of ovulation to the menstrual cycle became known. The fact that the rhythm method is not highly effective does not detract from its significance in having focused on ovulation as the key event. It was several decades more until a better understanding of endocrinology and physiology revolutionized the practice of contraception with the development in the early 1950's of synthetic steroids that could serve as oral contraceptive agents. The standard pill combines an estrogen with a progestin, a progesteronelike chemical. The two synthetic hormones have two major actions: they suppress the pituitary hormones through negative feedback and at the same time stimulate the endometrium and thereby simulate a menstrual cycle [*see illustration on opposite page*]. The combination of hormones is taken cyclically for 21 days each month. During this period the brain recognizes the elevated steroid levels in the blood. The resulting inhibition of the releasing factor in turn suppresses pituitary production of the gonadotropins LH and FSH and thus signals the cessation of further ovarian function. The endometrium, however, is spared the atrophy that would occur in the absence of ovarian steroids by the direct stimulatory action of the pill's steroids. On completion of a pill cycle endometrial breakdown ensues, with menstrual bleeding; the induced cycle can then be repeated.

With less public attention in the U.S. but with greater impact on the family-planning efforts of many underdeveloped countries, a second modernizing form of contraception was widely introduced at about the same time as oral contraceptives. This is intrauterine contraception. Unlike the development of oral contraceptives, the development of modern intrauterine devices (IUD's) began not with a logical sequence of fundamental chemical and biological discoveries but with the empirical observa-

tion in women that the presence of an intrauterine foreign body prevents pregnancy. The idea was buttressed by confirmation that the effect could be demonstrated in animals under controlled experimental conditions. The effect of an IUD is not to disrupt an established pregnancy. That is clear because the average cycle length in women using IUD's is not prolonged by even a day or two, nor is there the rise in the progesterone level that is characteristic of pregnancy. Observations in animals indicate that an IUD acts by preventing nidation but that it may do so by intervening at any postovulation step in the reproductive sequence. It acts by creating a uterine environment that is hostile to the metabolic processes of either the spermatozoa or the blastocyst, if one should be formed. Beyond this no precise mechanism can be defined.

Notwithstanding the development of oral contraceptives and IUD's, intensified research efforts are still required, based on considerations of safety and effectiveness and of the incomplete acceptance by the world's diversified population of the available techniques. Even the so-called modern methods require an advanced health establishment for effective implementation. The oral-hormone method is associated with troublesome minor side effects and rare but serious major risks. The IUD's in general use must be inserted by a skilled health worker, are frequently not tolerated by

women and in a small number of cases carry the risk of serious consequences.

Moreover, the success couples achieve with current contraceptives is far below their usual expectations. This is true even in countries with conditions of literacy, health services, transportation and communications that should facilitate proper utilization of present methods. In the U.S., for example, a third of the couples using contraceptives nevertheless have an unintended pregnancy within a five-year period, so that most couples depending on reversible contraceptive methods for many years after attaining the desired family size run a significant risk of an unwanted pregnancy. The limitations of contraceptive technology certainly contribute to the high rate of legal abortion in some countries and of illegal abortion in many others. In a sense research aimed at improved contraceptive technology is therefore a search for abortion-prevention therapy as well as an effort to provide more acceptable, effective and safe methods for voluntarily regulating fertility.

With the gradual elucidation of the normal hormonal requirements of the reproductive process it has become apparent that many steps in the sequence are vulnerable to controlled interference. Contraceptive development depends on an understanding of physiological mechanisms concerned with conception, on basic studies in animals and humans to establish effectiveness and safety and ultimately on acceptability studies un-

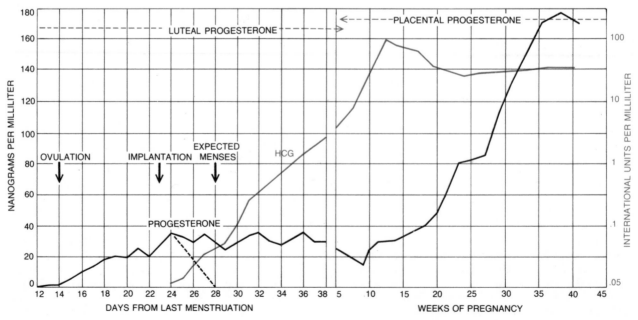

EFFECT OF PREGNANCY on the cycles illustrated on page 34 is essentially to maintain progesterone production, which would otherwise fall off (*broken line*), leaving the implanted blastocyst to be sloughed off with the menstrual flow. Instead the trophoblast (the outer cells of the fertilized egg) secretes the hormone HCG, which is similar to LH and causes the corpus luteum to keep secreting progesterone. Beginning at about the fifth week of pregnancy the placenta takes over the task of progesterone production.

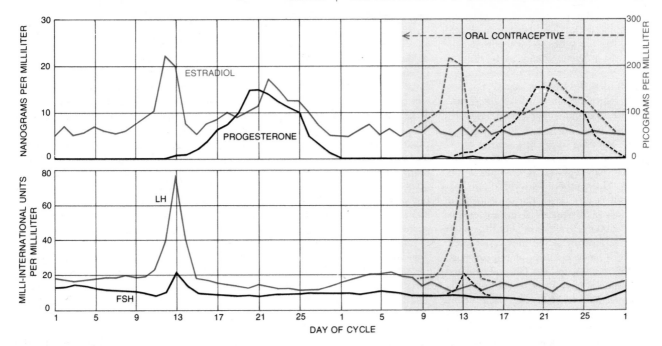

EFFECT OF ORAL CONTRACEPTIVE is to prevent ovulation by interfering with the normal cycle (*left and broken curves at right*). The pill contains synthetic steroids. Released into the circulation, they have a negative-feedback effect that inhibits pituitary secretion of the gonadotropins FSH and LH, which normally induce follicle development, ovulation and the secretion of gonadal steroids. In the absence of endogenous steroids the pill's synthetic steroids act on the endometrium so that a menstrual cycle is simulated.

der various social and cultural circumstances. The process is lengthy and complex, so that any new methods likely to emerge in the near future must now be at some advanced stage of development, with some testing in human subjects already under way. There are a number of such techniques that may be ready for general service within the next three to five years.

Several techniques for contraception in women involve new ways of delivering progestins. One method is injection. Two progestin compounds are being marketed in some countries as injections to be given every three months. They work by suppressing LH release and thereby preventing ovulation. They cause irregular bleeding, however, and there are questions as to their safety and reversibility that need to be resolved. The search goes on for other injectable compounds and inert carriers that will release them slowly and continuously. Progestin can also be released gradually from combination with a polymer that can be implanted under the skin. Subdermal implants—tubes or rods made of a rubberlike polymer into which the synthetic steroids have been introduced— are in an advanced stage of clinical investigation. There are also biodegradable implants; the steroid is incorporated in a polymer made, for example, of the biological molecule lactate, the polylactate is rolled into rods and implanted

under the skin and the hormone is released as the polymer gradually breaks down. Since progestins can be absorbed through the vaginal mucosa, it is also possible to incorporate the steroid in a plastic ring, about the size and shape of the rim of a diaphragm, that a woman can insert easily herself and leave in place a month or longer. This method is at the stage of product development.

A number of new kinds of IUD are under trial. Some of them are simply differently designed inert models but in other cases the IUD is primarily a carrier for an antifertility agent that acts locally in the uterus, either progesterone or a nonsteroid agent such as copper. Copper-carrying IUD's that are available in many countries need to be replaced after about two years; some newer models have a theoretical life span of 25 years. The progesterone-releasing IUD now being tested also has a limitation in effective time span, but its contraceptive effectiveness has been established as about the equal of other available devices.

Another approach is the induction of menstruation. Compounds are being tested that suppress the corpus luteum and thus bring about a menstrual discharge by eliminating the progesterone support the endometrium needs to sustain implantation. No single compound has met the test of effectiveness and safety but many are being synthesized and screened in animals for possible clinical trial. There was some hope that prosta-

glandin, a substance known to affect uterine muscle, could act systematically to suppress the human corpus luteum. Naturally occurring prostaglandins have been tried without success, and now various prostaglandin analogues are being synthesized and tested. Menstruation might alternatively be induced by giving synthetic progestins during the luteal phase of the cycle in doses sufficient to suppress progesterone production but not to maintain the pregnancy. Four synthetic progestins were tested in women and found to reduce luteal function but the effect was counteracted by HCG, which maintained luteal secretion. Nonetheless, the promise of a contraceptive method based on the principle of menstruation induction warrants an investigative effort of the highest priority. Such an approach could solve the problems of safety that appear to be associated with continuous-dosage hormones.

The rhythm method would be quite effective if the time of ovulation could be known precisely. An estrogenic fertility drug that acts through the hypothalamus to induce ovulation has been tested in normally ovulating women as a means of keeping ovulation on schedule. The test was not successful because in successive months of use the interval between drug ingestion and ovulation increased unpredictably. Now that the hypothalamic releasing factor (generally called LRF, for luteinizing-hormone releasing factor) has been isolated and synthesized, the prospect of regularizing ovulation with it has been put to clinical test. The few cases so far reported indicate the procedure may be feasible. A continuing program of synthesis and testing of modified LRF molecules might, on the other hand, find an LRF antagonist: a substance that would counteract LRF's gonadotropin-releasing action.

A "morning after" or "minutes after" pill to be taken after each coital exposure rather than regularly has certain attractions. The synthetic estrogen diethylstilbestrol is now available to reduce the chances of pregnancy following an isolated mid-cycle exposure, but its side effects and disruption of the ovarian cycle make it unacceptable for regular postcoital contraception. Several related compounds have been tested in women without success, and others are available for testing; one is on clinical trial in India. Two synthetic progestins have been tested experimentally but with poor effectiveness and considerable disruption of the bleeding pattern.

Still another possibility for contraception in women is immunization. A woman inoculated with purified human HCG develops antibodies to the hormone; later, when a blastocyst secretes HCG, the antibodies should interfere with the hormone's role in maintaining the corpus luteum so that menstruation takes place even in the event of a fertile cycle. A single inoculation should last indefinitely, but there are several possible ways to counteract the effect if desired. The method is promising and has been tested in a few volunteers, but several problems are still to be resolved.

For millenniums contraception was mainly left up to males. The diaphragm and the pill gave the responsibility (and more control) to females. Now there is revived interest in methods that involve the male, primarily by interfering with sperm production or development or by blocking the path of the sperm.

Progestin given orally can suppress gonadotropin release, and thus sperm formation, while testosterone is supplied to maintain normal secondary sex characteristics. Tests establishing that this combination of results can be achieved constitute a major advance, but the safety and side effects of the method and the specific agents and routes of administration require more investigation. What seems feasible is a biodegradable implant of testosterone that would last at least a year, supplemented by a weekly pill or a semiannual injection of progestin. There is also the possibility of inhibiting gonadotropin release by administering either progestin or testosterone alone by injection every three months. The difficulties are loss of libido from progestin and the danger of metabolic or cardiovascular disorders from the required high dosage of testosterone.

The vas deferens, which is easily accessible, may lend itself to reversible contraception as well as permanent sterilization. Several kinds of removable clip are under clinical study, as are small plastic plugs that can be removed and even a microvalve that can be closed or opened. So far all such devices that have been adequately tested either have failed to close the vas completely or have damaged the tissue. Another possibility is killing spermatozoa or rendering them immotile by putting a foreign body such as a silk filament in the vas without blocking it. The danger in all methods affecting sperm is the occurrence of congenital defects in a fetus that might be generated by a partially damaged sperm.

Judging by the number of leads that are known to be feasible and are being tested it seems likely that some effective new contraceptive methods will be generally available within a few years; it is possible, on the other hand, that all the innovations now being tested will prove to be too unsafe, ineffective or hard to design and produce. The continuous identification of new leads, through basic research providing better understanding of the normal reproductive process, remains critical to the development of better contraceptive techniques.

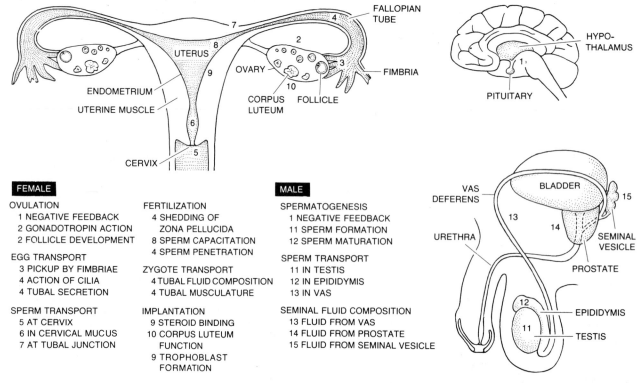

FEMALE		MALE	
OVULATION	FERTILIZATION	SPERMATOGENESIS	
1 NEGATIVE FEEDBACK	4 SHEDDING OF	1 NEGATIVE FEEDBACK	
2 GONADOTROPIN ACTION	ZONA PELLUCIDA	11 SPERM FORMATION	
2 FOLLICLE DEVELOPMENT	8 SPERM CAPACITATION	12 SPERM MATURATION	
	4 SPERM PENETRATION		
EGG TRANSPORT		SPERM TRANSPORT	
3 PICKUP BY FIMBRIAE	ZYGOTE TRANSPORT	11 IN TESTIS	
4 ACTION OF CILIA	4 TUBAL FLUID COMPOSITION	12 IN EPIDIDYMIS	
4 TUBAL SECRETION	4 TUBAL MUSCULATURE	13 IN VAS	
SPERM TRANSPORT	IMPLANTATION	SEMINAL FLUID COMPOSITION	
5 AT CERVIX	9 STEROID BINDING	13 FLUID FROM VAS	
6 IN CERVICAL MUCUS	10 CORPUS LUTEUM	14 FLUID FROM PROSTATE	
7 AT TUBAL JUNCTION	FUNCTION	15 FLUID FROM SEMINAL VESICLE	
	9 TROPHOBLAST		
	FORMATION		

VULNERABLE STEPS in the reproductive process suggest points at which contraceptive technology can intervene. One reason more attention has been paid to contraception in women in recent years is that there are so many potentially vulnerable links in the chain of reproductive events in the female. The numbers indicate the site in the male and female reproductive systems of each of listed steps.

Sex Differences in the Brain

by Seymour Levine
April 1966

*There is increasing evidence that mammalian behavior
patterns are basically female and that male patterns
are induced by the action of the sex hormone
testosterone on the brain of the newborn animal*

W hat makes a male mammal male and a female mammal female? We might sum up the answer in the word heredity, but this would evade the question. How is the genetic information translated into the differentiation of the sexes, as expressed in their physiology and behavior? Again we might summarize the answer in a single word: hormones. Recent investigations have revealed, however, that sexual differentiation in mammals cannot be explained solely in terms of hormones. There is now considerable evidence that the brain is also involved. According to this evidence there are distinct differences between the male brain and the female brain in a mammal, differences that determine not only sexual activity but also certain other forms of behavior.

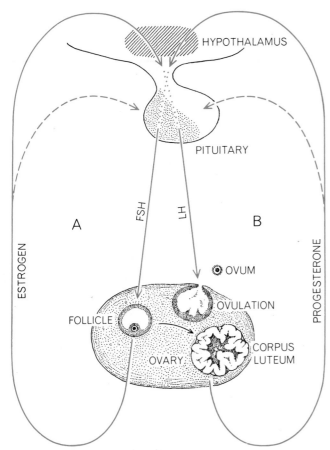

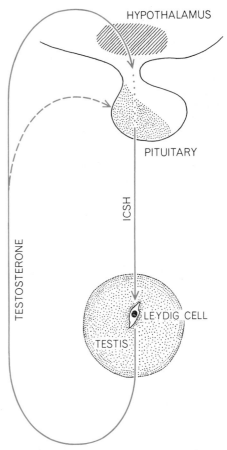

INTERPLAY OF SEX HORMONES differs in the female mammal (*left*) and the male (*right*). In the cyclic female system the pituitary initially releases a follicle-stimulating hormone (FSH) that makes the ovary produce estrogen (*colored arrows at A*): the estrogen then acts on the hypothalamus of the brain to inhibit the further release of FSH by the pituitary and to stimulate the release of a luteinizing hormone (LH) instead. This hormone both triggers ovulation and makes the ovary produce a second hormone, pro-gesterone (*colored arrows at B*). On reaching the hypothalamus the latter hormone inhibits further pituitary release of LH, thereby completing the cycle. In the noncyclic male system the pituitary continually releases an interstitial-cell-stimulating hormone (ICSH) that makes the testes produce testosterone; the latter hormone acts on the hypothalamus to stimulate further release of ICSH by the pituitary. Broken arrows represent the earlier theory that the sex hormones from ovaries and testes stimulated the pituitary directly.

Let us begin by examining one of the principal distinctions between males and females. In most species of mammals the female has a cyclic pattern of ovulation. The human female ovulates about every 28 days; the guinea pig, about every 15 days; the rat, every four to five days. The process is dominated by hormones of the pituitary gland. In cyclic fashion the anterior (front) part of the pituitary delivers to the ovary a follicle-stimulating hormone (FSH), which promotes the growth of Graafian follicles, and a luteinizing hormone (LH), which induces the formation of corpora lutea and triggers ovulation. The formation of corpora lutea is clear evidence that ovulation has occurred. The ovary in turn responds to FSH by releasing the female sex hormone estrogen and to LH by releasing the female sex hormone progesterone [see illustration on preceding page].

The male mammal shows no such cycle. Its testes continually receive from the pituitary the same hormone (LH) that stimulates formation of corpora lutea in the female's ovary; in the male, however, this hormone is known as the interstitial-cell-stimulating hormone (ICSH) because it causes the interstitial cells of the testes to secrete testosterone. Thus the patterns of pituitary effects on the sex organs are distinctly different in the two sexes: cyclic in the female, noncyclic in the male.

What might account for this difference? When the interaction of the pituitary and sex organs was discovered, it was natural to suppose that the sex hormones regulated the pituitary's secretions. In the female the pituitary hormones controlled the process that led to ovulation; the consequent output of estrogen and progesterone by the ovary caused the pituitary to cut down production of its stimulating hormones, and the cycle might therefore be described as a negative-feedback system.

Thirty years ago the endocrinologist Carroll A. Pfeiffer, then working at the Yale University School of Medicine, reported a series of studies unequivocally demonstrating that the process of sexual differentiation occurred very early in the course of a mammal's development. In these studies he undertook to exchange the sex organs in the formative period of early life. In newborn male rats he removed the testes and replaced them with transplanted ovaries; in newborn females he replaced the ovaries with testes; other animals in his experiments were provided with both organs—testes and ovaries. The

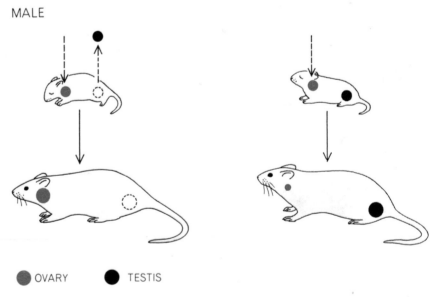

FEMALE

● OVARY   ● TESTIS

REVERSAL OF SEX in young female rats was achieved experimentally by Carroll A. Pfeiffer of the Yale University School of Medicine 30 years ago in proof of the action of the male sex hormone testosterone. When the ovaries of a young female (*at top left in color*) were removed and testes were implanted, the animal in effect became male (*gray*) and showed no estrus at maturity. Even when a female's ovaries were left intact (*top right*), the output of testosterone from the implant prevented normal functioning of the ovaries.

MALE

● OVARY   ● TESTIS

LACK OF TESTOSTERONE permitted a similar reversal of sex among young male rats in the Pfeiffer experiment. When the rat's testes were removed and an ovary was then implanted (*top left*), the ovary continued to function and the animal in effect became female (*color*). When an ovary was implanted in a normal male, however (*top right*), the male's output of testosterone kept the ovary from functioning and the rat remained male (*gray*).

main findings that emerged were these: Males with ovaries in place of testes showed the female capacity for producing corpora lutea in the ovarian tissues. Those that possessed testes as well as ovaries failed to form any corpora lutea in the implanted ovaries. Of the females that had testes implanted, many failed to show estrous cycles or any formation of corpora lutea in their ovaries if the ovaries were left intact.

From these results Pfeiffer deduced that, since the controlling factor seemed to be the presence or absence of testosterone, in the newborn rat testosterone acted to induce a permanent sexual differentiation of the pituitary. If testosterone was present during this critical early period, it would cause the pituitary to produce stimulating secretions thereafter in the noncyclic, male mode; if testosterone was absent, the pituitary would behave throughout life as if it belonged to a female.

Pfeiffer's hypothesis that the pituitary itself was sexually differentiated did not stand up, however. Direct evidence on this question was produced in the 1950's by Geoffrey W. Harris of the University of Oxford and investigators working with him at the Institute of Psychiatry in London. Harris and Dora Jacobsohn found that when the pituitary gland of a male rat was transplanted under the hypothalamus of a female, her reproductive functions and behavior remained entirely female and normal. The same absence of change was noted when pituitaries from female rats were implanted in males. Meanwhile the late F. H. A. Marshall of the University of Cambridge was able to demonstrate that a close relation exists between the external environment and reproduction. In many species of mammals the female cycle of ovulation is affected by light, diet, temperature and emotional stress. Moreover, electrical stimulation of the hypothalamus could induce ovulation, and lesions of the hypothalamus could block ovulation.

Reviewing Pfeiffer's findings and the other experimental evidence, Harris and another investigator, the late William C. Young of the University of Kansas, suggested that it was the brain (not the pituitary, as Pfeiffer had proposed) that was subject to differentiation by the action of hormones. According to this view, the brain of a mammal was essentially female until a certain stage of development (which in the rat came within a short time after birth). If testosterone was absent at this stage, the brain would remain female; if testosterone was present, the brain would develop male characteristics.

Under Harris' leadership the author and other investigators working in the department of neuroendocrinology at the Institute of Psychiatry started a systematic and extensive program of experiments to test this hypothesis. The

FEMALE

OVARY   TESTIS   FEMALE SEX HORMONE   MALE SEX HORMONE

MASCULINIZED FEMALE RATS were produced by injections of testosterone (*black syringe*) at birth. In Column 1 a normal female (*color*) is injected with male hormone when mature; the animal exhibits some male sexual behavior (*gray*). In Column 2 the female is injected with male hormone in infancy; when reinjected at maturity, it exhibits full male sexual behavior. In Column 3, in spite of an injection of female hormone (*colored syringe*) at maturity, the masculinized female fails to exhibit female sexual behavior.

program has been continued at the Stanford University School of Medicine. We worked mainly with rats, and the basic procedure entailed alteration of the newborn animal's normal exposure to sex hormones within the first four days after birth. Instead of transplanting organs we simply injected the hormone whose effects we wished to test; it was already known that a single injection of testosterone (in the form of the long-acting compound testosterone propionate) in a newborn female rat could produce the same effects as the implantation of male testes.

We found that females injected with testosterone in this critical early period did not develop the normal female pattern of physiology when they became adults. Their ovaries were dwarfed and they failed to produce corpora lutea or show the usual cycle of ovulation. On the other hand, males that were castrated (and thus deprived of testosterone) within the first days after birth did show signs of female physiology; when ovaries were implanted in them as adults, they developed corpora lutea. It was clear that a permanent control over the activity of the pituitary in the rat was established by the absence or presence of testosterone in the critical first few days after birth. In the absence of testosterone a pattern of cyclic release of FSH and LH by the pituitary was formed; if testosterone was present, it abolished the cycle.

Essentially the same effect has been demonstrated in guinea pigs and monkeys, but the critical period for these longer-gestating mammals occurs before birth. A series of injections of testosterone in the fetal stage of a female guinea pig or monkey produces permanent masculinizing effects such as we have observed in the female rat.

What are the effects of the early administration of testosterone on the rat's sexual behavior? In this area, as in physiology, there are measurable

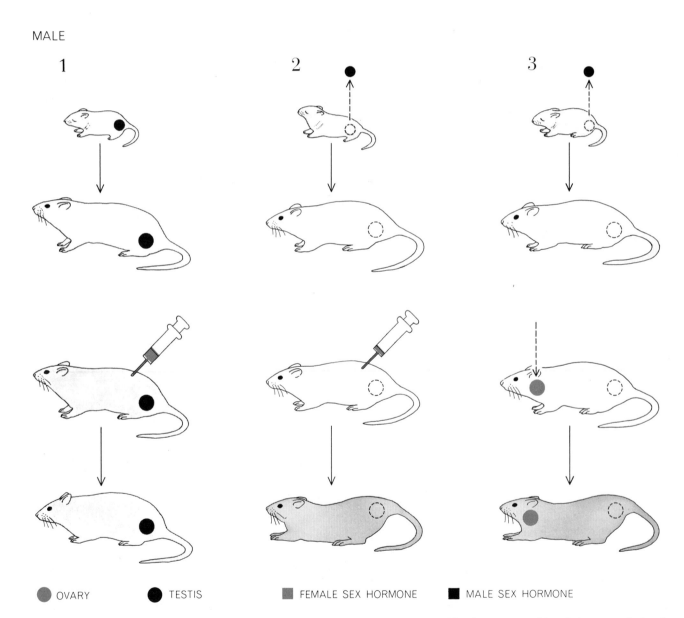

MALE

1   2   3

● OVARY   ● TESTIS   ■ FEMALE SEX HORMONE   ■ MALE SEX HORMONE

FEMINIZED MALE RATS were produced by injections of estrogen and progesterone or by ovary implants only when the males had been castrated at birth and thereby deprived of testosterone during the critical first days of life. In Column 1 a normal male (gray) is unaffected by the injection of female hormones (colored syringe) at maturity. In Column 2 a castrated male is similarly injected; it then assumes the female's permissive sexual posture. In Column 3 the same behavior is produced by implanting an ovary.

criteria for male and female behavior. The male goes through a complex pattern of behavior that begins with mounting of the female and proceeds through several stages to the final ejaculation. The female's display of sexual receptivity is marked by a "lordosis response" (which consists of arching the back and elevating the pelvis) ·when she is mounted by the male. Now, in most subprimate mammals, including the rat, the female's sexual behavior depends entirely on the hormones circulating in her bloodstream. Removal of the ovaries (and hence the elimination of estrogen and progesterone) will completely suppress her normal female sexual behavior, and conversely injections of estrogen and progesterone will restore it. Hence it was no surprise to find that the testosterone treatment of newborn female rats, which disrupted their normal secretion of sex hormones, affected their sexual behavior. The effects were marked, however, by several unusual features.

These masculinized females not only lost the usual female sexual receptivity, including the normal lordosis response to a male, but also failed to show the normal response even when they were given large replacement injections of estrogen and progesterone. Moreover, they showed male behavior that went beyond any previously observed. Male sex behavior is not uncommon even in normal female animals; they can often be observed going through the motions of mounting. A normal adult female rat, if injected with testosterone, will sometimes go so far as to mimic some components of the male's act of copulation. Some of our female rats that had been testosteronized at birth went further, however. Although such females lack any semblance of male genitalia, when they were given a new dose of testosterone as adults, they performed the entire male sexual ritual, including the motions that accompany ejaculation.

The male rats in our experiments showed a similarly striking change of sexual behavior as a result of hormonal alteration at birth. Normally it is extremely difficult to elicit female sexual behavior in an adult male merely by injecting him with female hormones. When, however, newborn male rats were castrated, so that they lacked testosterone at the critical stage of development occurring in the few days after birth, it was found that injection of very small doses of estrogen and progesterone in these males as adults caused them to display sexual behavior precisely like that of normal females. Clearly the

change in these animals involved the central.nervous system; the system's response to female hormones, as reflected in the animal's behavior, had been altered.

Thus all the experiments, both on males and on females, left little doubt that testosterone could determine the sexual differentiation of the brain in the first few days after birth. In some manner testosterone produced a profound and permanent change in the sensitivity of the brain to sex hormones. In the female it made the brain tissue much more sensitive to testosterone and insensitive to estrogen and progesterone, so that the animal did not display normal female behavior in response to these female hormones. In the male the absence of testosterone at the critical period caused the animal to be sensitive to estrogen and progesterone. To put it another way, the absence of testosterone at the differentiation stage would leave both males and females sensitive to the female hormones and capable of displaying female behavior; the presence of testosterone, on the other hand, would desensitize females as well as males, so that both sexes failed to display feminine behavior when they were challenged with female hormones.

That the sex hormones can act directly on the brain was clearly demonstrated in experiments by Harris and Richard Michael. They implanted a synthetic estrogen (stilbestrol) into the hypothalamus of female cats and found that the implant evoked full female sexual behavior although the cats did not show the usual physiological signs of estrus. In similar experiments with males Julian M. Davidson of Stanford University showed that implants of testosterone in the brain of a castrated male rat would elicit male sexual behavior, although again there was no sign of effects on the anatomy of the male reproductive system.

If the brain differentiates into male and female types, may not the difference be reflected in fields of behavior other than the sexual? A few experiments looking into this question have been conducted; they suggest that other forms of behavior can indeed be influenced by hormonal treatment during the critical period of sexual differentiation.

One of these studies involved a difference between male and female behavior that Curt P. Richter of the Johns Hopkins School of Medicine observed many

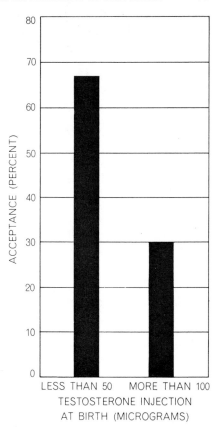

SEXUAL BEHAVIOR of female rats was substantially modified by the injection of male hormone at birth. Although dosed with female hormones at maturity, females that had received 100 micrograms or more of testosterone at birth were less than half as responsive to male sexual advances as rats that had received little or no male hormone.

years ago. He used an activity wheel that measured the amount of voluntary running activity an animal would perform each day. The activity of females, he found, went in cycles, rising to a peak at the time of ovulation; males, on the other hand, performed more uniformly from day to day. Harris recently applied this activity test to male rats that had been castrated shortly after birth and then implanted with an ovary as adults. They showed a cyclic pattern of running activity corresponding to the cycle of ovulation (covering four to five days) of the female rat.

Another test employed the open-field apparatus with which we have gauged animals' behavior in response to various emotion-evoking stimuli [see "Stimulation in Infancy," by Seymour Levine; SCIENTIFIC AMERICAN Offprint 436]. In this apparatus females tend to be more exploratory and to defecate less often than males. We found that female rats to which testosterone had been administered at birth displayed the male pattern of defecation behavior instead of the female pattern [*see illustration on this page*].

Analyzing the play of young monkeys before they reach sexual maturity, Young and his co-workers found that the juvenile male's behavior is distinctly different from the female's: the male is more inclined to rough-and-tumble play, more aggressive and more given to threatening facial expressions. Again experiments showed that injections of testosterone during the critical differentiation period (before birth in the monkey's case) caused females to display the male type of behavior in play.

Obviously the findings so far are only first steps in what promises to be an important new field of investigation. They invite a full exploration of the extent to which behavior, nonsexual as well as sexual, can be masculinized by testosterone treatment or feminized by castration at the critical stage of sexual differentiation. It presents a new biological mystery: If testosterone at the critical period does indeed produce sexual differentiation in the brain, by what mechanism does it do so? The studies on animals may well have clinical implications for human beings with respect to the problem of homosexuality. Human homosexual behavior undoubtedly involves many psychological factors that do not apply to the lower animals, but it may also depend in a fundamental sense on what the hormonal makeup of the individual happens to be during the development of the nervous system.

There are other questions of broader interest. Do the hormones of the thyroid gland, the adrenal cortex and other organs of the endocrine system exert differentiating effects on the developing brain? To what extent may the various hormones acting on the brain during infancy shape the future behavior of an individual? The artificially masculinized female rat and the feminized male have opened a wide field for speculation and research.

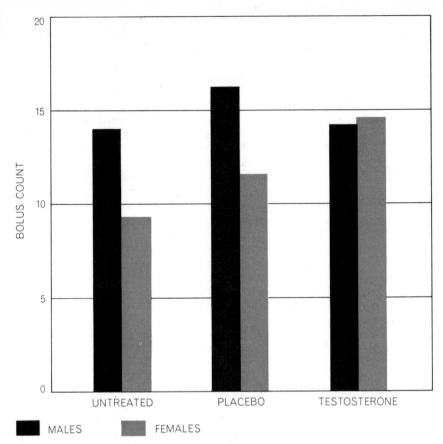

EXPLORATORY BEHAVIOR, more extensive among female rats than among males, was modified when the females were injected with male hormones at birth. The bar chart shows the frequency of defecation, which is inversely proportional to exploration, in three minutes' exposure in an open-field apparatus. When the females had not been injected at birth (*left and center*), their count was significantly lower than the males'. Females that had been masculinized (*right*), however, defecated at a rate insignificantly different from the males'.

III

TARGETS FOR STEROID HORMONE ACTION

III TARGETS FOR STEROID HORMONE ACTION

INTRODUCTION

The introduction to Section II stated that in the 1950s there was little understanding of the cellular bases of hormone actions. This topic is currently a very active area of research. The papers in this section address the problem of cellular effects with regard to the gonadal hormones. Eric H. Davidson's 1965 article cites the following theories of steroid hormone action: (a) hormones are cofactors in enzymatic reactions; (b) hormones activate enzymes; and (3) hormones modify cell membranes and affect the structure of intracellular organelles. A fourth and newer theory proposes that hormones regulate the genes.

This last idea received considerable impetus from E. V. Jensen's classic studies with radioactively labeled estrogen. Jensen found that when rats were injected with radioactive estrogen the uterus retained the radioactivity longer than many other tissues of the body. This prolonged estrogen retention was one characteristic of a target tissue for estrogen action. Later other tissues, such as the vagina, mammary gland, anterior pituitary, and hypothalamus, were also shown to retain estrogen for a prolonged period after it was administered. All of these target tissues for estrogen were shown to concentrate the steroid in the nuclear fraction of their cells.

In their article, Bert W. O'Malley and William T. Schrader discuss why certain steroid hormones are selectively retained in the nuclei of some cell types and not in others. It turns out that "target" cells possess receptor proteins in their cytoplasm. When a steroid enters a cell for which it is a target, the steroid and the receptor protein form a complex. This complex then enters the nucleus and binds to "acceptor" sites on the chromosomes of the target cell. When a steroid enters a cell for which it is not a target, receptors for it are absent and the steroid is not retained. Through a series of experiments with tissues rich in steroid receptors (e.g., the uterus and the oviduct) O'Malley and other researchers have shown that steroids step up the transcription of RNA, with consequent increases in the production of specific proteins.

Bruce S. McEwen's article documents the fact that particular brain regions are targets for steroid hormones. The pioneer work of W. E. Stumpf and D. W. Pfaff established the location of these target areas in the brain. From all available evidence, it appears that the same receptor mechanisms that operate in the uterus and the oviduct also operate in the brain. How the effect of a steroid on a brain cell's genetic apparatus is translated into a change in reproductive behavior is still not established, but McEwen suggests some possibilities. For example, steroids may alter the production rate of enzymes involved in the synthesis of substances that mediate communication among nerve cells (for a discussion of neurotransmitter substances, see Section IV).

The three papers that constitute this section emphasize one aspect of the action of steriod hormones—action on the genetic apparatus. Examination of this process has been the most exciting and fruitful avenue of steroid research at the cellular level, but other, nonnuclear mechanisms may also be important. A proper understanding of the molecular basis of steroid action is critical for the prevention and alleviation of pathologies of the reproductive system and for an appreciation of the ways in which chemical factors can affect our behavior and moods.

9　Hormones and Genes

by Eric H. Davidson

June 1965

One of the traditional questions of biology is: How do hormones exert their powerful effects on cells? Evidence is accumulating that many of these effects are due to the activation of genes

In the living cell the activities of life proceed under the direction of the genes. In a many-celled organism the cells are marshaled in tissues, and in order for each tissue to perform its role its cells must function in a cooperative manner. For more than a century biologists have studied the ways in which tissue functions are controlled, providing the organism with the flexibility it needs to adapt to a changing environment. Gradually it has become clear that among the primary controllers are the hormones. Thus whereas the genes control the activities of individual cells, these same cells constitute the tissues that respond to the influence of hormones.

New experimental evidence is now making it possible to complete this syllogism: it is being found that hormones can affect the activity of genes. Hormones of the most diverse sources, molecular structure and physiological influence appear able to rapidly alter the pattern of genetic activity in the cells responsive to them. The establishment of a link between hormones and gene action completes a conceptual bridge stretching from the molecular level to ecology and animal behavior.

In order to understand the nature of the link between hormones and genes it will be useful to review briefly what is known of how genes function in differentiated, or specialized, cells. One of the most striking examples of cell specialization in animals is the red blood cell, the protein content of which can be more than 90 percent hemoglobin. It has been shown that in man the ability to manufacture a given type of hemoglobin is inherited; this provides a clear case of a differentiated-cell function under genetic control. Hemoglobin also furnishes an example of another

principle that is fundamental to the study of differentiation: the specialized character of a cell depends on the type and quantity of proteins in it, and therefore the process of differentiation is basically the process of developing a specific pattern of protein synthesis. Some cells, such as red blood cells and the cells of the pancreas that produce digestive enzymes, specialize in synthesizing one kind of protein; other cells specialize in synthesizing an entire set of protein enzymes to manufacture nonprotein end products, for example glycogen, or animal starch (which is made by liver cells), and steroid hormones (which are made by cells of the adrenal cortex).

If one understood the means by which the type and quantity of protein made by cells was controlled, one would have taken a long step toward understanding the nature of the differentiated cell. Part of this objective has been attained: we now know something of how genes act and how proteins are synthesized. A protein owes its properties to the sequence of amino acid subunits in its chainlike molecule. The genes of most organisms consist of deoxyribonucleic acid (DNA), the chainlike molecules of which are made up of nucleotide subunits. The sequence of nucleotides in a single gene determines the sequence of amino acids in a single protein.

The protein is not assembled directly on the gene; instead the cell copies the sequence of nucleotides in the gene by synthesizing a molecule of ribonucleic acid (RNA). This "messenger" RNA moves away from the gene to the small bodies called ribosomes. On the ribosomes, which contain their own unique kind of RNA, the amino acids are assembled into protein. In the assembly

process each molecule of amino acid is identified and moved into position through its attachment to a specific molecule of a third kind of RNA: "transfer" RNA. It can therefore be said that the characteristics of the cell are determined at the level of "gene transcription"—the synthesis of messenger and ribosomal RNA.

Each differentiated cell in a many-celled organism contains a complete set of the organism's genes. It is obvious, however, that in such a cell only a small fraction of the genes are actually functioning; the gene for hemoglobin is not active in a skin cell and the assortment of genes active in a liver cell is not the same as the assortment active in an adrenal cell. The active genes release their information in the form of messenger RNA and the inactive genes do not. Exactly how the inactive genes are repressed is not clearly understood, but the repression seems to involve a chemical combination between DNA and the proteins called histones; it has been shown that histones inhibit the synthesis of messenger RNA in the isolated nuclei of calf-thymus cells, and similar results have been obtained with the nuclei of other kinds of cell. In any case it is clear that the characteristics of the cell are the result of variable gene activity. The prime question becomes: How are the genes selectively turned on or selectively repressed during the life of the cell?

Gene action is often closely linked to cell function in terms of time. It has been demonstrated that genes can exercise immediate control over the activities of differentiated cells—particularly very active or growing cells—and over cells that are going through some change of state. In many specialized cells at least part of the messenger RNA

HORMONE	SOURCE		CHEMICAL NATURE	FUNCTION
ECDYSONE	INSECT PROTHORACIC GLAND		STEROID	Causes molting, initiation of adult development and puparium formation.
GLUCOCORTICOIDS (CORTISONE)	ADRENAL CORTEX		STEROID	Causes glycogen synthesis in liver. Causes redistribution of fat throughout organism. Alters nitrogen balance. Causes complete revision of white blood cell type frequencies. Is required for muscle function. Alters central nervous system excitation threshold. Affects connective tissue differentiation. Promotes healing. Induces appearance of new enzymes in liver. Affects almost all tissues.
INSULIN	PANCREAS (ISLETS OF LANGERHANS)		POLYPEPTIDE	Affects entry rate of carbohydrates, amino acids, cations and fatty acids into cells. Promotes protein synthesis. Affects glycogen synthetic activity. Stimulates fat synthesis. Stimulates acid mucopolysaccharide synthesis. Affects almost all tissues.
ESTROGEN	OVARY		STEROID	Promotes appearance of secondary sexual characteristics. Increases synthesis of contractile and other proteins in uterus. Increases synthesis of yolk proteins in fowl liver. Increases synthesis of polysaccharides. Affects rates of glycolysis, respiration and substrate uptake into cells. Probably affects almost all tissues.
ALDOSTERONE	ADRENAL CORTEX		STEROID	Controls sodium and potassium excretion and cation flux across many internal body membranes.
PITUITARY ACTH	ANTERIOR PITUITARY		POLYPEPTIDE	Stimulates glucocorticoid synthesis by adrenal cortex. Stimulates adrenal protein synthesis and glucose uptake. Inhibits protein synthesis in adipose tissue. Stimulates fat breakdown.
PITUITARY GH	ANTERIOR PITUITARY		PROTEIN	Stimulates all anabolic processes. Affects nitrogen balance, water balance, growth rate and all aspects of protein metabolism. Stimulates amino acid uptake and acid mucopolysaccharide synthesis. Affects fat metabolism. Probably affects all tissues.
THYROXIN	THYROID		THYRONINE DERIVATIVE	Affects metabolic rate, growth, water and ion excretion. Promotes protein synthesis. Is required for normal muscle function. Affects carbohydrate levels, transport and synthesis. Probably affects all tissues.

HORMONES DISCUSSED IN THIS ARTICLE are listed according to their source, their chemical nature and their effects, which are usually quite diverse. Pituitary GH is the pituitary growth hormone. The steroid hormones share a basic molecular skeleton consisting of adjoining four-ring structures. The polypeptide hormones and the protein hormones consist of chains of amino acid subunits.

produced by the active genes decays in a matter of hours, and therefore the genes must be continuously active for protein synthesis to continue normally. Other differentiated cells display the opposite characteristic, in that gene activity occurs at a time relatively remote from the time at which the messenger RNA acts. The very existence of this time element in gene control of cell function indicates how extensive that control is. Furthermore, certain genes can be alternately active and inactive over a short period; for example, if a leaf is bleached by being kept in the dark and is then exposed to light, it immediately begins to manufacture messenger RNA for the synthesis of chlorophyll.

The sum of such observations is that the patterns of gene activity in the living cell are in a state of continuous flux. For a cell in a many-celled organism, however, it is essential that the genetic apparatus be responsive to external conditions. The cell must be able to meet changing situations with altered metabolism, and if all the cells in a tissue are to alter their metabolism in a coordinated way, some kind of organized external control is needed. Evidence obtained from experiments with a number of biological systems suggests that such control is obtained by externally modulating the highly variable activity of the cellular genetic apparatus. The studies that will be reviewed here are cases of this general proposition; in these cases the external agents that alter the pattern of gene activity are hormones.

Many efforts have been made to explain the basis of hormone action. It has been suggested that hormones are coenzymes (that is, cofactors in enzymatic reactions), that they activate key enzymes, that they modify the outer membrane of cells and that they directly affect the physical state of structures within the cell. For each hypothesis there is evidence from studies of one or several hormones. As an example, experiments with the pituitary hormone vasopressin, which causes blood vessels to constrict and decreases the excretion of urine by the kidney, strongly support the conclusion that the hormone attaches itself to the outer membrane of the cells on which it acts.

To these hypotheses has been added the new one that hormones act by regulating the genetic apparatus, and many investigators have undertaken to study the effects of hormones on gene activity. It turns out that the gene-regulation

hypothesis is more successful than the others in explaining some of the most puzzling features of hormone activity, such as the time lag between the administration of some hormones and the initial appearance of their effects, and also the astonishing variety of these effects [see illustration on preceding page]. There can be no doubt that some hormone action is independent of gene activity, but it has now been shown that a wide variety of hormones can affect such activity. This conclusion is strongly supported by the fact that each of these same hormones is powerless to exert some or all of its characteristic effects when the genes of the cells on which it acts are prevented from functioning.

The genes can be blocked by the remarkably specific action of the antibiotic actinomycin D. The antibiotic penetrates the cell and forms a complex with the cell's DNA; once this has happened the DNA cannot participate in the synthesis of messenger RNA. The specificity of actinomycin is indicated by the fact that it does not affect other activities of the cell: protein synthesis, respiration and so on. These activities continue until the cellular machinery stops because it is starved for messenger RNA. In high concentrations actinomycin totally suppresses the synthesis of messenger RNA; in lower concentrations it depresses this synthesis and appears to prevent it from developing at new sites.

So far the greatest number of studies of the effects of hormones on genes have been concerned with the steroid hormones, particularly the estrogens produced by the ovaries. This work has been carried forward by many investigators in many laboratories. It has been found that when the ovaries are removed from an experimental animal and then estrogen is administered to the animal at a later date, the synthesis of protein by cells in the uterus of the animal increases by as much as 300 percent. The increase is detected by measuring the incorporation of radioactively labeled amino acids into uterine protein, or by testing the capacity for protein synthesis of homogenized uterine tissue removed from the animal at various times after the administration of estrogen. Added proof that these observations have to do with the synthesis of protein is provided by the fact that the stimulating effects of estrogen are blocked by the antibiotic puromycin, which specifically inhibits protein synthesis.

In these experiments the principal rise in protein synthesis is first observed between two and four hours after estrogen treatment. Less than 30 minutes after the treatment, however, there is a dramatic increase in the rate of RNA synthesis. When actinomycin is used to block the rise in RNA synthesis, the administration of estrogen has no effect on protein synthesis! What this means is that since the diverse metabolic changes brought about in uterine cells by estrogen are all mediated by protein enzymes, none of the changes can occur unless the estrogen has induced gene action. Among the changes are the increased synthesis of amino acids from glucose, the increased evolution of carbon dioxide and the increased synthesis of the fatty lipids and phospholipids. It is not surprising to find that none of these metabolic changes in uterine cells can be detected when estrogen is administered to an animal that has first been treated with actinomycin.

The effect of estrogen on the synthesis of RNA is not limited to messenger RNA. There is also an increase in the manufacture of the other two kinds of RNA: transfer RNA and ribosomal RNA. The administration of estrogen first stimulates the production of messenger RNA and transfer RNA. The genes responsible for the synthesis of ribosomal RNA become active somewhat later, and the number of ribosomes per cell increases. One of the earliest changes brought about by estrogen, however, is an increase in the activity of the enzyme RNA-DNA polymerase. This enzyme appears to be responsible for all RNA synthesis in such cells.

Two main conclusions can be drawn from these various observations. First, there can be no reasonable doubt that treatment with estrogenic hormones results in activation at the gene level, and that many of the well-known effects of estrogen on uterine cells result from this gene activation. Second, it is clear that a considerable number of genes must be activated in order to account for the many different responses of the cells to estrogen. Consider only the fact that estrogen stimulates the production of three different kinds of RNA. At least two different genes are known to be associated with the synthesis of ribosomal RNA, and each cell needs to manufacture perhaps as many as 60 species of transfer RNA. As for messenger RNA, the variety of the changes induced by estrogen implies that under such influences it too must be produced

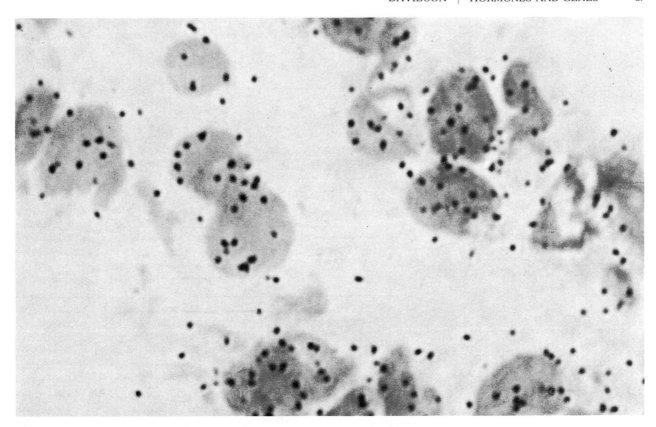

HORMONE IS LOCALIZED IN NUCLEI of cells in this radio-autograph made by George A. Porter, Rita Bogoroch and Isidore S. Edelman of the University of California School of Medicine (San Francisco). The hormone aldosterone was radioactively labeled and administered to a preparation of toad bladder tissue. When the tissue was radioautographed, the hormone revealed its presence by black dots. The dots appear predominantly in the nuclei (*dark gray areas*) of the cells rather than in the cytoplasm (*light gray areas*).

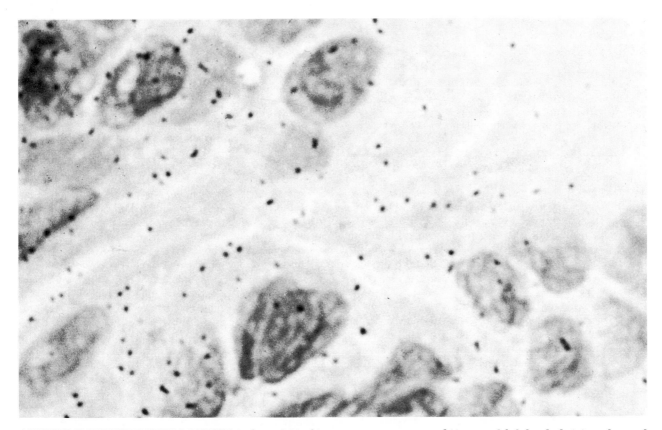

ANOTHER HORMONE IS NOT LOCALIZED in the nuclei in this radioautograph made by the same investigators. Here the hormone was progesterone, and it too was labeled and administered to toad bladder tissue. The dots are distributed more or less at random.

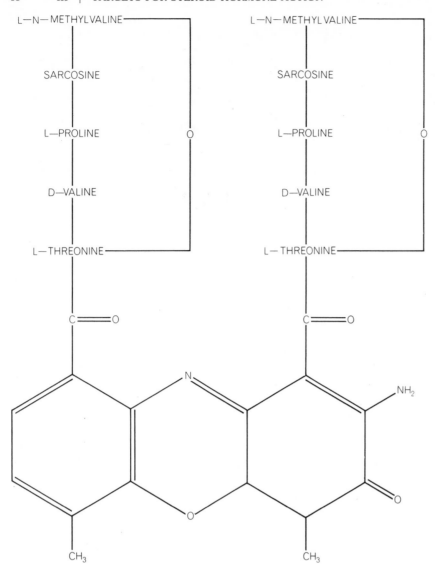

ANTIBIOTIC ACTINOMYCIN D has a complex chemical structure. The antibiotic blocks the participation of the genetic material in the synthesis of ribonucleic acid (RNA); thus it can be used in studies to determine whether or not a given hormone stimulates gene activity.

in a number of molecular species. We are therefore confronted with a major mystery of gene regulation: How can a single hormone activate an entire set of functionally related but otherwise quite separate genes, and activate them in a specific sequence and to a specific degree?

The question can be sharpened somewhat by considering the effect of estrogen not on uterine cells but on the cells of the liver. When an egg is being formed in a hen, the estrogen produced by the hen's ovaries stimulates its liver to produce the yolk proteins lipovitellin and phosvitin. Obviously a rooster does not need to synthesize these proteins, but if it is treated with estrogen, its liver will make them in large amounts! A more unequivocal example of the selective activation of repressed genes by a hormone could scarcely be imagined. What is more, experiments by E. N. Carlsen and his co-workers at the University of California School of Medicine (Los Angeles) have demonstrated that this gene-activating effect of estrogen is remarkably specific. Phosvitin is an unusual protein in that nearly half of its subunits are of one kind: they are residues of the amino acid serine. Carlsen and his colleagues found that estrogen most strongly stimulates liver cells to produce the particular species of transfer RNA that is associated with the incorporation of this amino acid into protein.

The effect of estrogen on liver cells is thus quite different from its effect on uterine cells. Indeed, it has long been recognized that hormonal specificity resides less in the hormone than in the "target" cell. We are now, however, able to ask new questions: How are the sets of genes that are activated by a given hormone selected? Are these genes somehow preset for hormonal activation? How does the hormone interact not only with the gene itself but also with the cell's entire system of genetic regulation?

The male hormone testosterone has also been shown to operate by gene activation. Like the estrogens, the male sex hormones can give rise to dramatic increases of RNA synthesis in various cells. In experiments on male and female rats it has been found that the effect of testosterone on the liver cells of a female is somewhat different from that on the liver cells of a castrated male. In both cases the hormone causes an increase in the *amount* of messenger RNA produced, but in the female it also brings about the synthesis of a new *variety* of messenger RNA. This effect, like the ability of estrogen to stimulate a rooster's liver cells to produce egg-yolk proteins, provides a new approach for examining the whole question of sexual differentiation.

Apart from the sex hormones, the principal steroids in mammals are those secreted by the adrenal cortex. One group of adrenocortical hormones is typified by cortisone; this hormone and its relatives are known for their quite different effects in different tissues. Only a fraction of these effects have been studied from the standpoint of gene activation, and there is much evidence to indicate that some of them are not mediated by the genes. Some responses to cortisone, however, do appear to be the consequence of gene activation.

If the adrenal glands are removed from an experimental animal and cortisone is administered later, the hormone induces in the liver cells of the animal the production of a number of new proteins. Among these proteins are enzymes required for the synthesis of glucose (but not the breakdown of glucose) and enzymes involved in the metabolism of amino acids. Moreover, cortisone steps up the total production of protein by the liver cells. The effect of cortisone on the synthesis of messenger RNA is apparent as soon as five minutes after the hormone has been administered; within 30 minutes the amount of RNA produced has increased two to three times and probably includes not

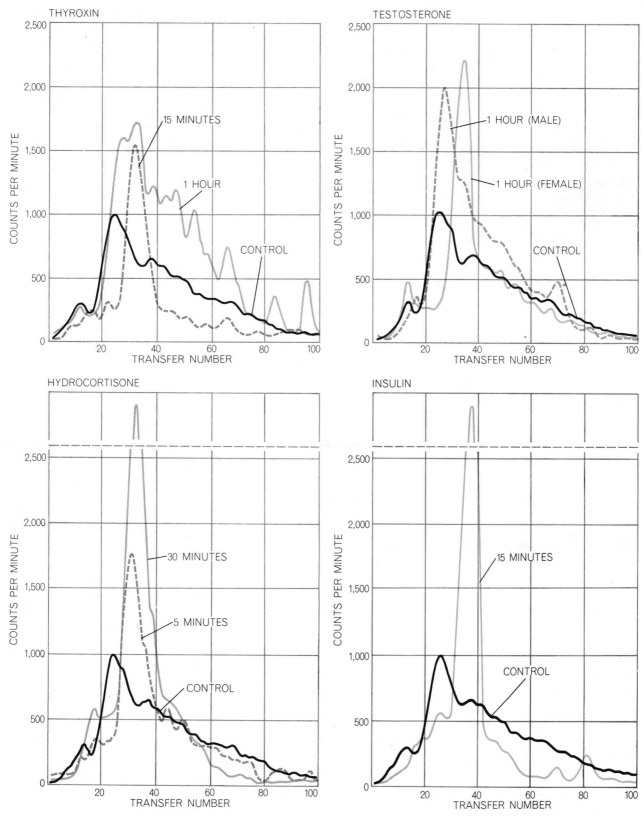

GENETIC ACTIVITY OF SEVERAL HORMONES is indicated by measurements made by Chev Kidson and K. S. Kirby of the Chester Beatty Research Institute in London. Their basic technique was first to administer to rats radioactively labeled orotic acid, which is a precursor of RNA. The tissues of the rat then incorporated the radioactive label into new RNA. Next liver tissue was removed from the rat and the species of RNA called "messenger" RNA was extracted from its cells. When the messenger RNA was analyzed by the method of countercurrent distribution, it gave rise to a charac-

teristic curve (*black "Control" curve in each graph*); "Transfer number" refers to a stage of transfer in the countercurrent-distribution process and "Counts per minute" to the radioactivity of the solution at that point. Then, in separate measurements, rats were first given one of a number of hormones (*top left of each graph*) and shortly thereafter radioactively labeled orotic acid. The curves (*color*) of the messenger RNA obtained from such rats were entirely different, depending on the time that had elapsed before the administration of the orotic acid or on the sex of the animal (*top right*).

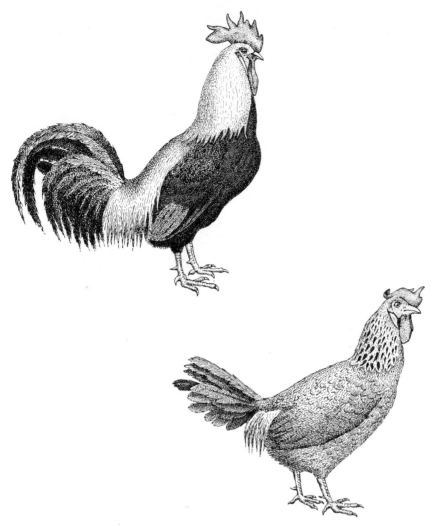

ROOSTER TREATED WITH ESTROGEN (*bottom*) is compared with a normal rooster (*top*). The signs of femaleness induced by estrogen include changes in comb and plumage.

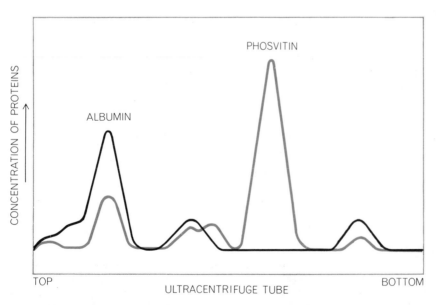

ULTRACENTRIFUGE PATTERNS show that phosvitin, a yolk protein found only in hens, is present in serum extracted from a bird that had been injected with estrogen (*colored curve*) but not in serum from a bird used as a control (*black curve*). Each curve gives the concentration of proteins as they are separated out of a mixture by an ultracentrifuge.

only messenger RNA but also ribosomal RNA. These events are followed by the increase in enzyme activity. Olga Greengard and George Acs of the Institute for Muscle Disease in New York have shown that if the animal is treated with actinomycin before cortisone is administered, the new enzymes fail to appear in its liver cells.

Another clear case of the activation of genes by an adrenocortical hormone has been demonstrated by Isidore S. Edelman, Rita Bogoroch and George A. Porter of the University of California School of Medicine (San Francisco). They employed the hormone aldosterone, which regulates the passage through the cell membrane of sodium and potassium ions. Tracer studies with radioactively labeled aldosterone showed that when the bladder cells of a toad were exposed to the hormone, the molecules of hormone penetrated all the way into the nuclei of the cells [*see illustrations on page* 87]. About an hour and a half after the aldosterone has reached its peak concentration within the cells the movement of sodium ions across the cell membrane increases. It appears that this facilitation of sodium transport is brought about by proteins the cell is induced to make, because it will not occur if the cells have been treated beforehand with puromycin, the drug that blocks the synthesis of protein. Moreover, treatment of the cells with actinomycin will block the aldosterone-induced increase in sodium transport through the membrane. Thus the experiments indicate that aldosterone activates genes in the nucleus and gives rise to proteins—that is, enzymes—that speed up the passage of sodium ions across the membrane.

Ecdysone, a steroid hormone of insects, is also believed to be a gene activator. The evidence for this conclusion has been provided by Wolfgang Beermann and his colleagues at the Max Planck Institute for Biology in Tübingen [see "Chromosome Puffs," by Wolfgang Beermann and Ulrich Clever, SCIENTIFIC AMERICAN Offprint 180]. If the larva of an insect lacks ecdysone, the development of the larva is indefinitely arrested at a stage preceding its metamorphosis into a pupa. Only when, in the course of normal development, the concentration of ecdysone in the tissues of the larva begins to rise does further differentiation take place; the larva then advances to metamorphosis. Ecdysone has been of especial interest to cell biologists because it has been observed

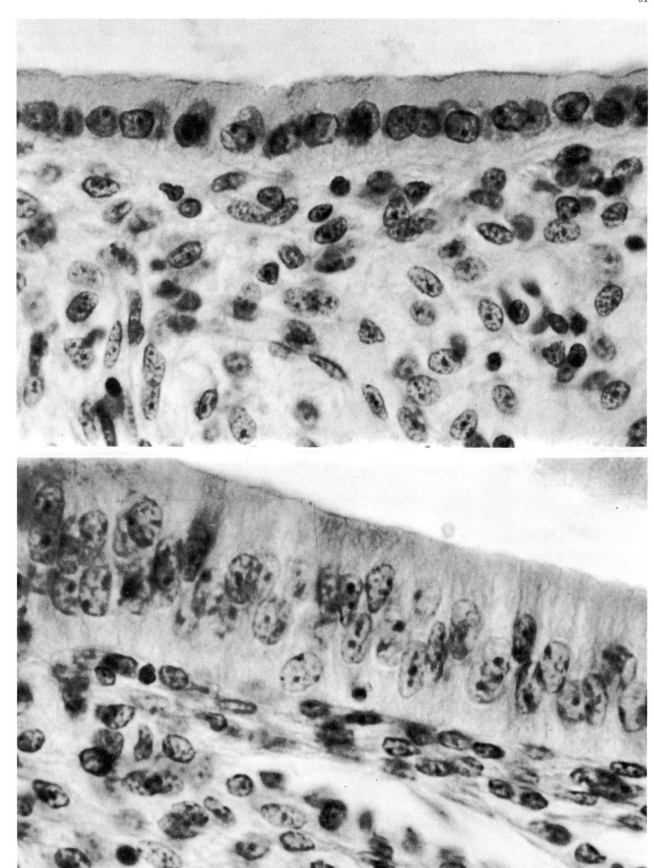

EFFECT OF ESTROGEN ON CELLS in the uterus of rats is demonstrated in these photomicrographs made by Sheldon J. Segal and G. P. Talwar of the Rockefeller Institute. The photomicrograph at top shows uterine cells from a rat that had not been treated with estrogen; the layer of cells at the surface of the tissue is relatively thin. The photomicrograph at bottom shows uterine cells from a rat that had been treated with the hormone; the layer of cells is much thicker. The effect involves enhanced synthesis of protein.

to cause startling changes in the chromosomes within the nuclei of the cells affected by it. Studies of this kind are possible in insects because the cells of certain insect tissues have giant chromosomes that can easily be examined in the microscope. These "polytene" chromosomes develop in many kinds of differentiated cell by means of a process in which the chromosomes repeatedly replicate but do not separate.

In some polytene chromosomes genetic loci, or specific regions, have a distended, diffuse appearance [see illustration below]. Biologists regard these regions, which have been named "puffs," as sites of intense gene activity. Evidence for this conclusion is provided by radioautograph studies, which show that the puffs are localized sites of intense RNA synthesis. In such studies a molecular precursor of RNA is radio-

actively labeled and after it has been incorporated into RNA reveals its presence as a black dot in the emulsion of the radioautograph. According to the view of differentiation presented in this article, different genes should be active in different types of cell, and this appears to be the case in insect cells with polytene chromosomes. In many different kinds of cell—salivary-gland cells, rectal-gland cells and excretory-tubule cells—the giant chromosomes have a different constellation of puffs; this suggests that different sets of genes are active, a given gene being active in one cell and quiescent in another.

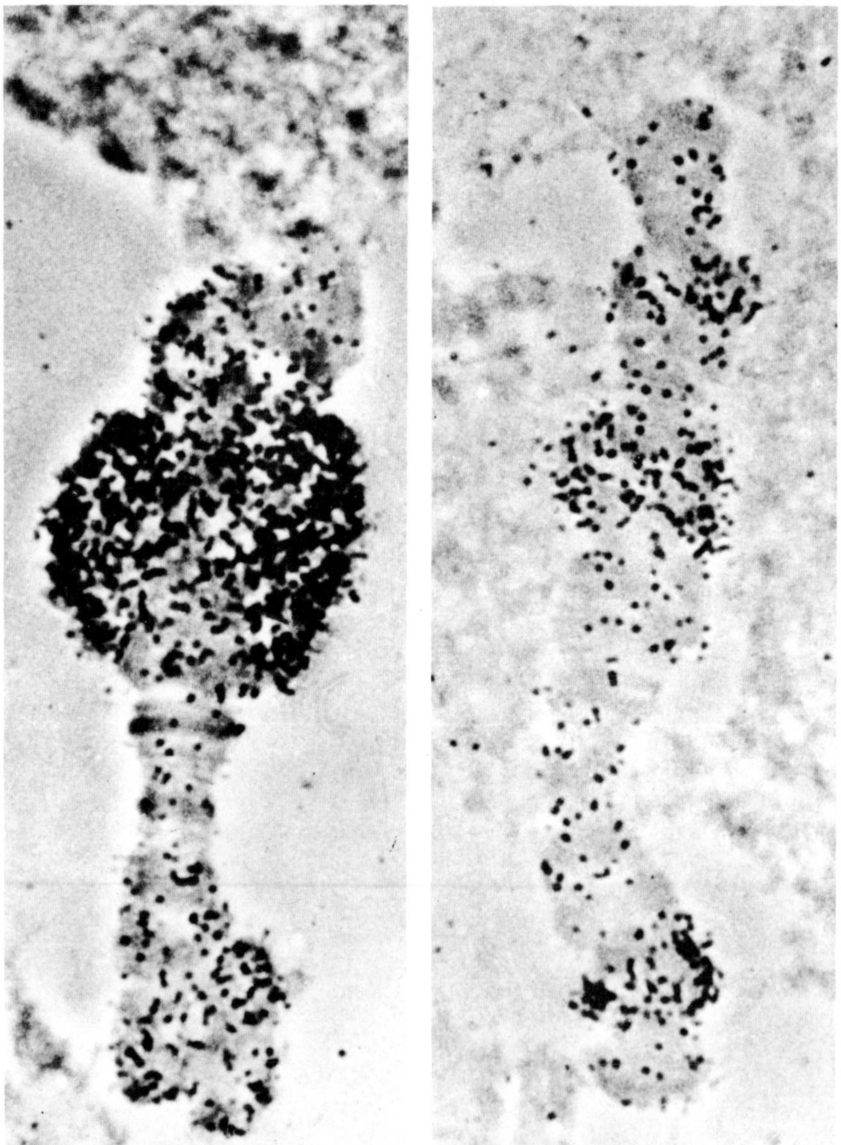

On the polytene chromosomes of insect salivary-gland cells new puffs develop as metamorphosis begins. This is where ecdysone comes into the picture: the hormone seems to be capable of inducing the appearance of specific new puffs. When a minute amount of ecdysone is injected into an insect larva, a specific puff appears on one of its salivary-gland chromosomes; when a slightly larger amount of ecdysone is injected, a second puff materializes at a different chromosomal location. In the normal course of events the concentration of ecdysone increases as the larva nears metamorphosis; therefore there exists a mechanism whereby the more sensitive genetic locus can be aroused first. This example of hormone action at the gene level, which is directly visible to the investigator, seems to have provided some of the strongest evidence for the regulation of gene action by hormones. The effect of ecdysone, which is clearly needed for differentiation, appears to be to arouse quiescent genes to visible states of activity. In this way the specific patterns of gene activity required for differentiation are provided.

What about nonsteroid hormones? Here the overall picture is not as clearcut. The effects of some hormones are quite evidently due to gene activation, and yet other effects of the same hormones are not blocked by the administration of actinomycin; a small sample of these effects is listed in the illustration on the opposite page. As for the hormonal effects that are quite definitely not genetic, they fall into one of the following categories.

(1) Some hormones act on specific enzymes; for example, the thyroid hormone thyroxin promotes the dissociation of the enzyme glutamic dehydrogenase. (2) Other hormones, for instance insulin and vasopressin, act on systems that transport things through cell mem-

"PUFF" ON A GIANT CHROMOSOME from the salivary gland of the midge *Chironomus tentans* appears after administration of the insect hormone ecdysone. In the radioautograph at left the round area at top center is a puff. The black dots result from the fact that the midge was given radioactively labeled uridine, which is a precursor of RNA. The concentration of dots in the puff indicates that it is actively synthesizing RNA. In the radioautograph at right is a chromosome from a fly that had been treated with actinomycin before receiving ecdysone. No puff has occurred and RNA synthesis appears to be muted. The radioautographs were made by Claus Pelling of the Max Planck Institute for Biology in Tübingen.

HORMONE	EVIDENCE FOR HORMONAL ACTION BY GENE ACTIVATION.	EVIDENCE THAT HORMONAL ACTION IS CLEARLY INDEPENDENT OF IMMEDIATE GENE ACTIVATION.
PITUITARY GROWTH HORMONE	General stimulation of protein synthesis. Stimulation of rates of synthesis of ribosomal RNA, transfer RNA and messenger RNA within 90 minutes in liver. Effect blocked with actinomycin.	
PITUITARY ACTH	Stimulates adrenal protein synthesis. Messenger RNA and total RNA synthesis stimulated.	Steroid synthesis in isolated adrenal sections is independent of RNA synthesis and is insensitive to actinomycin D.
THYROXIN	Promotes new messenger RNA synthesis within 10 to 15 minutes of administration, promotes stimulation of all classes of RNA by 60 minutes. Promotes increase in RNA–DNA polymerase at 10 hours, later promotes general increase in protein synthesis.	Causes isolated, purified glutamic dehydrogenase to dissociate to the inactive form. Affects isolated mitochondria in vitro.
INSULIN	Promotes 100 percent increase in rate of RNA synthesis. Causes striking change in messenger RNA profile within 15 minutes of administration to rat diaphragm; effect blocked with actinomycin. Actinomycin-sensitive induction of glucokinase activity.	Actinomycin-insensitive increase in ATP synthesis and in glucose transport into cells; mechanism appears to involve insulin binding to cell membrane, occurs at 0 degrees C.
VASOPRESSIN		Actinomycin-insensitive promotion of water transport in isolated bladder preparation under same conditions in which aldosterone action is blocked by actinomycin.

SUMMARY OF EXPERIMENTAL EVIDENCE is given in table. Facts indicating that hormones activate the genes (*middle column*) are compared with facts suggesting that hormonal action does not entail the immediate activation of the genes (*column at right*).

branes; indeed, it is believed that both of these hormones attach themselves directly to the membranes whose function they affect. (3) Still other hormones rapidly activate a particular enzyme; phosphorylase, a key enzyme in determining the overall rate at which glycogen is broken down, is converted from an inactive form by several hormones, including epinephrine, glucagon and ACTH.

This does not alter the fact that many nonsteroid hormones operate at the gene level. Some of the best evidence for this statement is provided by studies of several hormones made by Chev Kidson and K. S. Kirby of the Chester Beatty Research Institute of the Royal Cancer Hospital in London. They separately injected rats with thyroxin, testosterone, cortisone and insulin and then mea-

sured the synthesis of messenger RNA by the rats' liver cells [*see illustration on page 91*]. The most striking aspect of their measurements is the extremely short time lag between the administration of the hormone and the change in the pattern of gene activity. The activation of genes in the nuclei of the affected cells occurs so quickly that one is tempted to assume that it is an initial effect of the hormone.

Here, however, we come face to face with a basic problem that must be solved in any attempt to explain the exact molecular mechanism of hormone action. The problem is simply that of identifying the initial site of reaction in a cell exposed to a hormone. Does a hormone move directly to the chromosome and exert its effect, so to speak, "in person"? As we have seen, aldoste-

rone does appear to enter the nucleus, but there is little real evidence that other hormones do so.

For many years biologists have been looking for the "receptor" substance of various hormones. The discovery that hormones ultimately act on genes makes this search all the more interesting. The evidence presented here only goes as far as to prove that an early stage in the operation of many hormones is the selective stimulation of genetic activity in the target cell. The molecules of the hormones range in size and structure from the tiny molecule of thyroxin to the unique multi-ring molecule of a steroid and the giant molecule of a protein; how these various molecules similarly affect the genetic apparatus of their target cells remains an intriguing mystery.

10

The Receptors of Steroid Hormones

by Bert W. O'Malley and William T. Schrader
February 1976

*The cellular response to these hormones depends on
the presence of protein molecules called receptors. The
complex formed by the hormone and the receptor acts on
the genetic material of the cell*

Hormones secreted by the endocrine glands can influence the functioning of cells in distant and apparently unrelated tissues. In the subtle effects of these regulatory molecules there is a puzzling specificity: all cells are exposed to hormones, yet only a few respond to them. The effects of one class of hormones—the steroid hormones—have been particularly perplexing. The steroids are small molecules, and it is not obvious how they can incorporate enough information in their structure to ensure adequate specificity and to account for their diverse influences.

Interest in the steroid hormones extends beyond endocrinology because it has been found that the hormones stimulate cells by controlling the synthesis of particular proteins. Protein synthesis is a central process in the metabolism of the cell, and it directly expresses the information in the genes. One of the principal preoccupations of molecular biology has been the search for the mechanisms that control gene expression and thereby determine overall patterns of growth and development.

In recent years the part played by the steroid hormones in the regulation of protein synthesis has been worked out in considerable detail, although a few crucial events have remained obscure. The functioning of the hormones depends on their interaction inside the cell with protein molecules designated receptors. Each of the steroid hormones affects only a few tissues because only the cells of those tissues contain the appropriate receptor proteins. The complex formed by the hormone and its receptor controls protein synthesis by acting directly on the genetic material of the cell.

There are two large classes of hormones, the peptides and the steroids, and the two kinds of molecule seem to function through quite different mechanisms.

The peptide hormones can be regarded as small proteins; each consists of a sequence of amino acids linked by characteristic chemical bonds called peptide bonds. A typical peptide hormone is insulin, which is secreted by specialized cells in the pancreas; human insulin consists of 51 amino acid units.

The peptide hormones are comparatively large molecules, typically with a molecular weight of about 10,000. Because of their size they cannot readily pass through the plasma membrane that surrounds all cells, and indeed they probably never enter the cells they stimulate. Instead they act on molecules on the surface of the plasma membrane, which then transmit signals to the interior of the cell. The peptide hormones can influence a great variety of intracellular processes, but only indirectly.

The steroid hormones are the subject of the remainder of this article. They include the male sex hormones (collectively called the androgens), the female sex hormones (the estrogens and the progestins) and the hormones secreted by the cortex, or outer layer, of the adrenal glands (the corticosteroids). They typically have a molecular weight of about 300, which is roughly the same as that of common table sugar.

All the steroids are based on a common central structure of four interconnected rings of carbon atoms; three of the rings have six carbon atoms and the other ring has five atoms. The differences between the various steroids are determined by the pattern of chemical bonds within the rings and by the nature and orientation of the side groups attached to the rings [*see illustration on pages 96 and 97*]. Although the differences may appear to be superficial, they alter the molecules' shape and can thereby completely change their biological activity.

For example, testosterone and progesterone are identical except for one side group attached to one of the rings, yet the two hormones differ radically in function: testosterone governs the development of the male secondary sex characteristics and progesterone contributes to the maintenance of pregnancy.

The structural similarities of the steroid hormones are reflected in their origin. All of them are synthesized from the same chemical precursor, cholesterol. Although cholesterol has no known hormonal function, it is a steroid and has the characteristic four-ring structure. The hormones are manufactured by altering the side groups of cholesterol; the modifications are made by enzymes in the cells of endocrine glands.

Since the steroid hormones are small molecules, they can easily diffuse into cells of many kinds, and they can just as easily diffuse back out into the bloodstream. They are effective even in very small quantities; their concentration in the blood reaches only about 10^{-9} mole per liter. (One mole is an amount of a substance in grams equal to its molecular weight.) If the palate were as sensitive to flavors as the target cells are to hormones, we would be able to detect a pinch of sugar dissolved in a swimming pool.

Any theory explaining the action of the steroid hormones must account for their effectiveness in those minuscule concentrations. It must also explain how the relatively simple steroid molecules, which have few distinctive chemical groups and which resemble one another in structure quite closely, can have such a broad spectrum of biological effects. Finally, it must explain how molecules that enter virtually all cells can selectively stimulate a small population of them and pass through the rest with no apparent effect.

The first important clue to the functioning of the steroid hormones came from studies of bacteria. It was in bacteria that a mechanism regulating the expression of genes was first discovered.

The sequence of events in protein synthesis is essentially the same in bacteria and in higher organisms: it is the process in which information is transferred from the DNA, the genetic "master tape" of the cell, to a molecule of messenger RNA, a segment of "tape" carrying instructions for the synthesis of the protein. The DNA molecule, as is now well known, is a double-strand helix held together by bonds between pairs of nucleotide bases. The four kinds of base are always paired in the same way: adenosine bonds only to thymidine and guanosine bonds only to cytidine. The two strands are therefore complementary; given the sequence of bases in one strand, the sequence in the other is completely defined.

The genetic information is expressed when a segment of DNA representing a gene is transcribed to yield a corresponding length of messenger RNA, a process controlled by the enzyme RNA polymerase. The RNA, which is a single-strand molecule (and which also differs from DNA in that all the thymidine units are replaced by uridine), then becomes associated with the organelles called ribosomes. At the ribosomes the RNA is translated, each group of three bases specifying one amino acid, which is added to the protein molecule. Through that mechanism the sequence of bases in a segment of DNA specifies a sequence of amino acids, and this sequence determines all the properties of the protein.

The genetic code explains how a gene can specify the structure of a protein, but it cannot explain the particular assortment of proteins that is synthesized by a cell. In a bacterial cell there are thousands of genes, but only a few function at any given time. Systems regulating the expression of genes must therefore exist.

Our understanding of gene regulation is still far from complete, but one mechanism by which it is accomplished, at least in bacteria, was explicated in 1959 by the elegant studies of François Jacob and Jacques Monod of the Pasteur Institute in Paris. Working with the colon bacterium *Escherichia coli*, Jacob and Monod showed that a system of genes concerned with the metabolism of the sugar lactose is regulated by a specific protein. When the protein is present on the DNA, transcription is prevented: the synthesis of new messenger RNA from that gene cannot take place. They therefore called the protein a repressor. They found, however, that when lactose was added to the culture medium in which the bacteria were grown, the sugar in some way removed the repressor from the DNA, allowing transcription to begin. They called lactose an inducer for this system of genes, and called the regulatory process derepression.

The model devised by Jacob and Monod represents one system through

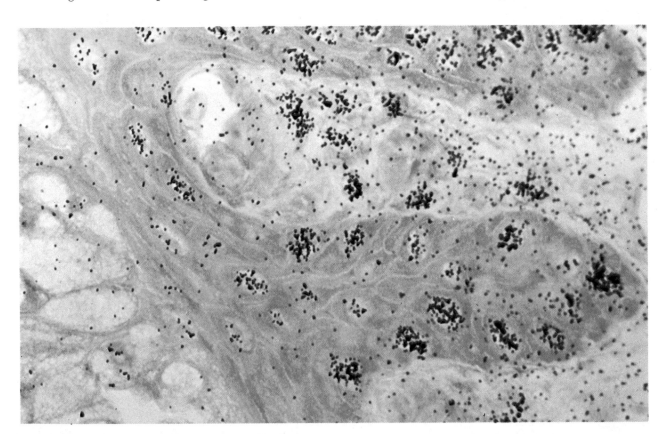

SPECIFICITY OF STEROID HORMONES for particular cells and the localization of the hormones within the nuclei of those cells are demonstrated by the technique of autoradiography. The black dots reveal the location of radioactively labeled molecules of the steroid hormone progesterone in a section of tissue from the uterine cervix of a guinea pig. The dots are clustered over the nuclei of cells and are sparsely distributed elsewhere. The effect is a result of the activities of progesterone receptor molecules. The hormone binds to the receptors in the cytoplasm of the cell, forming a complex that is then sequestered in the nucleus. In the making of the autoradiograph the guinea pig was first injected with progesterone labeled with tritium, the radioactive isotope of hydrogen. After 15 minutes the animal was killed and thin sections of frozen tissue were mounted on glass slides coated with a photographic emulsion. The slides were kept in darkness and cold for about three months, then the emulsion was developed and the tissue was stained. The radioactive decay of the tritium atoms exposed grains in the emulsion where the hormone was concentrated. The autoradiograph was made by Walter E. Stumpf and Madhabaranda Sar at the University of North Carolina at Chapel Hill.

which a relatively small and simple molecule (the inducer) can regulate the expression of a gene. The model is of particular interest to endocrinologists because there are a number of apparent similarities between the action of an inducer on a bacterial cell and the action of a steroid hormone on the cells of higher animals. In 1964 Peter Karlson of the University of Marburg made the comparison explicit: he proposed that the steroid hormones are in fact inducers and that they act by combining with repressor proteins. In the absence of hormone the repressors were supposed to block transcription.

It was soon confirmed that the administration of hormone to an animal results in an increase in the synthesis of RNA in the target cells, followed by an increase in protein synthesis. These findings were entirely consistent with the hypothesis that the steroid hormones act at the level of the gene [see the article "Hormones and Genes," by Eric H. Davidson, beginning on page 84]. It had not yet been demonstrated, how-

STEROID	PRINCIPAL SOURCE	PRINCIPAL TARGET TISSUES	HORMONAL FUNCTION	CHEMICAL FORMULA
ESTROGEN 18 CARBON ATOMS	OVARY	UTERUS, VAGINA, BREAST, HYPOTHALAMUS	DEVELOPMENT OF FEMALE SEX CHARACTERISTICS	
TESTOSTERONE 19 CARBON ATOMS	TESTIS	SEMINAL VESCICLES, PROSTATE, TESTIS	DEVELOPMENT OF MALE SEX CHARACTERISTICS	
PROGESTERONE 21 CARBON ATOMS	OVARY, PLACENTA	UTERUS, OVIDUCT	MAINTENANCE OF PREGNANCY	
HYDROCORTISONE 21 CARBON ATOMS	CORTEX OF THE ADRENAL GLAND	ALL CELLS	REGULATION OF ENERGY UTILIZATION	
ALDOSTERONE 21 CARBON ATOMS	CORTEX OF THE ADRENAL GLAND	KIDNEY	REGULATION OF ELECTROLYTE BALANCE	
CHOLESTEROL 27 CARBON ATOMS	DIET, LIVER	UNKNOWN	METABOLIC PRECURSOR OF ALL STEROIDS	

STEROID HORMONES are relatively small molecules, with a typical molecular weight of about 300. All of them share a common core structure, consisting of four interconnected rings of carbon atoms. They differ in the pattern of bonding within the rings, and in the side groups attached to them. The structural differences subtly alter the shapes of the hormone molecules, as is shown in the drawings at right; it is principally on the basis of shape that the hormones are recognized by their receptors. Only a few of the

ever, exactly how the hormones activate a gene. Were they inducers, strictly analogous to those discovered by Jacob and Monod in bacteria, or did they function through some more complicated mechanism?

In considering this question it is important to realize that although bacteria and higher organisms share the same ge-

MOLECULAR STRUCTURE

netic code, they differ fundamentally in organization. Bacteria are prokaryotic cells, that is, their genetic material is distributed throughout the cytoplasm. The cells of all the higher plants and animals are eukaryotic: they have a distinct nucleus, which confines the DNA within a specialized membrane. Within the nucleus the DNA is associated in a chemical complex with a number of proteins that are not found in prokaryotes. Moreover, in multicellular organisms the problem of gene regulation is intrinsically more complex than it is in bacteria. In the higher organisms each cell has an identical complement of DNA, but different cells make quite different kinds of protein. A cell in the pancreas, for example, might make insulin, whereas one in the blood-forming tissue might manufacture hemoglobin.

In view of these complications it seems reasonable to suppose the mechanisms of gene regulation in the higher plants and animals differ from those found in bacteria. In the case of the steroid hormones that supposition has been confirmed. Although the steroids do induce gene expression, they do not do so by combining with repressors of the kind described by Jacob and Monod and they do not cause derepression; on the contrary, they become coupled to receptor proteins that have a positive regulatory effect. In eukaryotic cells a gene is thought to be activated when a hormone-and-receptor complex binds to it, rather than when a repressor molecule is removed.

The first step in the investigation of the functioning of the steroid hormones was the demonstration that they have a particular affinity for their target cells. Since the hormones are present in such low concentration, the methods of conventional analytical chemistry are inadequate for the study of hormone physiology; instead it is necessary to employ hormones labeled with radioactive atoms. Highly radioactive steroid hormones were first prepared in the early 1960's by Elwood V. Jensen of the University of Chicago. By injecting female rats with a radioactive preparation of estrogen, Jensen and his colleagues showed that the hormone is retained longer in the uterus than it is in other tissues, such as muscle and blood. The uterus is considered a "target" organ of estrogen, whereas muscle and blood are not. Subsequently I. S. Edelman and his colleagues at the School of Medicine of the University of California at San Francisco demonstrated the retention of a steroid hormone at the cellular level. They em-

ployed the technique of autoradiography, in which a thin slice of tissue containing radioactively labeled molecules is coated with a photographic emulsion. The exposure of the emulsion by the radioactive molecules indicated that the hormone appears in the target tissues within minutes after it is administered to the animal. Moreover, it is retained there long after all the radioactive molecules have left the nontarget cells.

In 1968 Walter E. Stumpf, who is now at the University of North Carolina at Chapel Hill, proceeded one step further and showed that within the target cells the hormone tends to accumulate in the nucleus, providing additional evidence that the mechanism of steroid action is a genetic one. Stumpf too employed autoradiography, and he found that the movement of the hormone into the nucleus is extremely rapid: it precedes all other observable changes in the target cell.

The rapid movement of the steroid hormones does not necessarily imply that some mechanism exists to transport them specifically to the target cells; it is sufficient that the molecules be sequestered within those cells. In nontarget cells the hormone passes through the plasma membrane in both directions, and its concentration inside the cell cannot exceed the concentration in the bloodstream. In the target tissues the hormone molecules continue to diffuse into the cells but very few leave them, so that the concentration inside the cells increases [see illustration on next page].

These early investigations strongly suggested that some agent in the target cells binds to the steroid hormones and prevents their escape. Indeed, Jensen and his colleagues suggested in 1961 that such a receptor might be involved in the cellular response to steroid hormones. The hypothesis had the further advantage that it could explain how the relatively simple steroid molecules could exert such diverse effects; by forming a complex with a larger "helper" molecule they might become much more versatile. In the subsequent search for such a molecule two important criteria were established. First, any receptor molecule must be present in the target cells of the hormone but absent in all other cells. Second, the receptor molecule should have a high affinity for its particular hormone but low affinity for other steroids with different biological activity.

The identification of steroid receptor molecules was not an easy task, partly because the receptors are present in extremely small quantities (about 10,000

many steroids are shown. Cholesterol is not ordinarily considered a hormone, but it is the precursor from which all other steroids are synthesized in the endocrine glands.

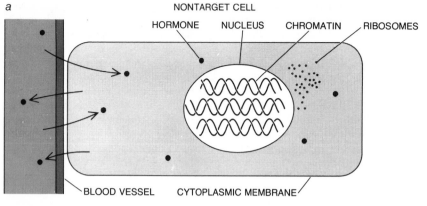

a

NONTARGET CELL

HORMONE   NUCLEUS   CHROMATIN   RIBOSOMES

BLOOD VESSEL   CYTOPLASMIC MEMBRANE

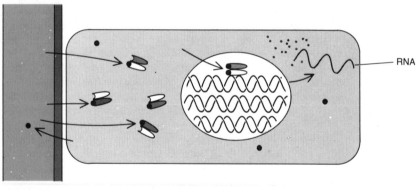

b

TARGET CELL

RECEPTOR MOLECULE   NUCLEUS   CHROMATIN   RIBOSOMES

BLOOD VESSEL   CYTOPLASMIC MEMBRANE

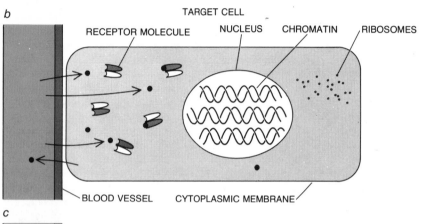

c

RNA

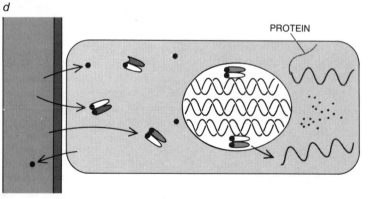

d

PROTEIN

ACTION OF STEROID HORMONES is mediated by receptor molecules found only in cells that respond to the hormone (target cells). In nontarget cells (*a*) the hormone diffuses freely into the cell and out of it, and the concentration remains quite low. In a target cell the hormone is sequestered by receptor molecules (*b*). Each receptor molecule binds two molecules of hormone, forming a complex that enters the nucleus (*c*) and becomes attached to the chromatin, the genetic material. The complex stimulates the transcription of particular genes, so that RNA encoding the information in those genes is synthesized. On the organelles called ribosomes the RNA is translated into proteins (*d*).

molecules per cell). They were ultimately identified in 1966 by David O. Toft and Jack Gorski of the University of Illinois. Toft and Gorski separated hormone-and-receptor complexes from other large molecules by centrifuging an extract from the target cells in a density gradient of sucrose. The method separates molecules on the basis of their molecular weight, yielding fractions containing progressively smaller molecules. By employing a radioactively labeled hormone, the fraction containing the hormone-and-receptor complex can be identified simply as a peak in radioactivity.

Toft and Gorski employed estradiol, a form of estrogen, labeled with tritium, the radioactive isotope of hydrogen. When they tested it in tissue from the rat uterus, they found that the hormone was bound selectively to a protein molecule with a molecular weight of about 200,000. The protein met the criteria established for a hormone receptor: it was present only in the target cells and it bound estradiol very tightly. The protein also displayed an affinity for steroids closely related to estradiol and for certain other nonsteroid substances that have a different structure but a similar molecular shape. Significantly all the substances that were shown to bind to the receptor protein mimic the biological activity of estradiol.

Similar receptor proteins have since been identified in the target tissues of all the known steroid hormones. Tissues that do not respond to a given hormone invariably lack receptors for that hormone. The receptors for estrogen, androgen and the corticosteroids have been characterized in several animals. One of the most difficult of the receptors to identify was the receptor for progesterone. It was eventually found in the chick oviduct, a known progesterone target tissue, by our research group at the Baylor College of Medicine. The progesterone receptor is similar in structure and function to the other steroid receptors.

The role of the receptor proteins was confirmed in the laboratories of Jensen, Gorski and Edelman when it was shown that the receptors not only sequester the hormone molecules in the target cells but also concentrate them in the cell nucleus. We observed the movement into the nucleus by administering a hormone, then after various intervals disrupting the cells and quickly separating the nuclei from the cytoplasm in a centrifuge. We observed a steady decline in the number of hormone-and-receptor complexes in the cytoplasm and a concomi-

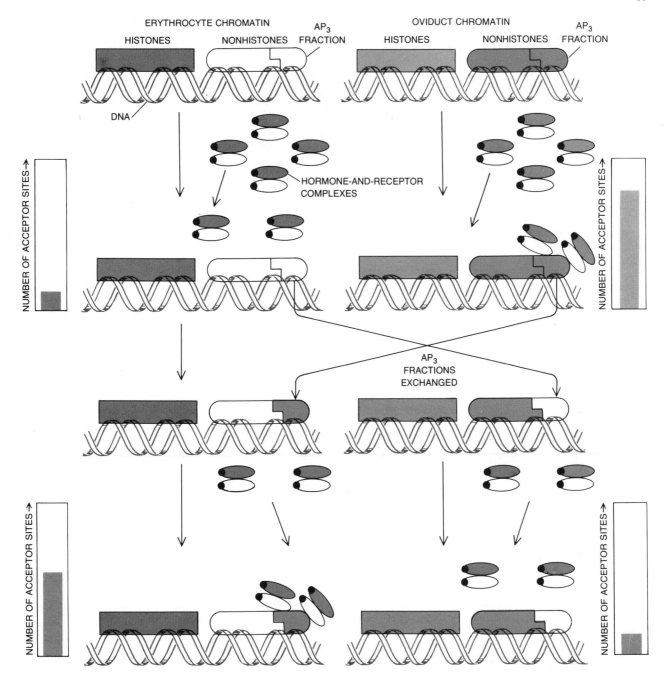

ACCEPTOR SITES for hormone-and-receptor complexes are observed only on the chromatin of target cells. Chromatin consists of DNA and two kinds of protein: the histones, which are much the same in all cells, and the nonhistone chromosomal proteins, which display much more diversity. The ability to bind the complexes resides in a particular fraction of the nonhistone proteins, designated the AP_3 fraction. Ordinarily the complexes bind to chromatin from target tissues, such as the oviduct, but do not bind to nontarget chromatin, such as that from chick erythrocytes. When the AP_3 fractions of the nonhistone proteins from each kind of chromatin are exchanged, the ability to bind hormone-and-receptor complexes migrates with the oviduct AP_3 fraction. The number of acceptor sites found on each kind of chromatin before and after the proteins are exchanged is indicated by the small bar graphs.

tant increase in their concentration in the nucleus. On the other hand, the receptor proteins could not be detected in the nucleus in significant quantity when the hormone was absent. Therefore the presence of the hormone somehow caused the receptors to be retained in the nucleus.

The mechanism by which the hormone-and-receptor complexes were retained in the nucleus was soon revealed.

In a series of experiments in our laboratory and in the laboratory of Shutsung Liao at the University of Chicago the complexes were combined in a cell-free system with nuclei isolated from target cells. When the complexes were absorbed into the nuclei from the incubation medium, it was found that they bind directly to the chromosomes. An analysis of the binding reaction suggested that in the nucleus of each target cell there are about 5,000 "acceptor" sites for hormone-and-receptor complexes. Of particular importance was the observation that when nuclei from nontarget cells were employed, the binding of the complexes was greatly diminished.

Although it had been shown that the steroid hormones form complexes with specific receptor proteins in their target cells and that those complexes

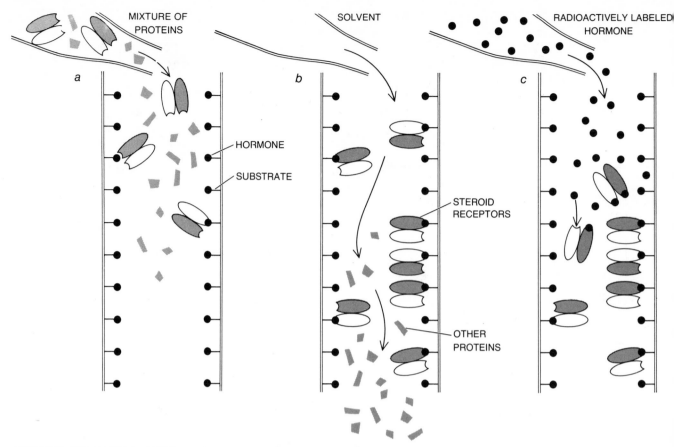

MIXTURE OF PROTEINS

SOLVENT

RADIOACTIVELY LABELED HORMONE

a

b

c

HORMONE

SUBSTRATE

STEROID RECEPTORS

OTHER PROTEINS

AFFINITY CHROMATOGRAPHY, a technique employed in isolating the receptors of steroid hormones, relies on one of the biological properties of the receptors: their affinity for the hormones. Hormone molecules are bound to an inert substrate in a glass column; then an extract from the cytoplasm of target cells is poured into the column (*a*). The receptors are detained by the fixed hormone molecules, whereas all other proteins are washed away (*b*). Finally, the receptors are freed from the substrate by incubating

enter the nucleus and bind to the chromosomes, it remained to be disclosed how the binding of the hormone-and-receptor complexes influences the expression of genetic information. The nature of the interaction must obviously depend not only on the activity of the hormone but also on the architecture of the chromosome.

The chromosomes of higher organisms incorporate both DNA and a variety of specialized proteins, organized in the complex substance called chromatin [see "Chromosomal Proteins and Gene Regulation," by Gary S. Stein, Janet Swinehart Stein and Lewis J. Kleinsmith; SCIENTIFIC AMERICAN, February, 1975]. There are two main classes of chromosomal proteins. The histones are highly alkaline proteins and are very similar from one tissue to another; indeed, they are very similar from one organism to another. The remainder, the nonhistone chromosomal proteins, are acidic.

In a series of studies conducted by us in collaboration with Thomas C. Spelsberg, we found that hormone-and-receptor complexes were able to bind directly to chromatin isolated from the nucleus.

Moreover, complexes of progesterone and their receptor proteins bound preferentially to chromatin from oviduct nuclei, compared with chromatin from other tissues. Receptor proteins without hormone were incapable of binding to chromatin.

We undertook to determine which elements of the chromatin participated in the binding of the complexes. Gordon M. Tomkins and his colleagues at the University of California at San Francisco had shown that hormone-and-receptor complexes will interact with DNA stripped of all its accompanying proteins. They found, however, that any DNA will suffice; it made no difference whether it was extracted from target cells or from other tissues. This was not a surprising result, since the DNA in all cells of an organism is identical. It seems unlikely for that reason that the DNA itself could regulate gene expression, and Tomkins' findings suggest in particular that the DNA cannot be directly responsible for the tissue specificity of the steroid hormones.

The binding sites were therefore sought among the chromosomal proteins. Because of their comparative uniformity the histones seemed to be unlikely candidates, and indeed Spelsberg found that chromatin from which all the histones had been removed bound the hormone-and-receptor complexes as effectively as intact chromatin. Furthermore, the histones could be removed from the chromatin of target cells and replaced with histones from other tissues or even from other organisms without affecting the binding of the complexes.

The nonhistones are much more heterogeneous than the histones; there may be more than 500 species of nonhistone proteins in a single nucleus, and they vary considerably from one tissue to another. By measuring the binding of receptor molecules to chromatin after removing selected groups of nonhistone proteins, Spelsberg revealed a selective affinity. The removal of two classes of nonhistones had no detectable effect, but when a third class, designated the AP_3 fraction, was extracted, the ability of' the residual chromatin to bind hormone-and-receptor complexes declined sharply. When the AP_3 fraction was replaced, binding activity was restored. Finally, in the most conclusive experiment, the AP_3 proteins from target cells were ex-

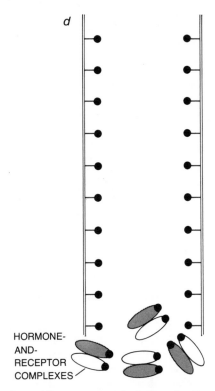

them with a concentrated solution of radioactively labeled hormone (*c*). The result is a virtually uncontaminated solution of radioactive hormone-and-receptor complexes (*d*).

changed with the same fraction from a nontarget tissue, yielding hybrid chromatins. The chromatin from the nontarget tissue was converted by the addition of target-cell AP_3 fraction into an efficient acceptor for hormone-and-receptor complexes. The target-cell chromatin, on

the other hand, lost its ability to bind to receptors when it was treated with the non-target-cell AP_3 fraction [*see illustration on page 99*]. The ability to bind the receptor complexes thus seems to depend on the presence of the AP_3 fraction on the DNA.

The progesterone receptor proteins employed in these experiments were merely crude extracts of hormone target cells from the chick oviduct; the receptor molecules constituted less than one ten-thousandth of the total protein. In order to characterize the receptor molecules more fully, and in order to ensure that the interactions we had observed were not modified by the presence of extraneous substances, we undertook to purify the receptor protein.

The principal method employed was affinity chromatography, a technique that isolates biological molecules by taking advantage of the specificity inherent in their own functioning. In this case progesterone molecules were chemically bonded to an inert, porous substrate, and the crude solution of proteins was then passed through the substrate. The receptor proteins bound to the hormone, whereas all the contaminants were readily washed away. Finally the receptors were freed from the bound hormone by incubating them with a comparatively concentrated solution of free progesterone. By that method the progesterone receptor was isolated from all other proteins; the purification was accomplished last year in our laboratory.

We found that the receptor molecule is a dimer, that is, it consists of two subunits (labeled *A* and *B*), each an independent strand of amino acids. The

subunits are not identical, but both have a molecular weight somewhat greater than 100,000. The subunits are roughly cigar-shaped; when they are bound together as a dimer, they probably lie side by side.

Each subunit has a single binding site for progesterone. No changes in the physical properties of the dissociated subunits have been detected when the hormone is bound to them, but the hormone has an important effect on the intact dimer: after the hormone has been bound, the receptor can be split into its two subunits by exposure to high temperature or to an elevated salt concentration. (In addition, of course, the hormone profoundly alters the biological activity of the molecule.)

When the purified receptors were incubated with oviduct nuclei or chromatin, they bound to acceptor sites on the chromatin just as the crude preparations had. It therefore appeared that no other cytoplasmic proteins were involved in the interaction. We were puzzled, however, to discover that the intact, dimeric receptors had no affinity for naked DNA, even though we had observed binding to DNA in crude preparations.

That paradox was resolved when we examined the behavior of the individual subunits. The *B* protein was able to bind to intact chromatin, and furthermore it showed the same tissue specificity for the AP_3 fraction of the nonhistone proteins. The *A* subunit did not bind to intact chromatin from oviduct tissues or from other tissues. On the other hand, the *A* subunit bound very strongly to naked DNA, whereas the *B* subunit showed no affinity for it. The binding to DNA observed in crude extracts was

		NAKED DNA		INTACT CHROMATIN	
		TARGET TISSUE	NONTARGET TISSUE	TARGET TISSUE	NONTARGET TISSUE
DIMERIC RECEPTOR					
A SUBUNIT					
B SUBUNIT					

RECEPTOR PROTEINS consist of two subunits, labeled *A* and *B*, with different capacities for binding to nuclear material. Although the subunits are not identical, they are about the same size, and each has a binding site for a single hormone molecule. The complete, dimeric receptor binds only to chromatin (made up of both DNA and the chromosomal proteins) from target cells. The *B* subunit displays the same specificity as the dimeric receptor. The *A* subunit does not bind to chromatin but does bind to "naked" DNA. Moreover, it has the same affinity for all DNA, whether it is derived from target cells or from cells of other tissues.

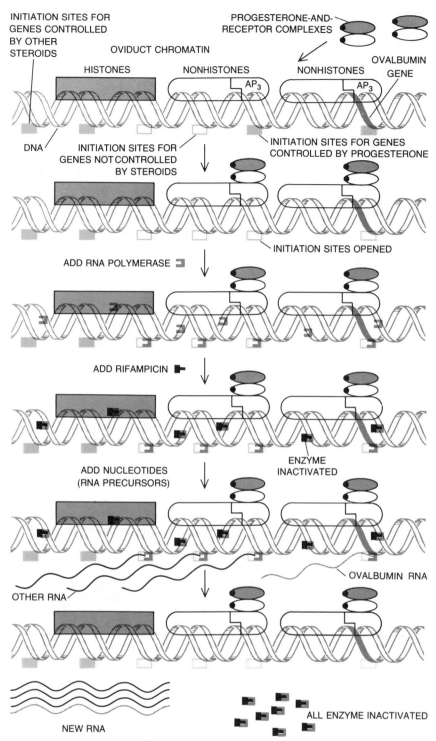

INITIATION SITES FOR GENES CONTROLLED BY OTHER STEROIDS

PROGESTERONE-AND-RECEPTOR COMPLEXES

OVIDUCT CHROMATIN

HISTONES

NONHISTONES

AP₃

NONHISTONES

AP₃

OVALBUMIN GENE

DNA

INITIATION SITES FOR GENES NOT CONTROLLED BY STEROIDS

INITIATION SITES FOR GENES CONTROLLED BY PROGESTERONE

INITIATION SITES OPENED

ADD RNA POLYMERASE

ADD RIFAMPICIN

ENZYME INACTIVATED

ADD NUCLEOTIDES (RNA PRECURSORS)

OVALBUMIN RNA

OTHER RNA

NEW RNA

ALL ENZYME INACTIVATED

EFFECT OF STEROID HORMONES on chromatin is to increase the number of initiation sites for the transcription of particular genes. The effect was demonstrated with chromatin from the chick oviduct, which is stimulated by progesterone to manufacture RNA coding for numerous proteins, among them the egg-white protein ovalbumin. After the chromatin had been exposed to hormone-and-receptor complexes the enzyme RNA polymerase was added to the solution. A few enzyme molecules occupied stable initiation sites in those regions on the DNA where transcription normally begins, but transcription was prevented by conducting the experiment in a medium that lacked the nucleotides needed for RNA synthesis. Initiation sites for genes controlled by other steroids remained unoccupied. The antibiotic drug rifampicin was then added, inactivating all RNA-polymerase molecules except those at initiation sites. Finally the nucleotide precursors of RNA were added, and at each initiation site a single molecule of RNA was produced. The RNA-polymerase molecules responsible for this transcription, having left their initiation sites, were then also inactivated. Treating the chromatin with hormone-and-receptor complexes increased the production of RNA, and specifically stimulated synthesis of messenger RNA for ovalbumin.

presumably caused by contamination with dissociated A subunits.

From that analysis it is possible to construct a hypothetical account of how a steroid hormone is directed to a gene in a target-cell nucleus. Initially the receptor molecule is in the cytoplasm, and it is in dimeric form. After binding two molecules of hormone the structure of the receptor is altered in some unknown way, and it becomes activated. The complex of hormone and receptor then enters the nucleus and binds to the chromatin at an acceptor site defined by the position of some specific protein in the AP_3 fraction of the nonhistone proteins. The binding of the receptor to the acceptor site takes place exclusively through the B subunit, since the A subunit is incapable of binding to intact chromatin. The dimer may then dissociate, liberating the A subunit, the only one that can interact directly with DNA. It is not yet clear whether the A protein is capable of recognizing specific nucleotide sequences of DNA, as the regulatory proteins of bacterial cells are. It is possible that the A protein merely binds to any nearby sequence of DNA, its location having been determined with sufficient precision by the specificity of the B subunit for the acceptor site on the nonhistone proteins.

Perhaps the most intriguing question raised by the steroid hormones pertains to the events after the hormone-and-receptor complex has bound to the chromatin. How is the selected segment of DNA activated by the binding of the receptor? How is the gene "turned on"? In order to answer these questions we must investigate the events that come immediately after the binding of the receptor molecules.

The first step in the sequence of events that leads eventually to protein synthesis is thought to be the binding of the enzyme RNA polymerase to the DNA. In bacteria the enzyme is bound at particular locations, called initiation sites, where the transcription of each gene begins. There is only one initiation site per gene, and hence by measuring the number of sites the number of active genes can be determined. In higher organisms the existence of initiation sites has not been proved, but the behavior of the gene is entirely consistent with the hypothesis that they do exist. We wished to monitor the number of initiation sites as an index of the number of genes expressed following hormone administration.

It was possible to estimate the number of initiation sites in oviduct chromatin by employing a system that produces one molecule of messenger RNA at each initiation site and then ceases transcription. The system is based on the properties of the antibiotic drug rifampicin, which permanently inactivates molecules of RNA polymerase unless they are occupying an initiation site. In this procedure excess RNA polymerase was added to oviduct chromatin, leading to the binding of enzyme molecules at all available initiation sites; transcription of the genes could not begin, however, because the incubation medium lacked the precursor nucleotides needed for RNA synthesis. Those precursors were then added to the solution, and simultaneously rifampicin was added. As a result all the RNA-polymerase molecules not occupying an initiation site were inactivated; those enzyme molecules at initiation sites each gave rise to a single molecule of messenger RNA, then they too were inactivated, so that all RNA synthesis stopped [see *illustration on opposite page*]. The number of RNA molecules produced is thus a measure of the number of initiation sites on the chromatin.

In our experiment progesterone or estrogen was administered to chicks for varying lengths of time, then the chromatin was isolated from oviduct cells. As in earlier experiments, a radioactively labeled hormone was employed, so that the number of hormone-and-receptor complexes in the cell nuclei could be estimated. The oviduct chromatin was then assayed for initiation sites by the addition of rifampicin. The results strongly supported the role of hormone-and-receptor complexes in gene regulation: the number of nuclear initiation sites per cell rose and fell in conjunction with the number of hormone-and-receptor complexes in the nuclei.

We have now employed the same techniques to demonstrate the hormonal regulation of transcription in an experiment performed entirely outside the living cell. Instead of injecting chicks with progesterone, we purified chromatin from the oviduct of chicks that had never been exposed to the hormone. We then added to the chromatin purified progesterone receptor molecules with bound hormone. RNA synthesis was initiated in the presence of rifampicin, and the number of RNA molecules produced was determined. Once again the number of initiation sites was dependent on the number of hormone-and-receptor complexes present. In this cell-free experiment the number of initiation sites produced was approximately equal to the number of hormone-and-receptor complexes bound to the chromatin. From this fact we concluded that the initiation

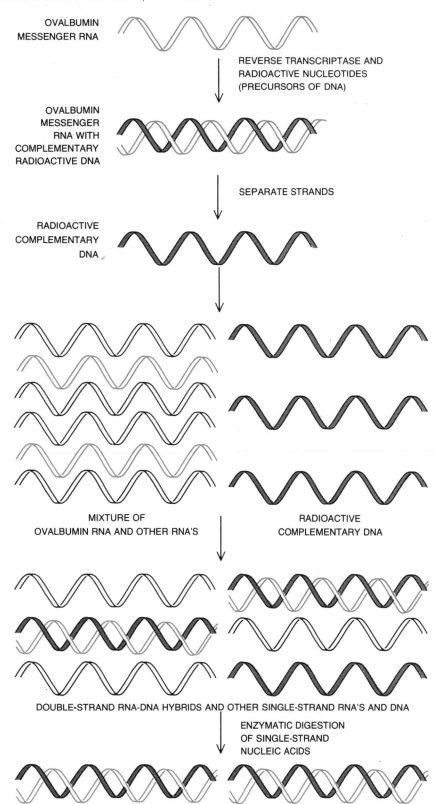

OVALBUMIN MESSENGER RNA

REVERSE TRANSCRIPTASE AND RADIOACTIVE NUCLEOTIDES (PRECURSORS OF DNA)

OVALBUMIN MESSENGER RNA WITH COMPLEMENTARY RADIOACTIVE DNA

SEPARATE STRANDS

RADIOACTIVE COMPLEMENTARY DNA

MIXTURE OF OVALBUMIN RNA AND OTHER RNA'S

RADIOACTIVE COMPLEMENTARY DNA

DOUBLE-STRAND RNA-DNA HYBRIDS AND OTHER SINGLE-STRAND RNA'S AND DNA

ENZYMATIC DIGESTION OF SINGLE-STRAND NUCLEIC ACIDS

RADIOACTIVE OVALBUMIN MESSENGER RNA-COMPLEMENTARY DNA HYBRID

IDENTIFICATION OF RNA coding for ovalbumin was accomplished through the technique called RNA-DNA hybridization. The procedure begins with the preparation of a pure specimen of the messenger RNA for ovalbumin. The enzyme reverse transcriptase is then employed to synthesize a strand of radioactive DNA with a sequence of nucleotides exactly complementary to that of the RNA. The complementary DNA is incubated with a mixture of RNA's, and because of its complementary sequence of nucleotides it forms double-strand molecules with ovalbumin messenger RNA but not with any other RNA. All single-strand nucleic acids are then digested, leaving only the double-strand RNA-DNA hybrids. The amount of ovalbumin messenger RNA is calculated from the rate and extent of hybridization.

reaction involves one hormone-and-receptor complex per chromatin acceptor site. The stimulation of transcription is dependent on the presence of the hormone; receptor proteins that lacked hormone had no effect. Furthermore, the extent of stimulation depended on the kind of tissue tested; target-cell chromatin was stimulated more than chromatin from other tissues.

The foregoing experiments demonstrated that hormone-and-receptor complexes can stimulate RNA synthesis. It remained to be shown that the particular genes transcribed were those coding for proteins known to be produced in response to the hormone. Making that determination requires an extraordinarily sensitive method for the detection and identification of specific messenger-RNA molecules. Such a method exists in the procedure called RNA-DNA hybridi-

zation. The procedure begins with the preparation of an exceedingly pure sample of the messenger RNA to be detected. We chose to employ the messenger RNA that codes for ovalbumin, an egg-white protein that is completely absent from chicks that have not been treated with estrogen or progesterone but that is produced copiously in the oviduct of chicks that have received either of these hormones. From the purified messenger RNA radioactive single-strand DNA is synthesized with the exactly complementary sequence of nucleotide bases. The synthesis is accomplished with enzymes of viral origin that reverse the normal flow of information in the cell, so that RNA becomes a template for the manufacture of DNA. The complementary strands of DNA are then isolated, and they can be employed as a molecular probe capable of recognizing any molecules identical with the original messenger-RNA template.

The RNA-DNA hybridization technique was first employed to assay the messenger RNA's produced in the chick oviduct in response to hormone. At various intervals after the administration of progesterone the messenger RNA was isolated from oviducts and incubated with single-strand DNA complementary to the ovalbumin messenger RNA. Because of the complementary sequences all the ovalbumin RNA formed double-strand hybrid molecules with the DNA; the remaining, extraneous RNA's remained as unpaired, single-strand molecules and could therefore be distinguished chemically and eliminated from the preparation. From the number of RNA-DNA hybrid molecules we were able to estimate the number of ovalbumin messenger-RNA molecules present in oviduct cells after hormone injection. The cellular content rose from zero to 10,000 molecules per cell in a matter of hours.

Finally, oviduct chromatin was incubated in a cell-free medium with purified progesterone hormone-and-receptor complexes. RNA was synthesized from these chromatin templates and assayed for ovalbumin messenger RNA by RNA-DNA hybridization. Only the RNA synthesized from chromatin exposed to receptors contained ovalbumin messenger RNA. Thus we concluded that hormone-and-receptor complexes have the capacity to bind to chromatin and to increase both overall gene transcription and the expression of DNA sequences coding for specific messenger-RNA molecules.

At physiological concentrations only the intact, dimeric receptors caused the proliferation of initiation sites and stim-

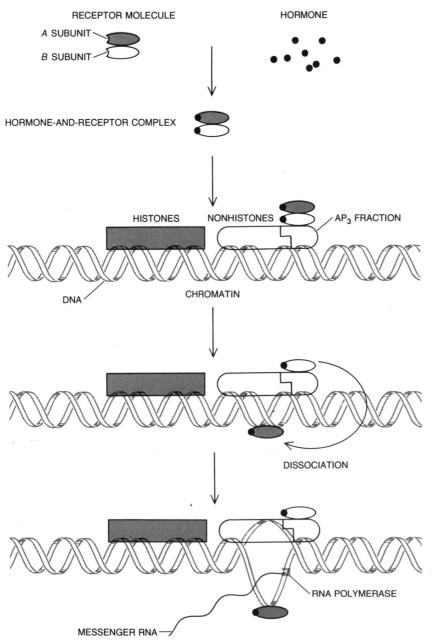

MECHANISM OF GENE ACTIVATION by the steroid hormones is thought to involve the separate interactions of both subunits of the hormone receptor molecule with chromatin. After a receptor molecule has bound two molecules of hormone and has entered the nucleus, it binds to the AP_3 fraction of the nonhistone chromosomal proteins. The binding takes place between the nonhistone protein and the *B* subunit of the receptor molecule, which thereby determines what genes will be activated. The subunits then dissociate, and the *A* subunit interacts with the DNA, enabling a molecule of RNA polymerase to occupy an initiation site or the DNA. A segment of DNA is then transcribed, producing a strand of messenger RNA that serves as a template for the construction of a protein.

ulated the synthesis of ovalbumin messenger RNA. The isolated *B* subunit was without effect regardless of the concentration. The *A* subunit did eventually increase the number of initiation sites, but only at concentrations about 50 times higher than the effective concentration of the dimer. That discovery supports the hypothesis that only the *A* protein interacts directly with DNA and stimulates the synthesis of messenger RNA. The *B* subunit apparently serves merely to designate the location of the gene to be expressed, a function accomplished through the binding of the *B* subunit at a position defined by certain of the nonhistone proteins. It is reasonable to suppose the genetic sequences controlled are adjacent to the corresponding acceptor sites on the chromosomal proteins.

The nature of the interaction between the *A* subunit and the DNA remains a topic of active investigation. It is still not known how the hormone-and-receptor complex alters a concealed or inactive initiation site to make it available to RNA polymerase. It is also not yet known how the regulated gene is turned off when enough RNA has been synthesized. The hormone and the receptor protein must eventually dissociate from each other and from the chromatin. The receptor molecule is apparently not destroyed in the process, and it may return to the cytoplasm, form another complex with additional hormone molecules and reenter the nucleus to continue hormonal stimulation. The hormone itself is probably altered in such a way that it becomes inactive, and it must eventually diffuse out of the cell.

All the effects of the steroid hormones can now be seen to be accomplished through specific protein receptor molecules; the absence of receptors precludes any response. It seems likely that this relation can be made quantitative: the magnitude of a cell's response appears to be related to the intracellular concentration of receptor proteins. Moreover, the concentration of receptors in a given tissue is not fixed: it can be altered by aging, by changes in the physiological state of development and even by the presence of other hormones. In the chick oviduct estrogen stimulates the production of progesterone receptors, and tissues treated with estrogen are therefore more responsive to progesterone. Conversely, in mammals progesterone depresses the level of estrogen receptors and makes the target tissue less responsive to estrogen. The stability of the hormone-and-receptor complex also influences the magnitude of a target

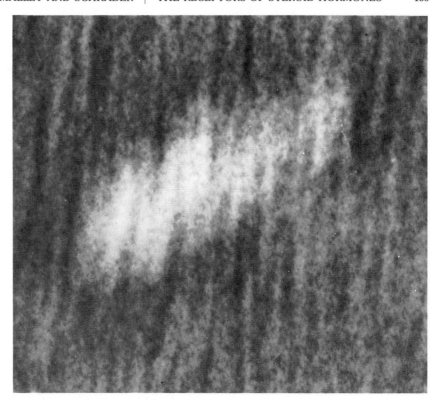

SHAPE OF THE RECEPTOR PROTEIN is revealed in an electron micrograph made by P. M. Conn of the Baylor College of Medicine. The protein is the light, oblong form in the center of the image; it is a *B* subunit of a progesterone receptor, with a hormone molecule bound to it. It is shown in its biologically active configuration; when the subunit is denatured, it assumes a globular form. The length of the protein is about 100 angstroms, and the magnification is roughly 700,000 diameters. The image is indistinct primarily because the specimen is destroyed by the intense electron beam as the micrograph is being made.

cell's response to a steroid hormone. Cells containing complexes that dissociate rapidly must be bathed continuously in a high concentration of hormone if the response is to be maintained.

The illumination of the molecular biology of the steroid hormones must ultimately reflect some light on clinical endocrinology. For example, the discovery of hormone receptors provides an explanation of an enigmatic syndrome called male pseudohermaphroditism. In that condition the male secondary sex characteristics fail to develop. The cause is not simply a deficiency of androgens, since the target tissues do not respond when additional androgens are administered. It results instead from a defect in the androgen receptor proteins. An entire series of steroid-unresponsiveness syndromes may be discovered, all of them caused by the absence of functioning hormone receptors.

The techniques devised for the investigation of the action of the steroids might also be applied to the identification of certain hormone-dependent cancers. A large proportion of breast cancers, for example, grow in response to estrogens circulating in the bloodstream,

and they can be treated by the surgical removal of the estrogen-secreting organs (the ovaries and the adrenal glands). The other breast tumors are unaffected by estrogens. Jensen and his colleagues at the University of Chicago and William L. McGuire and his colleagues at the University of Texas Health Science Center at San Antonio have recently shown that only the hormone-dependent tumors have receptors for estrogen. The distinction can now be employed as a diagnostic tool. Similar methods might be applied to the classification of prostate tumors whose growth is dependent on androgens and to lymphosarcomas dependent on corticosteroids.

A more precise understanding of how steroids bind to their receptor proteins could uncover methods for the sophisticated manipulation of the hormone response. For example, it should be possible to synthesize biologically inactive analogues of the natural hormones that would block the receptor binding sites and thereby suppress the hormonal response. Such "antihormones" could have therapeutic value, and perhaps even social consequences, since they might be safe and efficient contraceptives.

11

Interactions between Hormones and Nerve Tissue

by Bruce S. McEwen
July 1976

Steroid hormones secreted by the gonads and the adrenal cortex can be traced to target cells in the brain. In the newborn animal the sex hormones help to lay down brain circuits that control later behavior

The steroid hormones that are secreted by the cortex of the adrenal glands and by the gonads are potent substances. Throughout the body the adrenocortical hormones help to regulate the utilization of energy and the balance of electrolytes, such as sodium and potassium; they also affect mood by acting on certain areas of the brain. The gonadal steroids, secreted by the ovaries and the testes, act more specifically on tissues associated with sexual functions: in females the vagina, the uterus, the oviducts and the breasts, and in males the seminal vesicles and the prostate. The sex hormones also stimulate sexual behavior by acting on nerve cells in the brain.

Great progress has been made in identifying the target regions of such hormones in the brain. It has been established that the sex hormones directly influence sexual differentiation of the brain, that is, the pattern of nerve connections and hence the organization of nerve circuits in specific parts of the brain during embryonic and early postnatal development. The resulting neuronal pattern is thereafter not susceptible to permanent hormonal modification. Rather, in the adult animal the role of the sex hormones is limited to influencing the circuits' functional efficiency. Paradoxically the hormone that elicits the male brain pattern in newborn rats seems to be estradiol, one of the estrogens, or female hormones. Although the hormone that reaches the brain of the newborn male rat is testosterone, secreted in the testes, the male hormone is converted into estradiol by enzymes in the nerve cells that are the targets of sexual differentiation.

The first experiment to suggest that gonadal steroids directly affect brain function was reported in 1849 by Arnold A. Berthold of the University of Göttingen. Berthold found that roosters that had been castrated no longer crowed, fought or exhibited sexual behavior. He also found that if he transplanted testes into the abdominal cavity of the castrated roosters, the characteristic masculine behavior reappeared. Because the transplanted testes did not develop connections with the rooster's nervous system but did develop connections with its circulatory system, Berthold deduced that the behavioral signals dispatched by the testes reached the brain through the blood and not through the nerves.

We now know that in higher vertebrates the adult brain contains distinct populations of cells that are sensitive to different steroid hormones, some to estradiol and testosterone, which are secreted by the gonads, and some to the steroid hormones of the adrenal cortex. In our laboratory at Rockefeller University we have located various hormone-sensitive brain cells and have undertaken to establish how they fit into the nerve pathways that govern behavior and regulate the hormone-producing glands. Here I shall discuss our findings and also describe how the steroid products of the testes participate in the sexual differentiation of the developing brain.

Berthold's deduction that testicular hormones directly affect brain function was verified in 1969 by Ronald J. Barfield of Rutgers University, who restored sexual activity in castrated roosters by implanting tiny amounts of testosterone in the preoptic area of the brain. Barfield's work on the rooster was a continuation and extension of other work that showed the direct neural effects of gonadal steroids not necessarily related to sex behavior. In 1957 Bela Flerkó and János Szentágothai of the Medical University of Pécs in Hungary reported that when small fragments of ovarian tissue are implanted in the hypothalamic region of the brain of female rats, the rats' ovaries atrophy. In the early 1960's Robert D. Lisk of Princeton University reported similar results with hypothalamic implants of tiny amounts of the ovarian hormone estradiol. Both Lisk and Richard P. Michael of Emory University found that in female rats

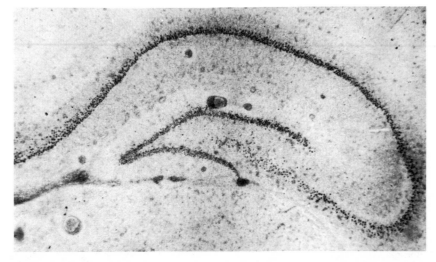

STEROID-HORMONE RECEPTORS IN RAT BRAIN can be located by administering a steroid labeled with tritium, the radioactive isotope of hydrogen. In this case the steroid was corticosterone, one of the principal hormones secreted by the adrenal cortex. One or two hours after administration of the labeled steroid frozen sections of the animal's brain are placed in contact with photographic emulsion and stored for several months. The decaying tritium atoms make black dots in the emulsion and reveal the presence of cells containing receptors for corticosterone. This low-power magnification of an autoradiogram of the hippocampus, which is a primitive region of the rat's brain, shows that nerve cells in the region are heavily labeled.

and cats such implants could also restore the sexual receptivity that had been lost after removal of the ovaries.

One can demonstrate that steroid hormones gain access to the brain from the blood by injecting radioactively labeled steroid hormones into the circulation and measuring the amount of radioactivity that appears in the brain tissue. Not only the brain but also virtually all the other tissues of the body are accessible to the circulating steroid hormones. Certain cells, the target cells, accumulate and retain the hormone by means of specific intracellular receptor proteins, which are believed to reside in the cytoplasm of the target cell. The hormone-protein complex is able to enter the cell nucleus and interact with the genes. The steroid hormone, coupled to its receptor protein, causes portions of the genetic material, DNA, to become accessible to the enzymes and substrates that can form new messenger-RNA molecules along one of the strands of DNA.

The messenger-RNA molecules bear the information necessary to direct the formation of new protein molecules in the cytoplasm of the cell. The new protein molecules enable the target cell to carry out its functional response to the hormone. Thus the oviduct of the hen responds to estradiol by manufacturing the protein ovalbumin, which is secreted into developing eggs. The uterus of female mammals responds to estradiol by synthesizing a great variety of cell proteins that enable its cells to grow, divide and prepare for the implantation of the fertilized ova [see the article "The Receptors of Steroid Hormones," by Bert W. O'Malley and William T. Schrader; beginning on page 94].

It is reasonable to assume that steroid

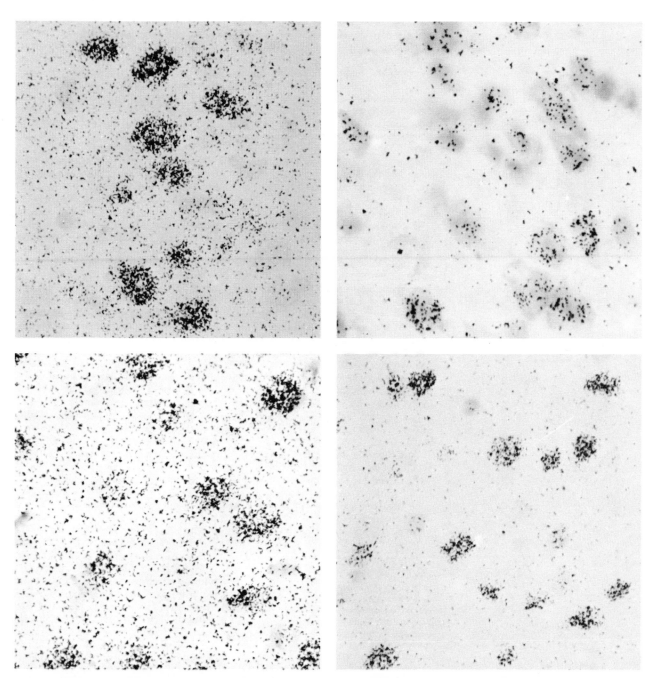

BRAINS OF RAT AND RHESUS MONKEY are compared in these autoradiograms for their ability to accumulate tritium-labeled estradiol, a major sex hormone, in nerve cells of the hypothalamus (*panels at top*) and tritium-labeled corticosterone, one of the adrenocortical hormones, in nerve cells of the hippocampus (*panels at bottom*). The two photomicrographs at the left represent the brain of a rat; the two at the right represent the brain of a rhesus monkey. In each case the most heavily labeled regions are the nuclei of the nerve cells, indicating that these are the ultimate target of the two kinds of steroid hormone. Autoradiograms, which were made by John L. Gerlach in the author's laboratory at Rockefeller University (corticosterone) and by Donald W. Pfaff (estradiol), are enlarged some 1,600 diameters.

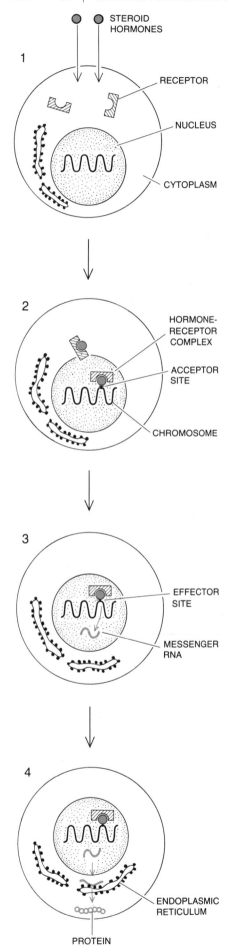

CELLULAR RESPONSE to steroid hormones is depicted schematically. Although steroids are presumably able to enter all cells, only certain target cells contain specific receptor proteins that bind the hormone (1). Receptor-hormone complexes are able to pass through the membrane that surrounds the cell nucleus and attach themselves to acceptor sites on the chromosome containing the genes (DNA) of the cell (2). The receptor triggers the synthesis of messenger RNA corresponding to the gene at an effector site (3), which may or may not be different from the acceptor site. Messenger RNA leaves nucleus and migrates to endoplasmic reticulum, where it presides over the synthesis of protein encoded by gene (4).

hormones affect the genetic material by similar molecular mechanisms in all target cells, wherever in the body they may be. Hence the brain, the most complicated organ of the body, should be amenable to the same kinds of biochemical investigation as those successfully pursued with the oviduct and the uterus. The principal limitations of such studies are the low concentration of hormone-sensitive cells in the brain and the large number of hormones capable of influencing brain function. Fortunately for the experimenter, cells sensitive to particular steroid hormones are commonly found in clusters in certain brain regions. The high density of the sensitive cells in such regions makes it possible to conduct the same kinds of biochemical investigation that can be conducted with more homogeneous tissues. By combining information on the localization of hormone-sensitive cells within the brain with information gathered from implanting hormones in specific brain regions, from electrical recordings of nerve-cell activity and from the administration of drugs that alter the electrical activity of the brain a picture can be formed of the circuits of nerve cells that may be involved in the control of particular hormone-sensitive behavior patterns.

Hormone-sensitive neurons are present only in certain distinct brain regions. The technique of autoradiography enables us to make these hormone-sensitive neurons visible under the microscope. In this procedure ovariectomized rats are injected intravenously with estradiol labeled with tritium, the radioactive isotope of hydrogen, and are killed one or two hours later. Their brains are removed, frozen and sectioned. The sections are then placed in contact with photographic emulsion and stored for three to 12 months. The radiation emitted by the decaying tritium atoms reveals quite precisely where the estradiol was deposited within the cell nucleus, even though the nucleus is only about five or 10 micrometers in diameter.

With the aid of autoradiography Donald W. Pfaff of Rockefeller University and Walter E. Stumpf of the University of North Carolina have found that in the brain of adult rats the highest density of estrogen-concentrating cells is in the preoptic area, the hypothalamus and an adjacent area, the

amygdala. These are all areas of the "primitive" brain, the archipallium, which has long been known to play a role in sexual behavior. Tiny implants of purified estradiol in two of these regions (the preoptic area and the hypothalamus) facilitate female sexual behavior and cause atrophy of the ovaries. Because the function of the amygdala in reproductive physiology is not well understood, a role cannot be assigned to the estrogen receptors in that area.

Estradiol appears to be bound to receptors in the cell nuclei of neurons. In 1970 Richard E. Zigmond in my laboratory found large amounts of tritium-labeled estradiol in cell nuclei isolated from the brain tissue of ovariectomized female rats to whom the steroid had been given an hour or two before they were killed. Other investigators, examining the cytoplasm of brain cells, have found estrogen-receptor sites, indicating the presence of molecules that can carry the hormone into the cell nucleus. Thus estrogen target cells in the brain conform to the general model of steroid target cells elsewhere in the body.

When it is loaded to full capacity with tritiated estradiol, each cell nucleus isolated from the preoptic area, the hypothalamus and the amygdala contains 3,000 to 5,000 molecules of hormone. Each cell nucleus isolated from the nearby pituitary gland, another important estrogen target, contains on the average 12,000 molecules of hormone. The receptor capacity of cell nuclei in the uterus is similar to that of cell nuclei in the pituitary. In the pituitary 80 percent of the cells are labeled, whereas in the samples of the preoptic area, the hypothalamus and the amygdala fewer than 50 percent of the cells contain estrogen receptors. It appears that there are also some differences in the number of receptors in individual target cells in these various tissues.

Recent work by Pfaff and Joan I. Morrell has shown that the localization of estradiol-sensitive neurons in the brain is remarkably constant in fishes, amphibians, birds and mammals. The most important finding in the effort to relate these observations to human physiology is that the brain of the rhesus monkey, which like man is a primate, has the same pattern of estradiol-concentrating neurons as the brain of the rat.

One of the major effects of estradiol on the brain of a female rat is to make the animal sexually receptive. It takes at least 20 hours, however, for a single injection of estradiol to bring about an increase in sexual receptivity in a female rat from which the ovaries have been removed. This time lag is independent of the dose of the hormone and is similar to the latency in the female rat's estrous cycle between the increase of estradiol secretion by the ovaries and the appearance of behavioral estrus. The time lag has enabled a number of laboratories to examine the intracellular events that may be involved in the effect of estradiol on sexual behavior. Administering a single behaviorally effective dose of tritium-labeled estradiol, we were able to show that receptors in the nuclei of cells in the pituitary and in the three most heavily labeled brain regions (the hypothalamus, the preoptic area and the amygdala) are occupied for less than 12 of the 20 hours. In fact, the maximum labeling of receptor sites comes within the first two hours. Thus the estrogen does not have to be present at the time of its behavioral effect. It would therefore seem that estradiol initiates metabolic changes within the target neurons, which in turn determine the readiness for the behavioral response.

Since the cell nucleus plays a role in the action of estradiol, the metabolic changes may involve the synthesis of RNA and protein. The hypothesis can be tested by seeing if estrogen action in the brain can be blocked by substances that inhibit the synthesis. Two such inhibitors are actinomycin D, an inhibitor of RNA synthesis, and cycloheximide, an inhibitor of protein synthesis. Roger A. Gorski of the University of California School of Medicine at Los Angeles, Richard E. Whalen of the University of California at Irvine and David M. Quadagno of the University of Kansas have shown that small implants of actinomycin D and cycloheximide in the preoptic area of the rat brain reversibly block the facilitation of female sexual behavior that is normally induced by estrogen. The inhibitors are only effective, however, if they are applied within 12 hours after the estrogen. The additional time lag before the appearance of behavioral estrus has not yet been accounted for in terms of other cellular events.

Estradiol also appears to play a role in the neural regulation of sexual behavior in adult male rats. Estradiol receptors are found in male and female brains in the same regions and in similar amounts. Moreover, the male hormone testosterone is transformed in the brain into one of two hormonal steroids: dihydrotestosterone and estradiol. The transformation into estradiol, which was discovered by Frederick Naftolin of McGill University and Kenneth J. Ryan of the Harvard Medical School, is not so surprising in view of the fact that the same conversion occurs in the normal biosynthetic pathway for estradiol in the gonads. Working in my laboratory, Ivan Lieberburg has recovered tritium-labeled estradiol from the brain-cell nuclei of rats after injecting tritium-labeled testosterone into the animals. The distribution of labeled estradiol derived from testosterone is not, however, like the pattern resulting from the administration of tritium-labeled estradiol itself. Testosterone-derived estradiol was not found, for example, in the pituitary gland, where estrogen receptors are abundant, because pituitary tissue lacks the converting enzymes. Testosterone-derived estradiol was recovered from receptors in the cell nuclei of the preoptic area, the hypothalamus and the amygdala. It is not clear what function, if any, testosterone itself has in the brain of the adult male rat. One possible function of the testosterone-derived estradiol is suggested by the work of Larry Christensen and Lynwood Clemens of Michigan State University. They showed

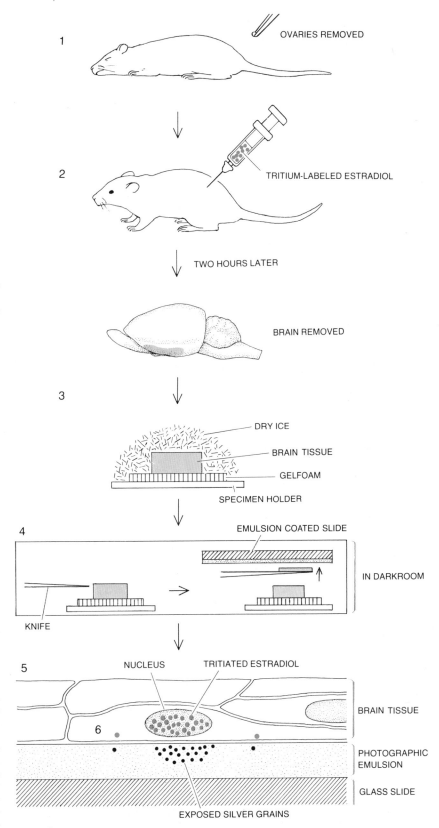

LOCATION OF STEROID TARGET CELLS is established by autoradiography. One begins by eliminating the animal's normal source of the steroid under investigation. Here the ovaries, the source of estradiol, are surgically removed (*1*). Estradiol labeled with tritium is injected (*2*). An hour or two later the animal's brain is removed and frozen (*3*). Sections of the brain are placed against a photographic emulsion on a microscope slide (*4*) and stored for several months. Electrons from the decaying tritium atoms expose silver atoms in the emulsion (*5*). Since the electrons travel only one or two micrometers in the emulsion, it is easy to tell by examining the developed autoradiogram what fraction of the tritiated estradiol molecules were delivered to the cell nucleus (which has a diameter of five to 10 micrometers) and what fraction of the molecules remained in the cytoplasm (*6*). The great majority of the molecules reach the nucleus.

that estradiol implants in the preoptic area are more effective than testosterone implants in restoring the male sexual behavior of castrated male rats.

The other major neural metabolite of testosterone, dihydrotestosterone, is relatively ineffective in restoring male sexual behavior even when it is implanted directly in the brain of castrated rats. Dihydrotestosterone does, however, increase the effectiveness of estradiol in restoring male sexual behavior when both are given to castrated male rats. Thus dihydrotestosterone may have a normal role in promoting male sexual behavior. It also appears to regulate the secretion of hormones by the hypothalamus and the pituitary, which in turn stimulates sperm formation and testosterone secretion by the testes. Receptors for dihydrotestosterone have been detected in the rat's brain and pituitary. They are less plentiful than those for estradiol. Their distribution within the brain also differs from the distribution of the estrogen receptors in that they are more plentiful in the septum and the hypothalamus than in other brain regions. Dihydrotestosterone receptors in the brain and the pituitary resemble those found in the prostate gland and the seminal vesicles, where dihydrotestosterone stimulates the growth and the secretory activity of those organs.

The second principal source of steroid hormones in man and other vertebrates is the adrenal cortex. The influence of adrenal steroids on the brain is not as well understood as the influence of estradiol and other sex hormones. Nevertheless, there are indications that adrenal steroids do significantly affect brain function. In human beings changes in mood are brought about by either an excess or an insufficiency of adrenal-steroid secretion. Such changes have been reported as a side effect of adrenal-steroid treatment of inflammation of the skin or the joints. Adrenal steroids have also been administered to regulate the ability of patients to detect sensory stimuli. Robert I. Henkin and his colleagues at the National Heart and Lung Institute find that people with Addison's disease (adrenal-steroid insufficiency) are more sensitive to sensory stimuli, such as sound and taste, than healthy people. On the other hand, they are less accurate than normal people in identifying the nature of the stimulus, for example in recognizing words or in distinguishing sweet solutions from sour ones. Both of these defects are corrected by therapy with adrenal steroids.

When the adrenal steroid corticosterone is labeled with tritium and injected into rats or monkeys from which the adrenals have been removed, the steroid turns up predominantly in two regions of the brain: the hippocampus and the septum, which also belong to the primitive brain. Steroid-receptor sites are found in both the cytoplasm and the nuclei of nerve cells in these two regions, indicating that corticosterone functions inside brain cells in the same way that other steroids do.

A potential role for adrenal steroids in the hippocampus can be inferred from experiments showing that the administration of adrenal steroids to human volunteers depresses the rapid eye movement (REM) that characterizes certain states of sleep. REM sleep seems to be associated with dreaming. In experimental animals the hippocampus shows a characteristic electrical activity, the theta rhythm, during REM sleep. It is therefore possible that corticosterone alters the characteristics of hippocampal nerve cells so that they become less sensitive to the neural stimuli that evoke the theta rhythm.

Not all adrenal steroids interact to the same degree with the same brain receptor sites. For example, tritium-labeled dexamethasone, a synthetic steroid, is selectively concentrated by the pituitary gland and becomes attached to receptor sites in the nuclei of pituitary cells. Although corticosterone also binds to such sites, dexamethasone binds much more readily, according to experiments conducted by my colleague Ronald de Kloet. (On the other hand, dexamethasone binds less effectively than corticosterone to receptor sites in the hippocampus.)

The output of steroids from the adrenal cortex is regulated by the amount of adrenocorticotrophic hormone (ACTH) secreted by the pituitary. It appears that through a feedback loop the production of ACTH in turn is regulated by the number of pituitary-cell receptor sites occupied by adrenocortical steroids. Patients whose adrenal cortex is overactive are frequently treated with adrenal steroids in an effort to reduce the pituitary's output of ACTH. The finding that pituitary receptor sites respond more strongly to dexamethasone than to corticosterone may explain why the synthetic steroid is more effective in suppressing ACTH output and thus in treating adrenal hyperfunction.

The neurons that respond to steroid hormones are part of complex circuits of nerve cells that connect stimuli from the senses with specific effectors of responses. To illustrate, let us return to the example of estradiol and reproduction in female rats. In the normal estrous cycle of the rat the pituitary secretes large amounts of luteinizing hormone (the "LH surge") in the afternoon of proestrus, approximately 30 hours after the initial increase in estradiol secretion by the ovaries. The LH surge causes ovulation to occur about 12 hours later. The LH surge does not take place if the ovaries are removed before the increase in estradiol secretion. If ovariectomized rats are given estradiol, however, the LH surge comes once again at the appropriate time.

The pituitary secretes some LH when estradiol has not been administered, but the amount is insufficient to cause ovulation. Although the effect of estradiol is to facilitate the secretion of LH, estradiol is not the true stimulus that initiates the LH surge. The stimulus for LH secretion arises from a biological clock in the brain, which is set to a specific 24-hour rhythm by the relative amounts of light and darkness detected by the eyes. The effector for LH secretion is a group of neurons that secrete a hormone consisting of 10 amino acid units from nerve endings in the base of the hypothalamus into the capillaries of the portal circulatory system of the hypothalamus and the pituitary. This short system of capillaries carries the hormone, called luteinizing hormone–releasing hormone (LH-RH), to the pituitary, where it stimulates the appropriate cells, the gonadotrophs, to release LH. The LH travels in the general circulation to the ovaries, where it induces the rupture of mature ovarian follicles, thereby releasing ova into the reproductive tract. Estradiol facilitates this sequence of events not only by increasing the amount of LH-RH secreted but also by elevating the sensitivity of the pituitary cells to release LH in response to LH-RH.

In the normal estrous cycle of rats the females exhibit their sexual behavior pattern every four days on the evening preceding ovulation. They exhibit it about 36 hours after the rise in estradiol secretion by the ovaries. If the ovaries are removed several days before testing females for sexual behavior, however, the female's response to the male is either to run away or to fight off the male's advances. If estradiol is given to ovariectomized female rats to replace the missing ovarian secretion, sensory stimuli, such as the male rat's grasping the female's flanks, cause her to assume the mating posture. The posture is called the lordosis response, from the Greek for "bending backward." Both the rump and the head of the female are raised and held rigid, making the back concave. The effector system in the brain for the lordosis response is a circuit of neurons that connects the sensory inputs from the flanks, the back and the pelvis with muscles in the back and the limbs. The incoming sensory information passes up the spinal cord and into the network of estradiol-sensitive neurons in the brain, which acts as a kind of switching mechanism that sends a return flow of information down another set of neurons in the spinal cord, causing the appropriate muscles to contract.

Neurons, including those that mediate the lordosis response, communicate with one another by means of specific chemical neurotransmitters, such as acetylcholine, norepinephrine and serotonin. The transmitters are released from synaptic endings and alter the electrical activity of adjacent neurons by way of specific receptor sites on their surfaces. At some of the receptor sites the transmitter is excitatory and increases the electrical activity of the responding neuron; at other sites the transmitter is inhibitory and decreases the activity. Therefore depending on which neurons are activated by specific stimuli, the outputs controlling the muscle contractions are either activated or inhibited. The action of estradiol in such neural networks may be to modify the capacity of some steroid-sensitive neurons for releasing their specific neurotransmitter and of others for responding to the transmitters released by adjacent neurons. There is little information on this important point, but the fact that hormone-sensitive cells in the brain have been localized should make it possible to obtain such information in the near future.

A possible model of how hormones modify the synaptic transmission of nerve impulses can be found in the ability of certain drugs to alter neurotransmitter function. For example, drugs that inactivate the serotonin system, which is itself inhibitory, have been observed to increase the lordosis response of spayed female rats primed with estradiol. On the other hand, inhibition of the noradrenergic system of the brain, which is itself also inhibitory, increases the output by the hypothalamus of corticotrophin-releasing factor (CRF), which in turn increases the secretion of ACTH from the pituitary. As I have mentioned, ACTH causes the adrenal glands to secrete adrenal steroids.

We can go one step further and consider

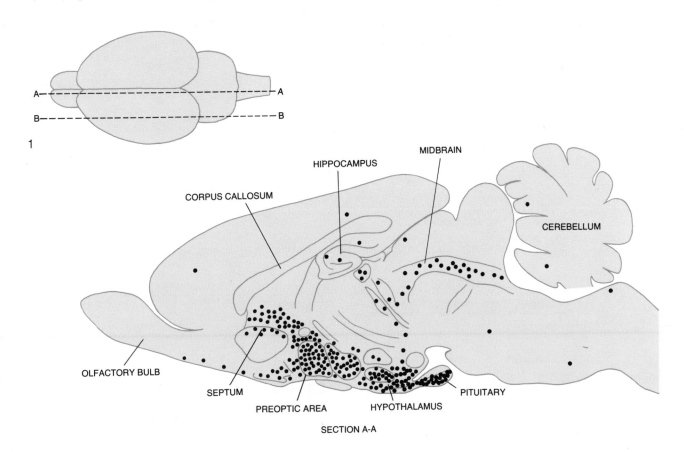

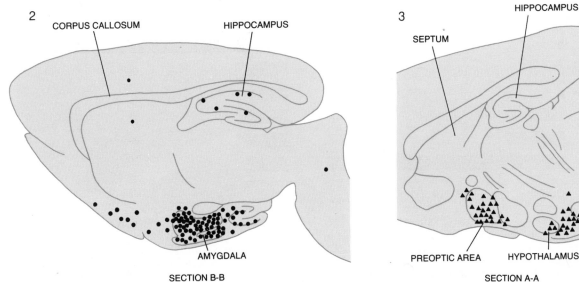

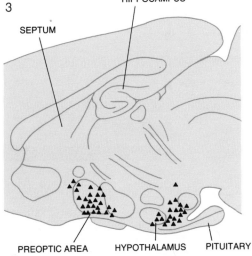

ESTRADIOL-SENSITIVE NERVE CELLS in the brain of the albino rat are concentrated in the preoptic area, the hypothalamus and the amygdala. The black dots in sectional maps No. 1 and No. 2 indicate regions in the brain that were made particularly radioactive when animals were given tritium-labeled estradiol. The experiments were conducted by Pfaff and Melvyn Keiner of Rockefeller University. In a related study Robert D. Lisk of Princeton University examined the effects of implanting tiny amounts of estradiol directly in the preoptic area and in the hypothalamus. Typical results are illustrated in sectional map No. 3. The triangles indicate sites of implantation that elicited female sexual behavior or suppressed secretion of neurotransmitters to anterior pituitary, which controls the function of the ovaries.

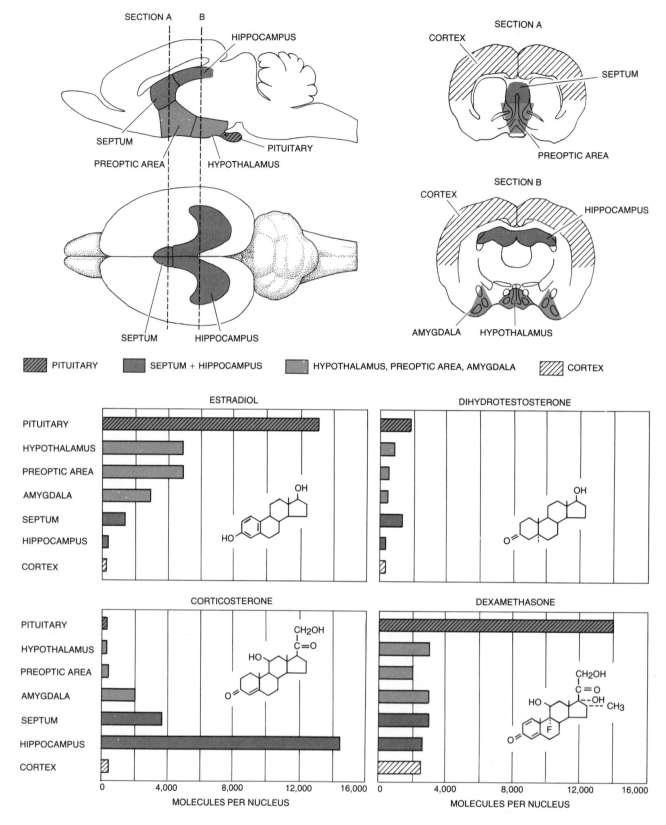

SECTION A   B

HIPPOCAMPUS

SEPTUM

PREOPTIC AREA   HYPOTHALAMUS   PITUITARY

SEPTUM   HIPPOCAMPUS

SECTION A

CORTEX   SEPTUM

PREOPTIC AREA

SECTION B

CORTEX   HIPPOCAMPUS

AMYGDALA   HYPOTHALAMUS

PITUITARY   SEPTUM + HIPPOCAMPUS   HYPOTHALAMUS, PREOPTIC AREA, AMYGDALA   CORTEX

ESTRADIOL

PITUITARY
HYPOTHALAMUS
PREOPTIC AREA
AMYGDALA
SEPTUM
HIPPOCAMPUS
CORTEX

DIHYDROTESTOSTERONE

CORTICOSTERONE

PITUITARY
HYPOTHALAMUS
PREOPTIC AREA
AMYGDALA
SEPTUM
HIPPOCAMPUS
CORTEX

0   4,000   8,000   12,000   16,000
MOLECULES PER NUCLEUS

DEXAMETHASONE

0   4,000   8,000   12,000   16,000
MOLECULES PER NUCLEUS

DIFFERING RESPONSE OF BRAIN CELLS to different kinds of steroid hormone has been studied by the author and his co-workers at Rockefeller University. They administered tritium-labeled hormones to male and female rats whose adrenals and gonads, the normal source of such steroids, had previously been removed. The animals were killed one or two hours later and their brains were dissected to remove the regions indicated in the diagrams at the top. The pituitary was also removed for study. The investigators isolated the cell nuclei from each sample and measured the amount of radioactive hormone present. The charts at the bottom show the number of hormone molecules per nu-

cleus, averaged for all nuclei in each tissue sample. Autoradiograms reveal that the female sex hormone estradiol is bound to receptors in about 80 percent of all pituitary cells. For the brain areas with the highest affinity for estradiol (the preoptic area, the hypothalamus and the amygdala) the hormone is found in fewer than half of the cells. Dihydrotestosterone, a steroid that closely resembles estradiol, gives rise to an uptake pattern that is quite different. The adrenocortical steroid corticosterone is found primarily in the hippocampus. The chemically similar synthetic steroid dexamethasone, however, mimics the estradiol more closely than it does the adrenocortical steroid.

the consequences of such drug-induced changes in adrenal-hormone secretion. Higher levels of steroids could interact with the brain to alter mood, perception and sleep. This is an important consideration because drugs that act on neurotransmitter systems are widely administered in the treatment and management of human emotional disturbances and mental illness. Not enough attention has been paid to the secondary effects of their action on the delicately balanced endocrine system.

Even in the absence of drugs, changes in behavior can influence neuroendocrine secretion. The familiar human experience described as stress (caused by many factors, including fear, physical trauma, severe heat or cold and even extreme joy) has as a common denominator an increased secretion of adrenal steroids directed by the increased release of CRF and ACTH. The neuroendocrine systems governing reproductive functions are also subject to behavioral modification. For example, male rhesus monkeys subjected to decisive defeat by dominant males show dramatically lower levels of testosterone, whose secretion is directed by a hypothalamic releasing factor. When defeated males are exposed to female companions, however, the testosterone levels are rapidly restored to normal.

Although the effects of steroid hormones on the adult brain are normally reversible, steroids are also capable of giving rise to effects that are permanent for the life of the individual and that result in sex differences in both behavioral and neuroendocrine function. Let us consider these effects, which are aspects of the process known as sexual differentiation, and the hormone receptors that may be involved in them.

If the hormone is to have a permanent effect, it must be present during a brief sensitive period of early brain development. The critical period in human beings is during fetal life. In laboratory rats, however, the critical period comes during the first week after birth, when the testes of the male secrete testosterone. The testosterone initiates events leading to the sexual differentiation of the brain.

Since the rat brain is undifferentiated until shortly after birth, it has been possible to experimentally dissect the phenomenon by which steroids of the testes cause sexual differentiation. The adult male rat continues to show strong male sexual behavior and exhibits the female lordosis response only slightly even when it is castrated and given estradiol. If the testes are removed from a newborn male rat, however, its brain retains a female pattern of differentiation. As an adult the animal will show only weak male sexual behavior even after treatment with testosterone, and it will display a strong lordosis response when it is given estradiol. The two kinds of response resemble those of spayed but otherwise normal female rats given similar hormone treatments.

In contrast, a female rat given testosterone on the fourth day after birth will as an

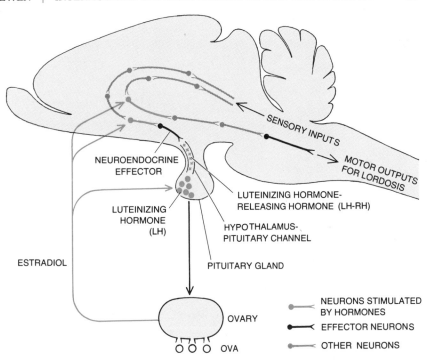

CONTROL SCHEME depicts the role of neural and chemical signals in regulating the production of a particular steroid hormone, estradiol, and in eliciting a specific form of sexual behavior, the lordosis response. The latter, observed in female rats, is a downward arching of the back that facilitates mating. At the base of the brain a group of nerve cells, known as neuroendocrine effectors, is influenced both by sensory inputs and by the level of estradiol circulating in the blood. The neuroendocrine effector secretes into a capillary bed at the base of the hypothalamus a small polypeptide molecule: luteinizing hormone–releasing hormone (LH-RH). When LH-RH, carried by the blood, reaches the pituitary gland, it triggers the release of luteinizing hormone (LH), another polypeptide. The blood carries LH to the ovary, where it stimulates the secretion of estradiol and, if the quantity of LH is enough, causes ovulation. Estradiol travels in the blood to the brain and the pituitary, where it acts on receptors in target cells to modify the neural circuits controlling LH-RH secretion and the lordosis response. An important stimulus for the secretion of LH-RH arises from a biological clock that is internal to the animal. The clock, not represented in the illustration, responds to relative amounts of light and darkness.

adult perform like a normal male in the tests for male and female sexual behavior. In other studies of early sexual differentiation it has been found that ovaries transplanted into a castrated newborn male rat or into a spayed newborn female rat will ovulate but that ovaries will not ovulate when they are implanted in a newborn female rat treated with testosterone or in a male castrated as an adult.

The permanent nature of sexual differentiation strongly suggests that testosterone influences the development of neurons and the formation of synaptic contacts with other neurons. These events may involve both cell replication (and therefore the synthesis of DNA) and the expression of genes (and therefore the synthesis of RNA and protein). A number of investigators report they have been able to block sexual differentiation with drugs that inhibit one or more of these synthetic events. Other workers, however, have been unable to get the same results. The discrepancy may be explained by the length of time the inhibitors are effective in relation to the duration of the exposure to testosterone. According to Gorski and his colleague Shinji Hayashi, microimplants of testosterone in the hypothalamic area of the brain must be left in place for 48 to 72 hours in order to bring about sexual differentia-

tion. Therefore if the inhibitors were to be effective, they too would have to be present for a similar period. It is doubtful that inhibitors have been active for the required time in any of the studies so far reported. An additional complication is the fact that the inhibitors of the synthesis of DNA, RNA and protein block the synthesis of substances other than those thought to be stimulated by testosterone. The longer the inhibitors are allowed to act, the greater the likelihood is that nonspecific brain damage will occur.

In spite of the difficulties with such experiments, the participation of the genetic material in the sexual differentiation of the brain is virtually assured by the fact that genes direct the growth and differentiation of all living matter. A more critical issue is the location of the cellular changes that underlie these phenomena. Independent studies by Ronald D. Nadler of Emory University and by Gorski and Hayashi show that a tiny amount of testosterone implanted in the preoptic region and the hypothalamus of newborn female rats is sufficient to give rise to sexual differentiation of the brain.

Detailed information regarding the intracellular consequences of sexual differentiation has been provided by Geoffrey Raisman and Pauline M. Field of the National

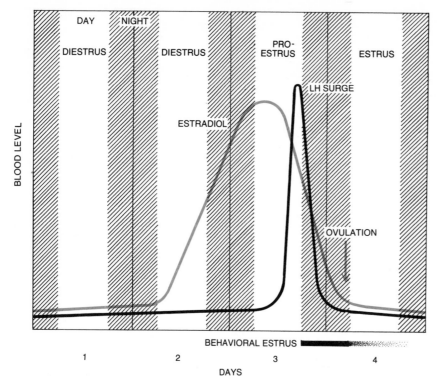

NORMAL ESTROUS CYCLE OF RAT causes females to exhibit estrus, or sexual, behavior every four days. Two days after estrus behavior, on diestrus Day 2, the estrogen level of the animal's blood begins to rise again, reaching a peak on the next day, proestrus, Day 3. The rising estrogen triggers a sharp rise in the level in the blood of luteinizing hormone (the "LH surge") on the afternoon of proestrus, causing ovulation to occur early in the morning of Day 4, estrus. Behavioral estrus, including lordosis response, which is also dependent on earlier estrogen secretion, can be stimulated by the male during the night between proestrus and estrus.

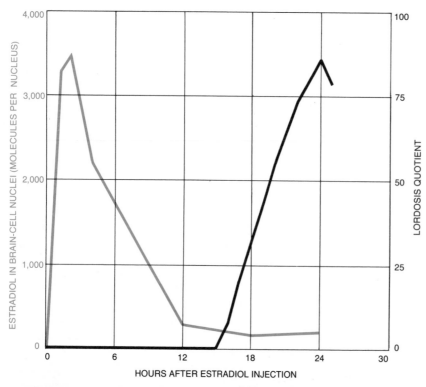

BRAIN ESTRADIOL LEVEL in female rats reaches a peak about 22 hours before the peak in lordosis behavior, according to the author's studies. The average number of molecules of tritium-labeled estradiol in the cell nuclei of the preoptic area, the hypothalamus and the amygdala is shown by the colored curve. Lordosis response (*black curve*) is expressed as the percentage of times a female rat facilitated a male's attempt to copulate by a downward arching of her back.

Institute for Medical Research at Mill Hill in London. When they compared the fine structure of the neural connections of the preoptic area in adult male and female rats, they found a difference in the distribution of specific types of synaptic contacts. Castration of newborn male rats during the critical period, but not later, prevented the male pattern from emerging. Treatment of female rats with testosterone during the sensitive period, but not later, induced a male pattern of synaptic contacts in the preoptic area.

Tissue from the preoptic area and the hypothalamus of fetal mice can be cultured outside the body under artificial conditions for several weeks. It has been shown by Dominique Toran-Allerand of Columbia University that such tissue is exceptionally sensitive to the application of testosterone and estradiol during a period in culture that corresponds to the sensitive period for sexual differentiation in the living animal. The major effect of the two steroids is to enhance the outgrowth of the fibers of developing neurons. This fits well with the observations of Raisman and Field, because the number and geometry of the growing fibers will help to determine the pattern of synaptic connections.

To recapitulate, newborn male rats deprived of testosterone by castration show a female pattern of brain organization as adults. If newborn female rats are given testosterone, they exhibit male sexual behavior as adults. Paradoxically the female steroid estradiol is at least as potent as testosterone, and perhaps more so, in giving rise to male sexual differentiation when it is administered to newborn female rats. As we have seen, the brain of the adult rat possesses enzymes for converting testosterone into estradiol and dihydrotestosterone. The administration of dihydrotestosterone to newborn rats has no effect on sexual differentiation. If the brain of the newborn rat also possesses the enzymes for converting testosterone into estradiol, one can conjecture that estradiol is the agent responsible for the brain differentiation associated with male sexual behavior.

Naftolin and his co-workers, and Judith Weisz and Carol Gibbs of the Hershey Medical Center in Hershey, Pa., have demonstrated that the brain of the newborn rat does possess the enzymes for converting testosterone into estradiol. My colleague Lieberburg gave tritium-labeled testosterone to newborn male and female rats and recovered tritium-labeled estradiol in purified cell nuclei from the preoptic area, the hypothalamus and the amygdala. The amount of testosterone-derived estradiol in the cell nuclei ranged between 30 and 50 percent.

Hence the brain of the newborn rat has the enzymes to convert testosterone to estradiol and it also has a receptor mechanism for the product: estradiol. Further studies in my laboratory have substantiated the existence of a receptor mechanism for estradiol in the cell nuclei of the brain of the newborn rat. We were able to obtain direct evidence for such receptors by injecting tritium-labeled derivatives of estradiol into newborn male and female rats. Such derivatives bind more effectively to the receptor sites in the animal than estradiol itself does. Cell nuclei isolated from newborn rats that had received the tritium-labeled derivatives contain large amounts of hormone attached to receptorlike proteins. In addition Michael Ginsburg and his co-workers at Chelsea College of the University of London and Linda Plapinger and Neil J. Maclusky in my laboratory have found a cytoplasmic estrogen receptor in the brain of the newborn animal and have shown that the receptor is depleted when radioactive estrogen is given to the animal. Evidently the cytoplasmic receptor migrates into the nucleus of the cell when it becomes loaded with the steroid.

The receptor system for estradiol in the brain of the newborn rat therefore resembles very closely, and may even be identical with, the receptor system in the brain of the adult rat, with the same anatomical distribution in the preoptic area, the hypothalamus and the amygdala. The major difference, according to our own work and that of Ginsburg's group in London, is the presence of estrogen receptors in the cerebral cortex of the newborn rat. These sites disappear between two and three weeks after birth and are virtually absent from the cerebral cortex of the adult rat. Their function remains obscure, but clearly it does not involve a response to estrogen derived from testosterone, because the cerebral cortex lacks the converting enzymes.

The hypothesis that the estrogen receptors of the preoptic area, the hypothalamus and the amygdala actually mediate sexual differentiation has stimulated a great deal of interest and research. Several reports from the laboratory of the late Peter McDonald of the Royal Veterinary College in London indicate that antiestrogens (drugs that compete with estradiol for the receptor sites and block its physiological actions) attenuate or prevent the sexual differentiation that is normally induced in newborn female rats by testosterone. Other published reports, however, fail to confirm this effect. Validation of the hypothesis thus awaits a conclusive experiment.

If estradiol administered to a female rat is so effective in giving rise to the male pattern of sexual differentiation, how is the female rat normally protected against its own estrogen and the estrogen of its mother? A major protective mechanism is an estrogen-binding blood protein, alpha-fetoprotein. Alpha-fetoprotein tends to keep the circulating estradiol from reaching the target neurons. Estradiol is able to reach its receptor sites in amounts sufficient to bring about sexual differentiation only if large amounts of it are given to the animal. Alpha-fetoprotein is manufactured by the fetal liver, and it persists, in declining amounts, during the first three weeks of postnatal life. My colleague Plapinger has found that alpha-fetoprotein is present in

the brain of both male and female newborn rats, not as a part of the brain itself but rather as a constituent of the cerebrospinal fluid. Since alpha-fetoprotein does not bind testosterone, the testicular testosterone of males has unhindered access to the brain, where it can be converted into the estradiol needed to give rise to sexual differentiation.

There are several synthetic estrogens that do not bind significantly to alpha-fetoprotein and therefore reach the estrogen-receptor sites in the brain of newborn rats even when they are administered in minute amounts. One of these estrogens, with the code name RU-2858, has been made available to us by Jean-Pierre Raynaud of the French pharmaceutical manufacturer Roussel-UCLAF. It is a form of estradiol with additional chemical groups added to the molecule. We find that RU-2858 is ef-

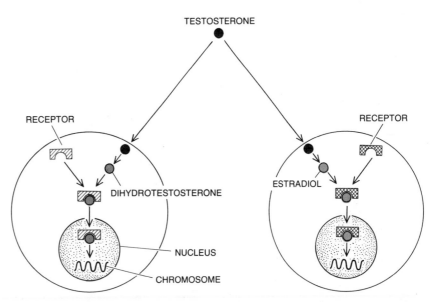

TRANSFORMATION OF TESTOSTERONE TO ESTRADIOL and another steroid, dihydrotestosterone, is accomplished by enzymes in many target cells, including those in the preoptic area, the hypothalamus and the amygdala, but not in the pituitary. This leads to the paradox that a "male" hormone, testosterone, is converted into a "female" hormone, estradiol, which then exerts strong male effects in particular cells where transformation occurs. Dihydrotestosterone increases effectiveness of estradiol in restoring male sexual behavior in castrated rats.

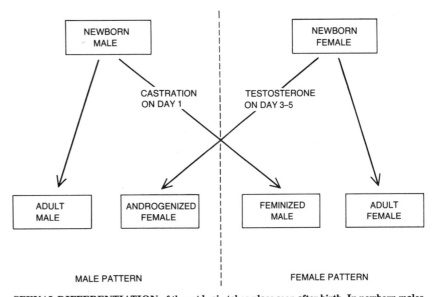

SEXUAL DIFFERENTIATION of the rat brain takes place soon after birth. In newborn males testosterone, secreted by the testes, is converted by target cells in the brain into estradiol, which gives rise to a permanent "male" pattern of brain structure. If the male is castrated at birth, however, the sexual differentiation of nerve circuits in the brain fails to take place and the brain retains a "female" pattern. Administration of testosterone to a newborn female rat evokes a "male" pattern of brain circuitry as a result of the testosterone's being converted intracellularly into estradiol. The female's own gonadal secretion of estradiol is prevented from reaching the estradiol-responsive brain cells by the mechanism depicted in top illustration on next page.

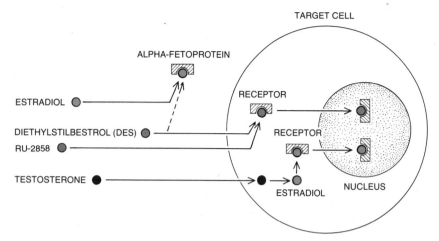

ACCESS OF ESTRADIOL TO BRAIN is blocked in newborn female rats by alpha-fetoprotein, a substance present in the newborn animal's blood and cerebrospinal fluid for about three weeks. Two synthetic estrogens, diethylstilbestrol and RU-2858, are able to reach receptors in target cells because they bind weakly or not at all to alpha-fetoprotein. Similarly, testosterone gains access to target cells and is converted into estradiol, which interacts with estrogen receptors. Evidently it is estradiol from testosterone that evokes "male" pattern in brain of males.

fective in loading the estradiol receptors in the brain of newborn rats at a dose less than a thirtieth of an effective dose of estradiol itself. Results obtained in McDonald's laboratory indicate that RU-2858 is also between 50 and 100 times more effective than estradiol in causing sexual differentiation in the rat brain. According to Raynaud, RU-2858 is also more effective than estradiol in stimulating the growth of the developing uterus in newborn rats. Hence its effects are by no means confined to the developing brain.

Synthetic estrogens such as RU-2858 have been made in an effort to find more effective means of controlling human fertility and of remedying the syndrome of inadequate estradiol secretion during pregnancy,

which can result in miscarriage. Their action on the developing brain of the rat has created an awareness of the possible deleterious effects of such synthetic estrogens on the human fetus. Another synthetic estrogen, diethylstilbestrol, has in fact become the object of concern because of the abnormal incidence of vaginal and cervical cancer in young women whose mothers had received the hormone during pregnancy. Like RU-2858, diethylstilbestrol is capable of causing sexual differentiation of the rat brain when it is administered during the sensitive period. Since information on the physiology of the human fetus is limited, it would be premature to conclude that sexual differentiation and protection from estrogenic effects on the sexual differentiation of

the brain operate identically in human beings and laboratory rats. Nevertheless, it is clear that synthetic estrogens present serious hazards to normal early development in both species.

Let me summarize briefly. Endocrinologists have discovered that steroid hormones have two quite different effects on the brain, both of them involving an action of steroids on the genetic material of the cell nucleus. On the one hand, hormones such as estradiol, normally regarded as being female hormones, are responsible for the reversible activation of the lordosis response and ovulation in adult female rats. On the other, when certain areas of the developing brain are exposed to hormones such as estradiol (or estradiol derived from the putative male hormone testosterone), there is a permanent change in the structure of the brain, resulting in a male pattern of behavior in the adult animal. If the developing brain of a newborn male is deprived of testosterone, say by castration, the animal's brain retains a female pattern of organization. The difference between the permanent responses to steroids in the newborn animal and the reversible responses in the adult must be due to the state of differentiation of the target neurons themselves at the time the hormone reaches them.

Since the genetic material, DNA, is the same in all cells of the body, the process of cell differentiation must involve the selective turning on of certain genes and the turning off of others. Under normal circumstances differentiation is irreversible for the lifetime of the tissue, that is, red blood cells do not begin to make neurotransmitters and brain cells do not begin to make hemoglobin.

According to this concept, testosterone or estradiol that reaches the nuclei of certain hormonally sensitive differentiating nerve cells during the critical period for the sexual differentiation of the brain provides a signal for activating certain genes and suppressing others. As a result the hormone may influence the pattern of the connections the affected nerve cells form with other nerve cells and thereby may determine the nerve circuits in part of the brain. Once these circuits are formed their basic structure is no longer susceptible to hormonal influence. During adult life the role of the hormone may be to alter the functional efficiency of the circuits. Hence even though certain genes may be turned on in a differentiated cell, they are not necessarily fully active at all times. Their activity may in some cases be modulated by hormones. On this view the estradiol that reaches the cell nuclei of adult neurons provides a signal for increasing or decreasing the activity of genes that are permanently expressed in that cell. In this way the hormone may be able to influence the functioning of developmentally fixed neural circuits that control, for example, sexual behavior. We must now discover what chemical properties of the target neurons are essential for the appearance of the behavioral response.

ESTROGEN-SENSITIVE NERVE CELLS in the brain of infant rats are revealed in these autoradiograms by the accumulation of tritium-labeled RU-2858, a synthetic estrogen, in the cerebral cortex (*left*) and hypothalamus (*right*). The experiment, conducted by Gerlach and Linda Plapinger in the author's laboratory, shows that in three-day-old female rats alpha-fetoprotein, which binds estradiol and therefore prevents it from reaching the cells that are responsive to estrogen, does not interfere with the access of RU-2858 to the two types of brain cell.

IV

HORMONES AND NEUROTRANSMITTERS

IV HORMONES AND NEUROTRANSMITTERS

INTRODUCTION

Section III introduced the idea that steroid hormones bind to intracellular receptors. Among the consequences of this reaction in the nervous system may be the "turning on" of enzyme systems involved in the production of neurotransmitters. That is, hormones may alter the amounts of neurotransmitter available in specific brain circuits.

Julius Axelrod's article tells us that neurotransmitters are chemicals that are released from nerve-cell endings and that cross the small gap between nerve cells (the synapse). Upon reaching the other side of the synapse, neurotransmitters are "recognized" and bound by receptors on the membrane of the postsynaptic nerve cell. This transaction somehow leads to a change in activity of the postsynaptic nerve cell. Thus, neurotransmitters serve as "messengers" between adjoining nerve cells. Axelrod, who won the Nobel Prize for his work, describes the criteria for calling a substance a neurotransmitter, enumerates the known (and putative) neurotransmitter substances, and details the mechanisms by which neurotransmitter systems regulate their own activity.

The article by James A. Nathanson and Paul Greengard illuminates precisely how a neurotransmitter from one nerve cell affects the activity of its neighbor. These authors present proof that the message carried by a neurotransmitter is translated by a "second messenger," cyclic AMP, within the postsynaptic nerve cell. An increase in the level of intracellular cyclic AMP, caused by a neurotransmitter, may then cause a change in the rate of protein synthesis that ultimately affects cell permeability to ions. A change in cell permeability to ions leads to a change in the electrical excitability of the cell.

With the introduction of the concepts of neurotransmission and "second messengers," we can piece together one way in which hormones and the nervous system are connected to form a circuit. A steroid hormone, produced by the ovary or testis, travels in the bloodstream and binds to intracellular receptors in a first set of nerve cells. This binding may ultimately change the rate of neurotransmitter synthesis and release. In turn, this change is relayed to a second set of nerve cells and is translated by cyclic AMP into an alteration in cellular activity. The second set of nerve cells relays this change in activity to a third set of nerve cells by means of neurotransmitters. The passing of information from one nerve cell to the next continues, and the information may eventually reach special nerve cells in the hypothalamus that produce releasing factors (see the article by Guillemin and Burgus in Section II).

Upon receiving appropriate neurotransmitter messages, these special hypothalamic cells may alter the rate of their production of releasing factors. The releasing factors then travel a short distance from the hypothalamus to the anterior pituitary. Here certain anterior putuitary cells have membrane receptors for particular releasing factors. The message is translated by "second messenger" cyclic AMP with a consequent alteration in the rate of production and release of protein hormones from the pituitary.

The pituitary hormones travel a long distance in the bloodstream to reach the ovaries or testis. Some cells of these glands contain specialized receptors on their membranes for appropriate pituitary hormones. The reception of a message from the pituitary is translated into a change in cyclic AMP production, and this is translated into an alteration in the rate of steroid hormone production. When the steroid hormone message reaches the brain, the circuit is complete.

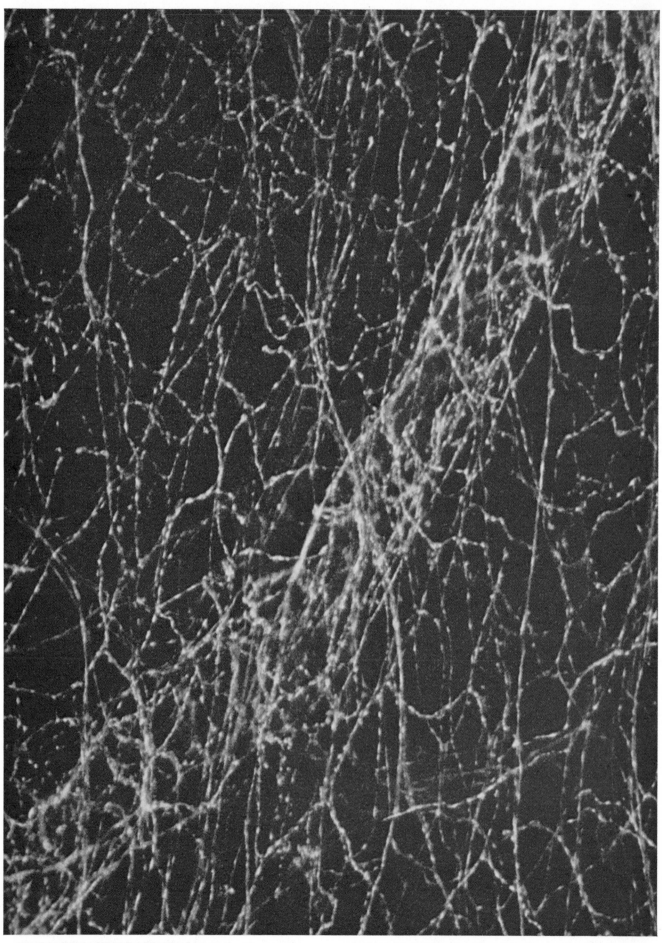

SYMPATHETIC-NERVE TERMINALS from the iris of a rat's eye emit a green glow after treatment with formaldehyde, showing that they contain noradrenaline, one of the neurotransmitters. The ter-

minals, studded with varicosities where the noradrenaline is stored, are enlarged 2,400 diameters in this fluorescence micrograph made by David Jacobowitz of the National Institute of Mental Health.

Neurotransmitters

by Julius Axelrod
June 1974

*These chemicals released from nerve-fiber endings
are the messengers by means of which nerve cells
communicate. Neurotransmitters mediate functions
ranging from muscle contraction to the control
of behavior*

In 1901 the noted English physiologist J. N. Langley observed that the injection of an extract of the adrenal gland into an animal stimulated tissues innervated by the sympathetic nerves: the nerves of the autonomic nervous system that increase the heart rate, raise the blood pressure and cause smooth muscles to contract. Just three years before that John J. Abel of Johns Hopkins University had isolated the hormone adrenaline from the adrenal gland, and so Langley's observation prompted T. R. Elliott, his student at the University of Cambridge, to inject adrenaline into experimental animals. Elliott saw that the hormone, like the crude extract, produced a response in a number of organs that was similar to the response evoked by the electrical stimulation of sympathetic nerves. He thereupon made the brilliant and germinal suggestion that adrenaline might be released from sympathetic nerves and then cause a response in muscle cells with which the nerves form junctions. Elliott thus first enunciated the concept of neural communication by means of chemical transmitters. A neurotransmitter is a chemical that is discharged from a nerve-fiber ending. It reaches and is recognized by a receptor on the surface of a postsynaptic nerve cell or other excitable postjunctional cell and either stimulates or inhibits the second cell. Today it is clear that many different neurotransmitters influence a variety of tissues and physiological processes. Neurotransmitters make the heart beat faster or slower and make muscles contract or relax. They cause glands to synthesize hormone-producing enzymes or to secrete hormones. And they are the agents through which the brain regulates movement and changes mood and behavior.

Elliott's concept of chemical neurotransmission was accepted slowly. Langley, who disliked theories of any kind, discouraged further speculation by Elliott until more facts were available. That took time. The first definite evidence for neurochemical transmission was obtained in 1921 by Otto Loewi, who was then working at the University of Graz in Austria, through an elegant and crucial experiment. Loewi put the heart of a frog in a bath in which the heart could be kept beating. The fluid bathing the heart was allowed to perfuse a second heart. When Loewi stimulated the first heart's vagus nerve (a nerve of the parasympathetic system that reduces the heart rate), the beat of the second heart was slowed, showing that some substance was liberated from the stimulated vagus nerve, was transported by the fluid and influenced the perfused heart. The substance was later identified by Sir Henry Dale as acetylcholine, one of the first neurotransmitters to be recognized. In a similar experiment the stimulation of the accelerans nerve (the sympathetic nerve that increases the heart rate) of a frog heart speeded up the beat of an unstimulated perfused heart. In 1946 the Swedish physiologist Ulf von Euler isolated the neurotransmitter of the sympathetic system and identified it as noradrenaline.

The Transmitters

To be classed as a neurotransmitter a chemical should fulfill a certain set of criteria. Nerves should have the enzymes required to produce the chemical; when nerves are stimulated, they should liberate the chemical, which should then react with a specific receptor on the postjunctional cell and produce a biological response; mechanisms should be available to terminate the actions of the chemical rapidly. On the basis of these criteria two compounds are now estab-lished as neurotransmitters: acetylcholine and noradrenaline. Nerves that contain them are respectively called cholinergic and noradrenergic nerves. There are a number of other nerve chemicals that meet many of the listed criteria but have not yet been shown to meet them all. These "putative" transmitters are dopamine, adrenaline, serotonin, octopamine, histamine, gamma aminobutyric acid, glutamic acid, aspartic acid and glycine.

This article will deal mainly with one class of neurotransmitters, the catecholamines, since more is known about these compounds than about some other transmitters and since many of the principles governing their disposition appear to govern those of transmitters in general. The catecholamines include noradrenaline (also known as norepinephrine), dopamine and adrenaline (or epinephrine). They have in common a chemical structure that consists of a benzene ring on which there are two adjacent hydroxyl groups and an ethylamine side chain. Noradrenaline is present in peripheral nerves, the brain and the spinal cord and in the medulla, or inner core, of the adrenal gland. In peripheral tissues and in the brain noradrenaline acts as a neurotransmitter, that is, it exerts most of its effect locally on postjunctional cells. In the adrenal medulla it functions as a hormone, that is, it is released into the bloodstream and acts on distant target organs. Dopamine, once thought to be simply an intermediate in the synthesis of noradrenaline and adrenaline, is also a neurotransmitter in its own right in the brain, where it functions in nerves that influence movement and behavior. The third catecholamine, adrenaline, is largely concentrated in the adrenal medulla. It is discharged into the bloodstream in fear, anger or other stress and acts as a hormone on a number of organs, including the heart, the liver and the intestines. Just in the past year it has developed that adrenaline is probably also a neurotransmitter, since it is found in nerves in the brain.

Techniques developed a decade ago in Sweden made it possible to visualize catecholamines in neurons directly, by the fluorescent glow they emit after treatment with formaldehyde vapor. Fluorescence photomicrography, electron microscopy and radioautography have revealed the structure and functioning of the sympathetic nerve cell in great detail [see illustration below]. The neuron has a cell body and a long axon, or main fiber, that branches into a large number of terminals. Each nerve ending is studded with varicosities, or swellings, that look like beads on a string, so that a single sympathetic neuron can innervate thousands of other cells: "effector" cells.

In 1960 Georg Hertting, Gordon Whitby and I were able to show that radioactive noradrenaline (noradrenaline in which tritium, the radioactive isotope of hydrogen, has been substituted for some of the hydrogen atoms) is taken up selectively and retained in sympathetic nerves. In my laboratory at the National Institute of Mental Health we went on to find out where the neurotransmitter is stored within the nerve cell. Electron

micrographs of sympathetic-neuron varicosities reveal large numbers of vesicles with dark, granular cores. When photographic film was exposed to tissues from rats injected with labeled noradrenaline, the silver grains developed by the radiation from the radioactive hydrogen atoms were strikingly localized over the granulated vesicles [see illustrations on opposite page]. This indicated that it is in those vesicles that noradrenaline is stored within the nerve.

Synthesis and Release

The process leading to the synthesis of catecholamine transmitters begins in the cell body, which has the machinery for making the four enzymes needed for their formation: tyrosine hydroxylase, dopa decarboxylase, dopamine beta-hydroxylase (DBH) and phenylethanolamine N-methyltransferase (PNMT). The enzymes synthesized in the cell body are carried down the axon by a natural flowing process to the nerve endings, where the synthesis of the catecholamines is achieved.

The discharge of neurotransmitter from the nerve endings caps a complex series of events. When a nerve is stimulated, its membrane is depolarized, with sodium moving into the nerve as potassium comes out; the nerve signal propa-

gates as a wave of depolarization that moves along the nerve axon to the endings. As Bernhard Katz of University College London first showed for acetylcholine, the depolarization causes a quantum—a packet or spurt, as it were—of the transmitter to be discharged from the nerve ending into the synaptic cleft.

Biochemical evidence recently obtained in our laboratory and others shows that noradrenaline is released from nerves in much the same way. The vesicles in the endings contain not only noradrenaline but also the enzyme, DBH, that converts dopamine into noradrenaline. When the sympathetic nerve is stimulated electrically, noradrenaline and the enzyme are released in about the same proportions in which they are present in the vesicles. The only way that could happen would be through the fusion of the vesicle with the outer membrane of the nerve, followed by the formation of an opening large enough to allow molecules of noradrenaline to be extruded along with the much larger molecules of the enzyme. Such a release mechanism is called exocytosis. The detailed events whereby the vesicle fuses with the neural membrane and makes an opening to discharge its soluble contents are uncertain, as is the subsequent fate of the vesicle. We do know that certain conditions prevent the release of noradrenaline and DBH. One is the presence of vinblastin, a compound that breaks down the protein structures in nerve cells called neurotubules. Another is the presence of cytocholasin-beta, a substance that disrupts the function of the contractile filament system in cells. A third is the absence of calcium. These findings suggest that the long, tubelike protein structures may orient the vesicles to a site on the neuronal membrane from which the release occurs. It is well known that microfilaments in cells other than nerves, such as muscle cells, can be activated by calcium so that they contract. It is therefore possible that depolarization causes calcium to activate a contractile filament on the neural membrane, which thereupon contracts to make an opening large enough so that the soluble contents of the vesicle can be discharged.

The observation that DBH is released from nerves suggested to Richard Weinshilboum, a research associate in my laboratory, that the enzyme might find its way into the bloodstream. We devised a sensitive assay for the enzyme and found it is indeed present in the blood, and we and others went on to measure the amount of the enzyme (which is found specifically in sympathetic nerves) in a

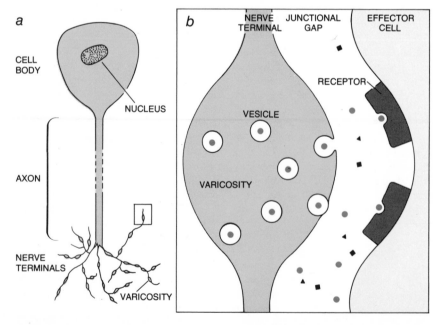

SYMPATHETIC NEURON, or nerve cell (a), consists of a cell body, a long axon and numerous nerve terminals studded with varicosities. Enzymes involved in the synthesis of the transmitters are made in the nucleus and transported down the axon to the varicosities, where the transmitters are manufactured and stored. A varicosity and its junction with another cell are enlarged (b). The transmitter (colored dots) is stored in vesicles. When the nerve is excited and depolarized, vesicles move to the cell membrane and fuse with it, releasing transmitter into the junctional gap. The transmitter reaches receptors on the effector cell that recognize only it, not any other chemicals (black shapes) that are present in the gap.

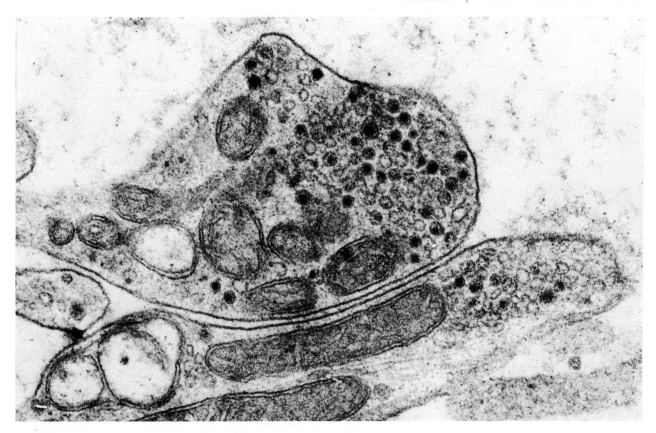

VARICOSITIES on noradrenaline-containing nerve endings from a rat pineal gland are enlarged 90,000 diameters in an electron mi- crograph made by Floyd Bloom of the National Institute of Mental Health. The varicosities contain vesicles, many with dense cores.

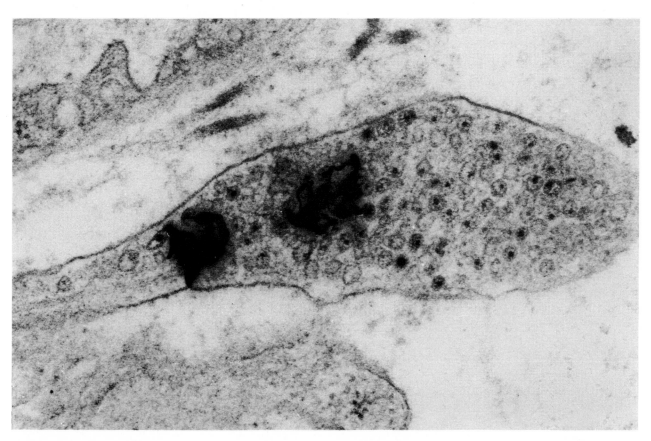

RADIOACTIVE NORADRENALINE is shown by radioautogra- phy to be localized in the vesicles. A pineal-tissue sample was tak- en from rats injected with labeled noradrenaline. The radioactivity developed silver grains (black blots) in a photographic film laid on the sample. The developed grains were strikingly localized over the vesicles, which were thus identified as sites of transmitter storage.

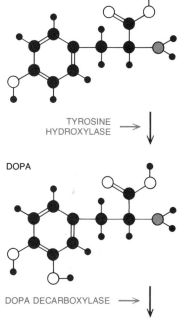

TYROSINE

TYROSINE
HYDROXYLASE →

DOPA

DOPA DECARBOXYLASE →

DOPAMINE

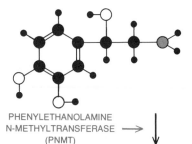

DOPAMINE
BETA-HYDROXYLASE
(DBH) →

NORADRENALINE

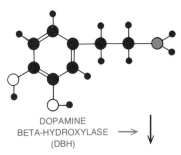

PHENYLETHANOLAMINE
N-METHYLTRANSFERASE →
(PNMT)

ADRENALINE

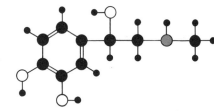

● HYDROGEN

○ OXYGEN

◉ NITROGEN

● CARBON

PRODUCTION of catecholamine transmitters is accomplished by four enzymes (*color*) in sympathetic-nerve terminals and in the adrenal gland. Tyrosine, an amino acid, is transformed into the intermediate dopa. Removal of a carboxyl (COOH) group forms dopamine, which is itself a transmitter and is also the precursor of the transmitter noradrenaline. In the adrenal gland the process continues with the addition of a methyl (CH_3) group to form adrenaline.

variety of disease states. It is low in the hereditary disorder of the autonomic system called familial dysautonomia and in Down's syndrome (mongolism), and it is high in torsion dystonia (a neurological disease involving muscle spasticity), in neuroblastoma (a cancer of nervous tissue) and in certain forms of hypertension. The findings suggest that in each of these diseases there are abnormalities in the functioning of the sympathetic nervous system.

Action and Inactivation

Once the neurortansmitter is liberated it diffuses across the cleft between the nerve terminal and adjacent cells. The capacity of a neighboring effector cell to respond to the transmitter then depends on the ability of a receptor on the postjunctional cell's surface to selectively recognize and combine with the neurotransmitter. When the receptor and transmitter interact, a series of events is triggered that causes the effector cell to carry out its special function. Some of these responses occur rapidly (in a fraction of a second), as in the propagation of nerve transmission across a synapse; others occur slowly, in minutes or sometimes hours, as in the synthesis of intracellular enzymes. There are two receptors that recognize noradrenaline, alpha and beta adrenergic receptors, and there is one for dopamine. These receptors can be distinguished from one another by the specific response each elicits and by the ability of specific drugs to block those responses.

The beta adrenergic receptors turn on an effector cell, and they do so by means of adenosine 3'5' monophosphate, or cyclic AMP, the universal "second messenger" that mediates between hormones and many cellular activities elicited by those hormones [see "Cyclic AMP," by Ira Pastan; SCIENTIFIC AMERICAN Offprint 1256]. Investigators have traced several of the steps in the activation of the receptor by noradrenaline by studying the interaction of noradrenaline and fat cells or cells of the liver or of the

pineal gland. We have found the pineal, which makes a hormone called melatonin that inhibits the activity of sex glands, particularly suitable because it is heavily supplied with nerves containing noradrenaline [see "The Pineal Gland," by Richard J. Wurtman and Julius Axelrod; SCIENTIFIC AMERICAN Offprint 1015]. Melatonin is synthesized in a number of steps, one of which, the conversion of serotonin to N-acetylserotonin, is catalyzed by the enzyme serotonin N-acetyltransferase. It is that enzyme's synthesis that is controlled by the beta adrenergic receptor. When noradrenaline is released from a nerve innervating the pineal, it interacts with beta adrenergic receptors on the outside of the membrane of a pineal cell. Once a receptor is occupied by noradrenaline, the enzyme adenylate cyclase, on the inner surface of the cell membrane, is activated. The adenylate cyclase then converts the cellular energy carrier ATP to cyclic AMP, which in turn stimulates the synthesis of serotonin N-acetyltransferase [*see illustration on opposite page*]. This complex series of events can be turned off by propranolol, a drug that prevents the noradrenaline from combining with the beta adrenergic receptor.

The adenylate cyclase system is involved in scores of biological actions. The ability of the pineal cell to carry out its special function, the manufacture of melatonin, by utilizing the almost universal adenylate-cyclase system depends on the presence of receptors on the cell surface that can specifically recognize noradrenaline and of the enzyme hydroxyindole-O-methyltransferase, uniquely present in the pineal cell, that can convert N-acetylserotonin to melatonin.

Once the neurotransmitter has interacted with the postjunctional cell, its actions must be rapidly terminated; otherwise it would exert its effects for too long and precise control would be lost. In the cholinergic nervous system the acetylcholine is rapidly inactivated by the enzyme acetylcholinesterase, which metabolizes the transmitter. In the past 10 years it has become clear that the inactivation of neurotransmitters through enzymatic transformation is the exception rather than the rule. Catecholamine neurotransmitters are metabolized by two enzymes, catechol-O-methyltransferase (COMT) and monoamine oxidase (MAO); the latter is a particularly important enzyme that removes the amino (NH_2) group of a wide variety of compounds, including serotonin, noradrenaline, dopamine and adrenaline. There are enzyme-inhibiting chemicals that

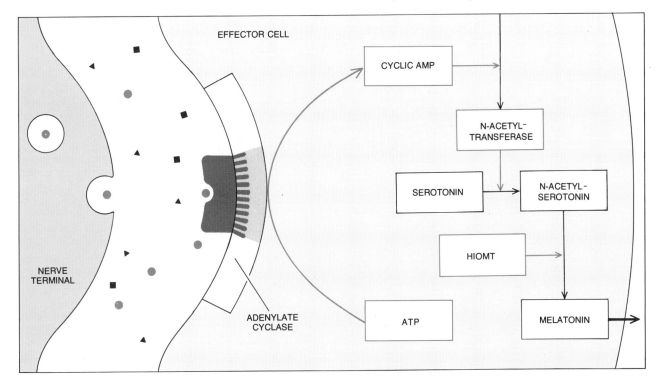

MODE OF ACTION of a transmitter is exemplified by the effect of noradrenaline on a pineal cell. Noradrenaline (*colored dots*) released from a nerve ending binds to a beta-adrenergic receptor on the pineal-cell surface. The receptor thereupon activates the enzyme adenylate cyclase on the inside of the pineal-cell membrane. The activated adenylate cyclase catalyzes the conversion of adeno-sine triphosphate (ATP) into cyclic adenosine monophosphate (AMP). The cyclic AMP stimulates synthesis of the enzyme N-acetyltransferase; the enzyme converts serotonin into N-acetyl-serotonin. This is transformed in turn by the pineal cell's specific enzyme, hydroxyindole-O-methyltransferase (HIOMT), to form melatonin, the pineal-gland hormone that acts on the sex glands.

can prevent COMT and MAO from carrying out their biochemical transformations; when such inhibitors were administered, the action of noradrenaline was found still to be rapidly terminated. There had to be a method of rapid inactivation other than enzymatic transformation.

In order to track down such a mechanism we injected a cat with radioactive noradrenaline. The labeled transmitter persisted in tissues that were rich in sympathetic nerves for many hours, long after its physiological actions were ended, indicating that radioactive noradrenaline was taken up in the sympathetic nerves and held there. My colleagues and I designed a simple experiment to prove this. Sympathetic nerves innervating the left salivary gland in rats were destroyed by removing the superior cervical ganglion on the left side of the neck; about seven days after this operation the noradrenaline nerves of the salivary gland on the right side were intact, whereas the nerves on the left side had completely disappeared. When radioactive noradrenaline was injected, the transmitter was found in the right salivary gland but not in the left one. We also found that in cats injected with radioactive noradrenaline the transmitter was re-leased when the sympathetic nerves were stimulated electrically. The experiments clearly demonstrated that noradrenaline is taken up into, as well as released from, sympathetic nerves. As a result of these experiments we postulated that noradrenaline is rapidly inactivated through its recapture by the sympathetic nerves; once it is back in the nerves, of course, the neurotransmitter cannot exert its effect on postjunctional cells. Leslie L. Iversen of the University of Cambridge has since shown that this neuronal recapture by sympathetic nerves is highly selective for noradrenaline or compounds resembling it in chemical structure. Recent work indicates that uptake by nerves may be the most general mechanism for the inactivation of neurotransmitters.

Regulation

Chemical transmitters in sympathetic nerves (and presumably in other nerves) are in a state of flux, continually being synthesized, released, metabolized and recaptured. The activity of nerves can also undergo marked fluctuation during periods of stress. In spite of all these dynamic changes the amount of catecholamines in tissues remains constant. This is owing to a variety of adaptive mechanisms that alter the formation, release and response of catecholamines. There are fast regulatory changes that require only fractions of a second and slower changes that take place after minutes or even hours.

When sympathetic nerves are stimulated, the conversion of tyrosine to noradrenaline in them is rapidly increased. The increased nervous activity specifically affects tyrosine hydroxylase, the enzyme that converts tyrosine to dopa, because its activity is inhibited by noradrenaline and dopamine. Any increase in nerve-firing brought on by stress, cold and certain drugs lowers the level of catecholamines in the nerve terminals. This reduces the negative-feedback effect of noradrenaline and dopamine on tyrosine hydroxylase, so that more tyrosine is converted to dopa, which in turn is converted to make more catecholamines. Conversely, when nerve activity is decreased, the catecholamine level rises, slowing down the conversion of tyrosine to dopa by once again inhibiting the tyrosine hydroxylase.

Another rapid regulation is accomplished at the nerve terminal itself, where the alpha adrenergic receptors are situated. When the alpha receptors are activated, they diminish the release of noradrenaline from nerve terminals into the synaptic cleft. When too much noradrenaline is released, it accumulates in the synaptic cleft; when the catecholamine level is high enough, it activates the alpha receptors on the presynaptic nerve terminals and shuts off further release of the neurotransmitter.

A slower regulatory process is brought on by prolonged firing of sympathetic nerves, which can step up the manufacture of the catecholamine-synthesizing enzymes tyrosine hydroxylase, DBH and (to a lesser extent) PNMT; the rise in the enzyme level enables the nerves to make more neurotransmitter. We discovered this phenomenon of increased enzyme synthesis when we gave animals reserpine, a versatile drug that lowers the blood pressure and incidentally increases sympathetic-nerve firing (which tends to raise the pressure) by a reflex action. The reserpine brought about a gradual increase in tyrosine hydroxylase and DBH in sympathetic nerves and the adrenal gland and of PNMT in the adrenal gland. Increases in these enzymes were also found in animals exposed to stress, cold, physical restraint, psychosocial stimulation or insulin injection. When the synthesis of proteins was prevented by drugs, on the other hand,

there was no elevation in enzyme activity after reserpine was given. This indicated that increased nerve activity stimulates the synthesis of new molecules of tyrosine hydroxylase, DBH and PNMT; with a greater need for neurotransmitters there is a compensatory increase in the synthesis of enzymes that catalyze the making of these transmitters.

In order to learn whether the command for increased synthesis of new tyrosine hydroxylase and DBH molecules can be transmitted from one nerve to another we cut the nerve innervating certain noradrenaline cell bodies—the superior cervical ganglia—on one side. When nerves were then stimulated reflexly by reserpine, there was an elevation of tyrosine hydroxylase and DBH levels in the innervated ganglia but not in the denervated ones. The experiment showed that one nerve can transmit information to another nerve (presumably by means of a chemical signal) that causes the postsynaptic nerve to make new enzyme molecules.

Sensitivity

In 1855 the German physiologist J. L. Budge observed that when the nerves leading to a rabbit's right eye were destroyed, the pupil of that eye became

more dilated than the left pupil. The phenomenon was later explained by the American physiologist Walter B. Cannon, who postulated that as a result of denervation the effector cells somehow become more responsive. He called this effect the "law of denervation supersensitivity." Subsequent work showed that denervation supersensitivity is caused by two separate mechanisms, one presynaptic and the other postsynaptic. When nerves are destroyed, presynaptic inactivation by recapture is abolished, thereby leaving the neurotransmitters to react with the postsynaptic site longer.

Denervation also causes a profound change in the degree of activity of the postjunctional cell. Recent work with the pineal gland in our laboratory has suggested a hypothesis for supersensitivity, and also for subsensitivity, in postjunctional cells. As we have seen, noradrenaline stimulates the synthesis of the enzyme serotonin N-acetyltransferase through a beta adrenergic receptor in the postjunctional pineal cell. When the nerves to pineal cells are destroyed (or depleted of noradrenaline by the administration of reserpine), the pineal cells become 10 times as responsive to noradrenaline; that is, when the postjunctional cell is deprived of its neurotransmitter for a period of time, it takes just

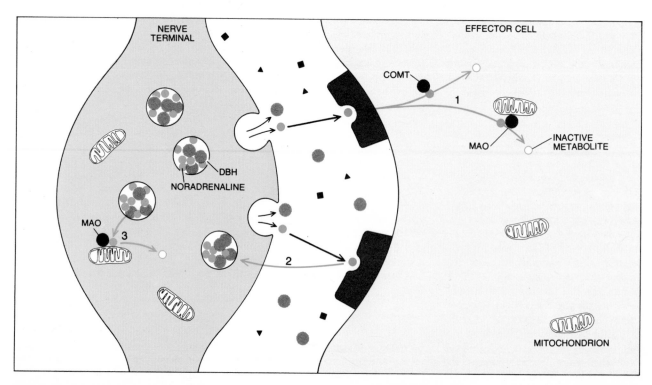

RELEASE AND INACTIVATION of the neurotransmitter noradrenaline is shown in more detail. The enzyme DBH is stored in the noradrenergic nerve terminals along with the transmitter and is released with it into the junctional gap. The noradrenaline binds to the receptors on the effector cell, eliciting that cell's response as shown in the illustration on the preceding page. Then the norad-

renaline's action is terminated either through metabolism (1) by the enzymes catechol-O-methyltransferase (COMT) and/or monoamine oxidase (MAO), or by recapture and storage (2) in the presynaptic sympathetic-nerve terminal; the latter is the more important process. MAO, stored in the membrane of mitochondria, also inactivates noradrenaline that leaks out of vesicles (3).

one packet of catecholamines to cause the same increase of N-acetyltransferase in the cell as 10 packets of transmitters would cause in a normally innervated cell. If, on the other hand, the pineal cell is exposed to an excessive amount of catecholamines for a period of time, it becomes less responsive: a larger amount of the transmitter is required to produce the same increase in N-acetyltransferase.

These experiments suggest that changes in the responsiveness of excitable cells are the result of an alteration in the "avidity" with which the receptor binds the neurotransmitters. If the receptor is exposed to small amounts of catecholamine for some time, it reacts with the neurotransmitter easily; if too many neurotransmitter molecules bombard the receptor, it becomes less responsive. Depending on the tissue, this change in sensitivity can come within hours or days, so that it is an effective adaptive mechanism for excitable cells. It is possible that the tolerance that is often developed to a drug taken in excess may reflect subsensitivity on the part of cells that respond to the drug.

Role in the Brain

The brain has billions of nerves that talk to one another by means of neurotransmitters. Neurobiologists are just beginning to unravel the complex biochemistry and physiology of chemical transmission in the brain. Many different neurotransmitters function in brain neurons, but because there are more precise methods of measuring catecholamines and drugs are available that perturb their formation, storage, release and metabolism, we know more about brain catecholamines than about the other neurotransmitters. Fluorescence photomicrography and drugs that selectively destroy catecholamine-containing nerves have made it possible to locate the noradrenaline, dopamine and serotonin cell bodies and trace the pathways of their axons and nerve endings [see illustrations on page 129]. The cell bodies of the dopamine-containing nerves are in the area of the brain stem called the substantia nigra, whence the dopaminergic axons course through the brain stem, many of them terminating in the caudate nucleus. The dopamine-containing tracts in the caudate nucleus play an important role in the integration of movement.

The elucidation of the biochemistry and pharmacology of dopamine in the brain has led to the development of a powerful treatment of a crippling disease, Parkinsonism. The Swedish pharmacologist Arvid Carlsson noted in 1959

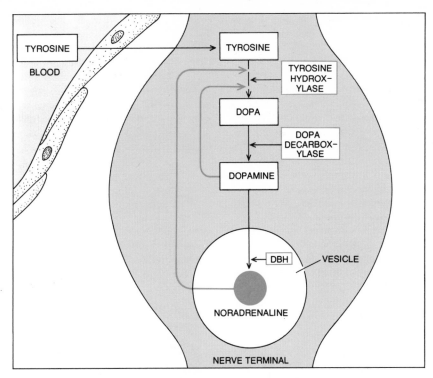

RAPID REGULATION of catecholamine synthesis is accomplished by a feedback mechanism: a buildup of dopamine and noradrenaline inhibits (*colored arrows*) the activity of tyrosine hydroxylase, which catalyzes the first step in the synthesis. An increase in nerve activity reduces the amount of dopamine and noradrenaline in the terminal, removing the inhibition; tyrosine hydroxylase activity increases and more transmitter is synthesized.

that when reserpine was given to rats, it sharply reduced the dopamine content of the caudate nucleus in the brain and also caused a Parkinson-like tremor. The administration of dopa, a dopamine precursor that can get from the blood into the brain more easily than dopamine, reversed the tremors. These findings prompted Oleh Hornykiewicz, who was then working at the University of Vienna, to measure the content of dopamine in the brain of patients who had died of Parkinson's disease. He found that there was virtually no dopamine in the caudate nucleus. The finding led directly to a major therapeutic advance by George C. Cotzias of the Brookhaven National Laboratory: when dopa, the dopamine precursor that can cross the blood-brain barrier, is administered, it makes up the dopamine deficiency and effectively relieves the symptoms of Parkinson's disease. This is a good example of how basic research can sometimes lead rapidly to a new treatment for a disease.

There are two main nerve tracts containing noradrenaline in the brain, the dorsal and ventral pathways. The cell bodies of the noradrenaline-containing tracts are found in the lower part of the brain in the area called the locus ceruleus, or "blue place." Noradrenaline-containing nerve tracts are highly branched

and reach many parts of the brain. Among the areas they innervate are the cerebellum and the cerebral cortex, which are concerned with the fine coordination of movement, alertness and emotion. Another part of the brain innervated by noradrenaline neurons is the hypothalamus, which controls many visceral functions of the body such as hunger, thirst, temperature regulation, blood pressure, reproduction and behavior. Manipulation of the noradrenaline levels in the brain can change many of the functions of the hypothalamus, particularly the "pleasure" centers. Noradrenaline tracts also appear to be involved in mood elevation and depression. Recently nerves containing adrenaline have also been observed in the brain stem. The next few years should show whether these adrenaline-containing tracts also control emotion, mood and behavior.

Drugs have been powerful tools for probing the action of neurotransmitters. As our knowledge concerning neurotransmitters has broadened, so has our understanding of the action of drugs on behavior and on the cardiovascular and motor systems; the two trends have interacted nicely. In the early 1950's pharmacologists recognized that the hallucinogenic agent lysergic acid diethylamine (LSD) not only resembles serotonin in chemical structure but also counteracts some of its pharmacologic actions (by occupying sites intended for serotonin). Several workers therefore proposed that serotonin must have something to do with insanity. Other hallucinogenic agents such as mescaline and amphetamine, on the other hand, are related in structure to noradrenaline. In the mid-1950's clinical investigators were learning that chemicals such as chlorpromazine could mitigate psychotic behavior, and that monoamine oxidase inhibitors and imipramine and related drugs could relieve depression. At about the same time it was observed that reserpine, which was proving valuable not only for hypertension but also for schizophrenia, markedly reduced the levels of noradrenaline and serotonin in the brain. The observations combined to suggest that these drugs exerted their actions on the brain by interfering with neurotransmitters. When my colleagues and I found that radioactive noradrenaline can be taken up and released from nerves, we were in a good position to investigate how a drug influences the disposition of injected radioactive transmitters.

Effect of Drugs

The first compound we examined was cocaine, a potent stimulant that can produce psychosis and that also intensifies the action of noradrenaline. When radioactive noradrenaline was injected into cats that had been given cocaine, the uptake of catecholamines by the sympathetic nerves was prevented, demonstrating that cocaine magnifies the effect of noradrenaline by preventing its capture and inactivation and leaving larger amounts of the catecholamine to react with the effector cell. Antidepressant drugs such as imipramine had the same effect: they blocked the uptake of noradrenaline into sympathetic nerves. By using radioactive noradrenaline we found that amphetamine, which is both a stimulant and a mind-altering drug, affects noradrenergic nerves in two ways: it blocks the uptake of noradrenaline and also promotes the release of the neurotransmitter from nerves.

Many drugs that are effective in the treatment of hypertension affect the

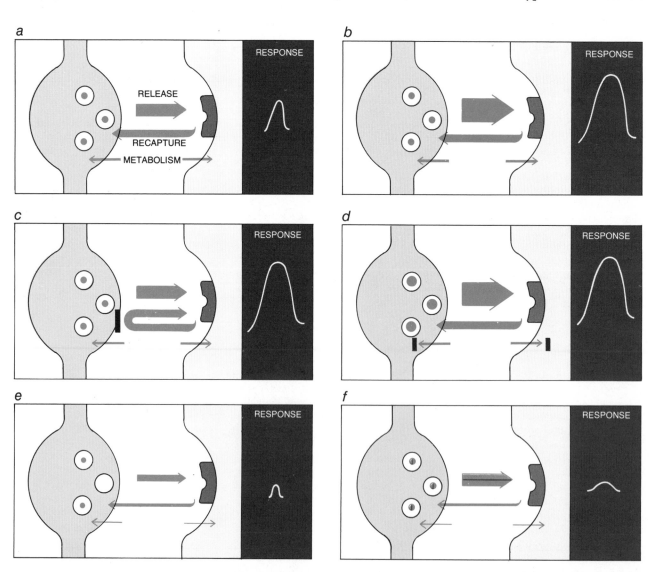

CERTAIN ADRENERGIC DRUGS increase or decrease the availability of noradrenaline at the adrenergic receptor. Normal release, recapture and metabolism (*colored arrows*) are illustrated, with a curve representing the normal response of a postjunctional cell (*a*). Antidepressant drugs enlarge that response in several ways, all of which increase the availability of noradrenaline at the synapse. Amphetamine does so by promoting the release of noradrenaline (*b*). Amphetamine and imipramine and related drugs block recapture (*c*); the monoamine-oxidase inhibitors interfere with inactivation through metabolism (*d*). Conversely, reserpine, which reduces blood pressure and may induce depression, reduces the response by depleting the noradrenaline in storage (*e*); alphamethyldopa and other "false transmitters" are stored in the vesicles with noradrenaline and released with it, diluting its effect (*f*).

storage and release of noradrenergic transmitters. Reserpine and guanethidine reduce blood pressure by preventing the nerves that raise the pressure from storing noradrenaline. Antihypertensive drugs such as alpha methyl dopa, on the other hand, are transformed by enzymes in the nerve into substances that resemble the noradrenaline chemically. The "false transmitters" are stored and released along with natural neurotransmitters, diluting them and thus reducing their effect.

In the past 10 years many psychiatrists and pharmacologists have been struck by the fact that drugs that relieve mental depression also interfere with the uptake, storage, release or metabolism of noradrenaline. Whereas imipramine blocks the uptake of noradrenaline by nerves and amphetamine both releases noradrenaline and blocks its uptake, monoamine oxidase inhibitors, as their name implies, prevent the metabolism of the catecholamine. In other words, all these antidepressants produce similar results by different mechanisms: they increase the amount of catecholamine in the synaptic cleft, with the result that more transmitter is available to stimulate the receptor. Conversely, reserpine, a compound that decreases the amount of the chemical transmitters, sometimes produces depression. These considerations led to the proposal of a catecholamine hypothesis of depressive states, which holds that mental depression is associated with the decreased availability of brain catecholamine and is relieved by drugs that increase the amount of these transmitters at the adrenergic receptor. Although the hypothesis is not yet entirely substantiated, it has provided a valuable framework within which new approaches to understanding depression can be sought.

The introduction in the 1950's of antipsychotic drugs such as chlorpromazine and haloperidol revolutionized the treatment of schizophrenia, dramatically reducing the stay of schizophrenics in mental hospitals and saving many billions of dollars in hospital care. Research in the past decade has shown that antipsychotic drugs also exert their effect on the catecholamine neurotransmitters. Carlsson had observed that antischizophrenic drugs caused an increase in the formation of catecholamines in the rat brain, and he formed the hypothesis that this was owing to the drug's ability to block dopamine receptors. Work by other investigators has confirmed and extended this hypothesis. Antipsychotic drugs do block dopamine receptors in the brain, and there is a strong associa-

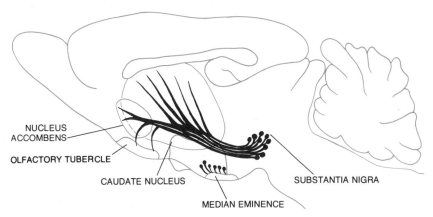

DOPAMINE TRACTS, the main bundles of nerves containing dopamine, are shown (*black*) in a drawing of a longitudinal section along the midline of the rat brain. The cell bodies are concentrated in the substantia nigra, and the axons project primarily to the caudate nucleus. A dopamine deficiency in that region causes Parkinsonism, which can be treated with dopa.

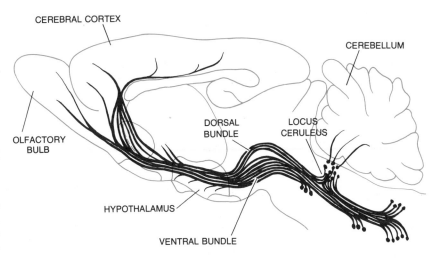

NORADRENALINE TRACTS arise primarily in the locus ceruleus and reach many brain centers, including the cerebellum, cerebral cortex and hypothalamus. Illustrations on this page are based on maps made by Urban Ungerstedt of Royal Caroline Institute in Sweden.

tion between the blocking ability of various drugs and their capacity to relieve schizophrenic symptoms. These findings point clearly to the involvement of the dopaminergic nerves in schizophrenia.

Amphetamine has also helped to clarify the nature of schizophrenia. Taken repeatedly in large amounts, amphetamine produces a psychosis manifested by repetitive and compulsive behavior and hallucinogenic delusions that are indistinguishable from the symptoms exhibited by paranoid schizophrenics. Amphetamine releases catecholamines from nerves in the brain to stimulate both noradrenergic and dopamine receptors. After doing experiments with two forms of amphetamine Solomon H. Snyder of the Johns Hopkins University Medical School hypothesized that the schizophrenia-like psychosis the drug induces is due to excessive release of dopamine.

The ability of antischizophrenia drugs, which block dopamine receptors, to relieve symptoms of amphetamine psychosis is consistent with this hypothesis.

Although there have been rapid advances in our knowledge of neurotransmitters in the past 20 years, much remains to be discovered about these compounds. Only a few of the chemical transmitters of the brain neurons have even been characterized. The role of neurotransmitters in behavior, mood, reproduction and learning and in diseases such as depression, schizophrenia, motor disorders and hypertension is beginning to evolve. If only the present trend toward reducing the funds committed to research support can be reversed, exciting new discoveries about neurotransmitters should soon be made, many of which will surely contribute directly toward the treatment or cure of some of man's most tragic afflictions.

13

"Second Messengers" in the Brain

by James A. Nathanson and Paul Greengard
August 1977

Nerve cells communicate by secreting neurotransmitters. These chemical messages are translated by second messengers within the cell into transient and longer-lasting physiological actions

For a multicellular organism to survive and function effectively its component cells must act in a coordinated fashion. Such coordination necessitates the transfer of information between cells in widely separated parts of the organism, and in most higher animals there are two major pathways of intercellular communication: the endocrine system and the nervous system. In the endocrine system specialized cells secrete hormones, which are carried in the bloodstream to distant parts of the body and influence the activity of specifically responsive target cells. In the nervous system a network of nerve cells with elongated processes communicate with one another by secreting neurotransmitters, which traverse the tiny gap between two nerve cells and produce a change in the electrical activity of the receiving cell.

Both systems involve messenger molecules that are released from one cell, travel a certain distance and interact with the surface of a second cell to modify its activity. In view of this similarity and assuming that nature functions economically one can postulate that some types of chemical transmission between nerve cells might be mediated by mechanisms similar to those mediating the physiological effects of certain hormones. This point of view has led to new perceptions of the biochemical organization of the brain and the mechanism of action of many drugs that affect behavior.

To provide background for a discussion of the molecular mechanisms of nerve transmission, let us first review some current concepts of the mechanism of hormone action. Hormones regulate an enormous range of biochemical processes in their target cells by influencing the rate at which enzymes and other proteins are manufactured, by affecting the activity of enzymes in key metabolic pathways or by altering the permeability of cell membranes. Because these processes operate in the interior of the target cell, the hormone itself or the information conveyed by it must somehow be made available inside the cell.

The delivery of a hormonal message to the interior of the cell appears to be achieved in one of two ways. Steroid hormones, which are derived from cholesterol, are easily soluble in fat and hence can pass through the fatty outer membrane of the target cell and directly influence processes inside it. Hormones of this type include cortisone and the sex hormones estradiol and testosterone. Peptide and amino-acid-derived hormones such as insulin and adrenalin (epinephrine), however, are not able to penetrate the cell membrane because of their size or molecular structure. Instead they attach themselves to specialized receptor sites on the surface of the cell and influence the biochemical machinery from the outside.

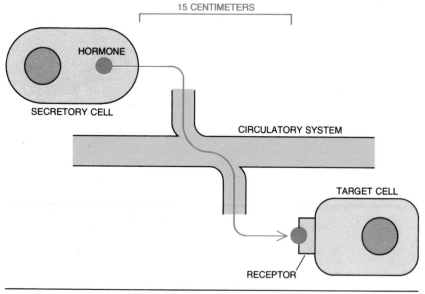

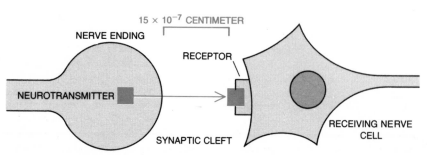

ANALOGOUS MECHANISMS underlie communication in the endocrine system (*top*) and the nervous system (*bottom*). In both chemical messengers (respectively hormones and neurotransmitters) are released from one cell, travel through the extracellular medium and bind to receptors on the surface of a second cell to modify its activity. The intracellular effects of many hormones and neurotransmitters appear to be mediated by the second-messenger cyclic AMP.

The hormone receptors—large protein molecules embedded in the cell membrane—are quite selective in their ability to bind the hormone for which they were designed, presumably because the molecular configuration of the receptor allows the hormone molecule to fit the receptor quite precisely. The forces that hold the hormone to the receptor are not the covalent ones that bind the atoms in a molecule; they are weaker forces that soon release the hormone, leaving the receptor free to accept additional molecules of the same hormone. Thus the extent to which a hormone influences its target cell depends on the concentration of the hormone in the fluid outside the cell and the affinity of the hormone for the membrane receptor.

Once a hormone has bound to a receptor, how does it convey its message to the interior of the cell? Earl W. Sutherland and his colleagues at Case Western Reserve University first addressed this question some 20 years ago. At that time they were studying the mechanism by which the hormone adrenalin causes liver cells to release the sugar glucose into the bloodstream when the body is under stress. The released glucose comes from the breakdown of glycogen (animal starch), which is held in reserve by the liver. Sutherland and his colleague Theodore W. Rall found that when they exposed to adrenalin cell membranes isolated from liver cells, an unidentified factor was produced that, when it was mixed with the cytoplasm of the liver cells, mimicked the action of adrenalin in causing the conversion of glycogen to glucose. Hence it seemed that the response to the hormone had at least two stages: the interaction of the

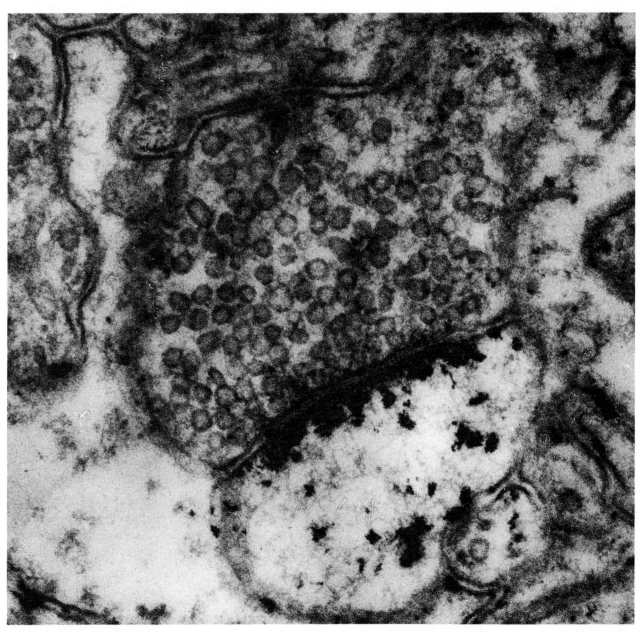

SECOND-MESSENGER FUNCTION of cyclic AMP in nerve-cell communication is suggested by the localization of phosphodiesterase, the enzyme that degrades cyclic AMP, at the synaptic junction between two nerve cells where chemical transmission occurs. Noel T. Florendo and Russell J. Barrnett, in collaboration with the authors at the Yale University School of Medicine, localized the enzyme by applying chemicals to brain tissue that reacted with the enzyme's product to form a dense precipitate. They then examined the tissue in the electron microscope. In the micrograph of a single synaptic junction shown here, the precipitate marking the location of phosphodiesterase is associated with the region of the receiving cell membrane possessing neurotransmitter receptors. This finding supports the hypothesis that the neurotransmitter molecules released from the circular vesicles in the nerve terminal (*top*) bind to the receptors and induce the manufacture of cyclic AMP, which then mediates a variety of actions inside the cell. Magnification is 138,000 diameters.

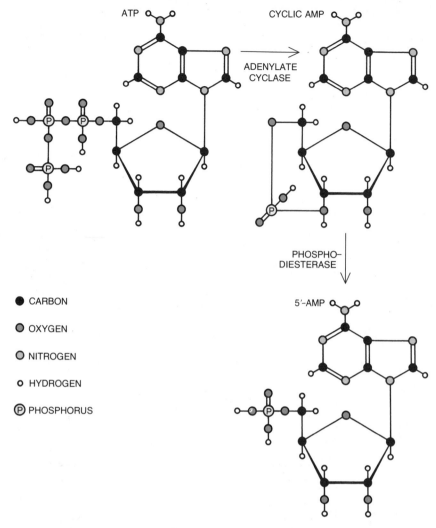

- ● CARBON
- ◉ OXYGEN
- ◎ NITROGEN
- ○ HYDROGEN
- Ⓟ PHOSPHORUS

SYNTHESIS AND DEGRADATION of cyclic AMP are accomplished by two enzymes associated with the outer membrane of certain hormone-sensitive or neurotransmitter-sensitive cells. Adenylate cyclase converts the energy-carrier adenosine triphosphate (ATP) into cyclic AMP by removing two phosphate groups from the molecule and joining the remaining phosphate with the molecule's carbon backbone to form a ring. Phosphodiesterase inactivates cyclic AMP by opening the phosphate ring, converting the molecule into an inert form of AMP.

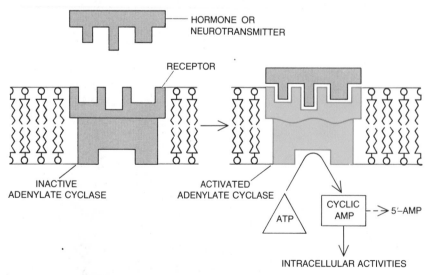

ADENYLATE CYCLASE IS ACTIVATED by the binding of a hormone or a neurotransmitter to its receptor on the cell membrane. The enzyme then converts some of the ATP in the cytoplasm into cyclic AMP, which relays the signal from the membrane to interior of the cell.

hormone with the membrane to form the unidentified factor, followed by the factor's activation of the biochemical mechanism in the cytoplasm.

Subsequent experiments identified the factor as cyclic adenosine monophosphate (cyclic AMP), one of the class of small molecules called nucleotides. It is related in structure to adenosine triphosphate (ATP), the universal currency of chemical energy in the cell. The "cyclic" in cyclic AMP refers to the fact that the single phosphate group (PO_4) in the molecule forms a ring with the carbon atoms to which it is attached.

Sutherland and his co-workers soon found that the membranes of liver cells (and many other cells) contain an enzyme, adenylate cyclase, that converts ATP into cyclic AMP. Because ATP is located almost exclusively in the cytoplasm, Sutherland and his colleagues G. Alan Robison and Reginald W. Butcher reasoned that at least part of the adenylate cyclase molecule must face inward and that the cyclic AMP manufactured by the enzyme is released into the interior of the cell. When they exposed liver cells to adrenalin, the rate at which adenylate cyclase converted ATP into cyclic AMP was substantially increased, indicating that there was a functional link between the binding of hormone to the receptor on the outside of the membrane and the activation of adenylate cyclase on the inside. Such a connection was subsequently shown to exist for a wide variety of hormones that bind to membrane receptors, although since different kinds of cells possess receptors for different hormones, a given hormone will increase the level of cyclic AMP in its target cells but not in other cells.

It is now generally accepted that the cyclic AMP generated by adenylate cyclase in response to the binding of a hormone to the receptor acts as a "second messenger" to relay the message of the hormone (the first messenger) from the membrane to the cell's biochemical machinery. In this way the low-level signal represented by the hormone can be amplified many thousands of times by the manufacture of cyclic AMP.

Up to this point we have discussed the interactions among hormones, receptors and cyclic AMP in cells outside the nervous system. Can analogous mechanisms help to explain how nerve cells communicate? The nerve cell, or neuron, is the basic structural and functional unit of the central nervous system; behavior is the net result of the complex interaction of many nerve cells. Information is conveyed along the elongated fiber of a neuron in the form of an electrochemical impulse. The impulse stops, however, when it reaches the tiny synapse, or gap, that separates the fiber terminal from its receiving neuron. To bridge the synapse and reinitiate electrochemical transmission, neurotransmitter is released and travels across the gap between one cell and the next. Like the hormones we have been discussing, neurotransmitters do not enter the receiving cell but interact with receptors on the outside of the cell membrane, leading to a change in the electric potential across the membrane.

The first connection between cyclic AMP and brain function was made when Sutherland and his co-workers found a large amount of the enzyme adenylate cyclase in the brain of vertebrate animals, indicating that cyclic AMP was being actively manufactured there. In 1967 Eduardo De Robertis, working in collaboration with Butcher and Sutherland, found that when brain tissue was disrupted by homogenization and the resulting subcellular components were separated according to their density by spinning them in a centrifuge, those fractions containing the largest amount of pinched-off nerve endings also showed the highest level of adenylate cyclase activity. This finding was interesting because many of the nerve-ending particles include fragments of membrane from both sides of the synaptic junction and hence represent the precise areas of the brain where nerve cells communicate. The fact that adenylate cyclase was specifically associated with those areas suggested that cyclic AMP might somehow be involved in synaptic transmission.

In the same experiments it was found that the nerve-ending particles also contained high levels of phosphodiesterase, an enzyme that degrades cyclic AMP into a physiologically inactive form of adenosine monophosphate. Somewhat later Noel T. Florendo and Russell J. Barrnett, working in collaboration with our laboratory at the Yale University School of Medicine, developed a cytochemical procedure to determine the location of phosphodiesterase within individual cells with the aid of the electron microscope. Using this technique, they demonstrated that the phosphodiesterase activity in the synaptic region was localized in the part of the membrane of the receiving cell thought to possess neurotransmitter receptors. This localization further suggested a role for cyclic AMP in synaptic transmission, since phosphodiesterase at the postsynaptic site would have access to, and hence be able to degrade, cyclic AMP that had been synthesized as a result of the stimulation of adenylate cyclase by a neurotransmitter.

At about this time several experiments demonstrated that electrical or neurotransmitter-induced stimulation of nerve tissue could result in large increases in cyclic AMP. In our laboratory Donald A. McAfee and Michel Schorderet, working with a sympathetic-nervous-system ganglion from the neck of rabbits and cattle, showed that electrical stimulation of the nerves innervating the ganglion, resulting in synaptic transmission, was associated with an elevation in cyclic AMP levels. McAfee and John W. Kebabian then showed that the application of the neurotransmitter dopamine to these ganglia mimicked the effect of electrical stimulation in elevating cyclic AMP levels, and conversely that the application of cyclic AMP could reproduce some of the electrophysiological effects of dopamine. Meanwhile Shiro Kakiuchi and Rall at Case Western Reserve, and somewhat later John W. Daly and his co-workers at the National Institute of Arthritis, Metabolism, and Digestive Diseases, reported that chopped pieces of brain tissue show large increases in cyclic AMP content when they are exposed to solutions containing various neurotransmitters such as norepinephrine or histamine.

Although all these experiments indi-

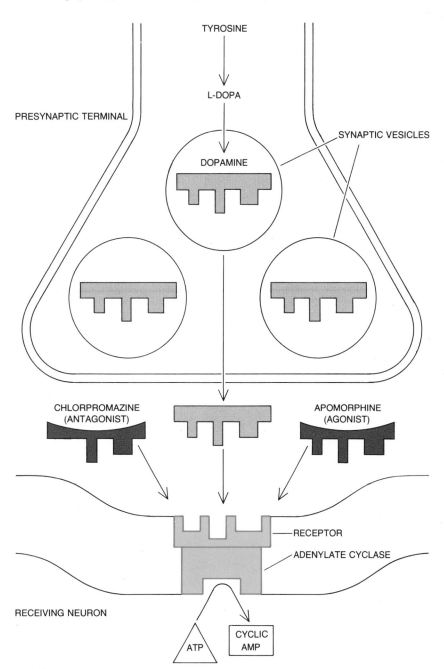

DOPAMINE-SENSITIVE ADENYLATE CYCLASE mediates the postsynaptic effects of the neurotransmitter dopamine and is the site of action of certain drugs that affect behavior. In this illustration dopamine released by the activity of presynaptic nerve terminals traverses the synaptic space and binds to a postsynaptic dopamine receptor, resulting in the activation of adenylate cyclase and the synthesis of cyclic AMP within the postsynaptic cell. The activity of the dopamine-sensitive adenylate cyclase is influenced by drugs known to bind specifically to dopamine receptors. Antagonist drugs such as the antischizophrenic agent chlorpromazine (Thorazine) block the receptor and prevent its activation by dopamine. Agonist drugs such as apomorphine, on the other hand, mimic the action of dopamine by activating the receptor.

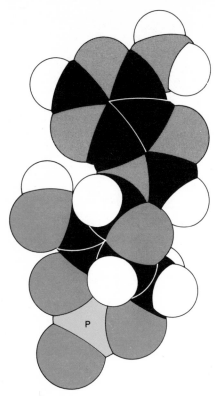

● CARBON

◉ OXYGEN

◉ NITROGEN

○ HYDROGEN

Ⓟ PHOSPHORUS

SPACE-FILLING MODEL of cyclic AMP shows that the molecule is compact. It consists of a five-carbon sugar to which are attached an adenine ring (*top*) and a phosphate group.

cated that there was some kind of association between neurotransmitter receptors and cyclic AMP levels, they left unanswered the question of whether the effects of any particular neurotransmitter were coupled directly to the activation of adenylate cyclase. In order to prove a functional link between the binding of a particular neurotransmitter to its receptor and the subsequent synthesis of cyclic AMP it was necessary to demonstrate the presence of a specific neurotransmitter-sensitive adenylate cyclase, that is, an enzyme whose activity is largely dependent on the presence of a particular neurotransmitter. Before describing this enzyme in more detail it is worth discussing briefly how a neurotransmitter receptor is linked to the action of drugs that affect behavior.

Since nerve cells communicate primarily by releasing neurotransmitters at synaptic junctions, it follows that anything that interferes with the binding of a neurotransmitter to its receptor will disrupt normal nerve-cell communication and thereby alter behavior. Such interference can be produced by foreign

substances, for example drugs, that have been introduced into the bloodstream. If a particular drug has a molecular configuration similar to that of a native neurotransmitter, it may be able to bind to the membrane receptor for that neurotransmitter and mimic the neurotransmitter's action. Drugs of this type are called receptor agonists. If the drug has a configuration similar to that of a neurotransmitter but not quite as similar as that of a receptor agonist, it may be able to bind to the receptor without activating it. In that case the drug will prevent the activation of the receptor by a neurotransmitter. Drugs of this type are called receptor antagonists. Other drugs that influence behavior are neither agonists nor antagonists. Some may have a mixed action by binding to the neurotransmitter receptor and causing partial activation; some may affect the receptor indirectly by altering the amount of neurotransmitter available for binding. Over the past several years this relatively simple concept of the relations among drugs, receptors and behavior has led to substantial advances in our understanding and treatment of disorders of the nervous system and has focused attention on the role cyclic AMP may play in both normal and abnormal brain function.

For example, it is generally accepted that the symptoms of Parkinson's disease, or shaking palsy, result from the degeneration of a group of neurons whose fibers project to the basal ganglia near the center of the brain from a region at the base of the brain known as the substantia nigra. These neurons secrete the neurotransmitter dopamine at their fiber terminals, and their degeneration reduces the amount of dopamine available to interact with the receptors on the receiving cells in the basal ganglia. As a result the receiving cells begin to function abnormally and cause the symptoms characteristic of Parkinson's disease: tremor, rigidity and a delay in the initiation of movement. Although dopamine is depleted in the brains of patients with the disease, the dopamine receptors in the basal ganglia appear to be undamaged.

These facts, set forth in large part by Arvid Carlsson of the University of Göteborg, Oleh Hornykiewicz of the University of Vienna and the late George C. Cotzias of the Brookhaven National Laboratory, have led to a dramatic new treatment for Parkinson's disease: the administration of the drug *levo*-dihydroxyphenylalanine (L-DOPA), the amino acid precursor of dopamine. When L-DOPA is given orally, it enters the bloodstream and travels to the brain, where it is taken up and converted to dopamine. (The neurotransmitter itself cannot enter the brain from the circulation.) The newly manufactured dopamine can then act as an

agonist: it stimulates the dopamine receptors in the basal ganglia. By making up for the lack of native dopamine in this way, L-DOPA is able to reverse some of the symptoms of the disease.

Drugs that act as antagonists of the dopamine receptor are also of therapeutic value. Such drugs include the phenothiazine tranquilizer chlorpromazine (Thorazine), which is widely used in the treatment of schizophrenia. Psychotic patients treated with chlorpromazine often show a dramatic improvement in their mental symptoms, but the side effects of the drug limit its clinical usefulness. For example, after prolonged treatment patients may begin to manifest tremors and other abnormal movements similar to those seen in Parkinson's disease. When administration of the tranquilizer is stopped, the abnormal movements usually disappear.

NEUROTRANSMITTER	TYPE OF RECEPTOR
DOPAMINE	dopamine
NOREPINEPHRINE	alpha-adrenergic
	beta-adrenergic
SEROTONIN	serotonin
HISTAMINE	H$_1$
	H$_2$
ACETYLCHOLINE	muscarinic (slow)
	nicotinic (fast)
ENKEPHALIN	opiate

DRUGS AFFECTING BEHAVIOR can be conveniently separated into two categories: those that interact directly with the neurotransmitter receptor and those that affect the

Hence it seems that chlorpromazine brings on a drug-induced Parkinson's disease by blocking dopamine receptors in the basal ganglia, thereby mimicking the symptoms of dopamine depletion even though normal amounts of the neurotransmitter may be present.

Besides being a troublesome side effect of antipsychotic drug treatment, drug-induced Parkinson's disease has shed some light on the biochemical abnormalities that may underlie schizophrenia. If drugs that appear to block dopamine receptors alleviate the symptoms of schizophrenia, then perhaps schizophrenia results from an overactivity of dopamine-containing neurons in certain parts of the brain. The overactivity of these cells would cause an excessive release of dopamine from their nerve endings, leading to an overstimulation of postsynaptic dopamine recep-

tors. By blocking these receptors chlorpromazine apparently prevents this overstimulation and so diminishes the symptoms of schizophrenia.

These two findings—that dopamine-receptor agonists are useful agents against Parkinson's disease and that dopamine-receptor antagonists are effective agents against schizophrenia—made it highly desirable to further understand the biochemical nature of the dopamine receptor in the brain of mammals. The work of Kebabian, McAfee and Schorderet described above had suggested that cyclic AMP might play an important role in mediating neuronal responses to dopamine. In order to show that neurotransmitter binding and cyclic AMP synthesis were functionally linked, however, it was necessary to identify an adenylate cyclase that would

synthesize cyclic AMP from ATP in the presence of dopamine.

In 1972 Kebabian, together with Gary L. Petzold of our laboratory, obtained experimental evidence demonstrating the presence of a dopamine-sensitive adenylate cyclase in the caudate nucleus, one of the basal ganglia of the brain and a region rich in dopamine receptors. The enzyme was located in synaptic membranes and bore a remarkable similarity to the dopamine receptor. Its activity was stimulated by very low concentrations of dopamine and was strongly inhibited by two classes of antischizophrenic drugs known to block the dopamine receptor. These results strongly suggested that the dopamine receptor in the caudate nucleus and in certain other areas of the mammalian brain might in fact be a component of the dopamine-sensitive adenylate cyclase, and that cy-

EVIDENCE FOR MEDIATION BY A CYCLIC NUCLEOTIDE		DRUGS ACTING AT THE NEUROTRANSMITTER RECEPTOR		DRUGS AFFECTING THE LEVEL OF NEUROTRANSMITTER AVAILABLE TO THE RECEPTOR	
CYCLIC AMP	CYCLIC GMP	AGONISTS (ACTIVATE RECEPTOR)	ANTAGONISTS (BLOCK RECEPTOR)	INCREASE LEVELS	DECREASE LEVELS
yes	no	apomorphine alpha-bromcryptine	antischizophrenics (Thorazine, Haldol)	levo-dihydroxyphenylalanine (L-DOPA) amantadine amphetamines (Dexedrine) methylphenidate (Ritalin)	alpha-methyl-para-tyrosine
no	yes (?)	phenylephrine (Neosynephrine)	phentolamine (Regitine)	tricyclic antidepressants (Elavil, Tofranil) MAO inhibitors (Parnate) amphetamines cocaine	reserpine (Serpasil) alpha-methyl-dopa (Aldomet)
yes	no	epinephrine (adrenalin) isoproterenol (Isuprel)	propranolol (Inderal)		
yes	no	5-methoxy-N,N-dimethyltryptamine	lysergic acid diethylamide (LSD) methysergide (Sansert)	tricyclic antidepressants (Elavil, Anafranil) tryptophan	para-chloro-phenylalanine
no	yes (?)	2-methyl-histamine	diphenhydramine (Benadryl) dimenhydrinate (Dramamine)	histidine amodiaquine	alpha-hydrazino-histidine brocresine
yes	no	betazole (Histalog)	metiamide cimetidine		
no	yes (?)	pilocarpine carbachol bethanechol (Urecholine)	scopolamine atropine (belladonna) propantheline (Pro-Banthine)	insecticides (Parathion, Malathion) nerve gas (DFP) pyridostigmine (Mestinon)	botulinus toxin
no	no	nicotine	d-tubocurarine (curare) succinylcholine (Anectine)		
yes	?	morphine heroin methadone meperidine (Demerol)	naloxone (Narcan)		

receptor indirectly by altering the amount of neurotransmitter available for binding. Drugs affecting neurotransmitter levels work in various ways, such as increasing the synthesis of a neurotransmitter (L-DOPA), inducing the release of preexisting neurotransmitter (am-

phetamine) or blocking the breakdown or sequestration of neurotransmitter (certain antidepressants). Cyclic AMP and a related compound, cyclic GMP, appear to mediate the actions of several neurotransmitters and to play a role in the action of many behavioral drugs.

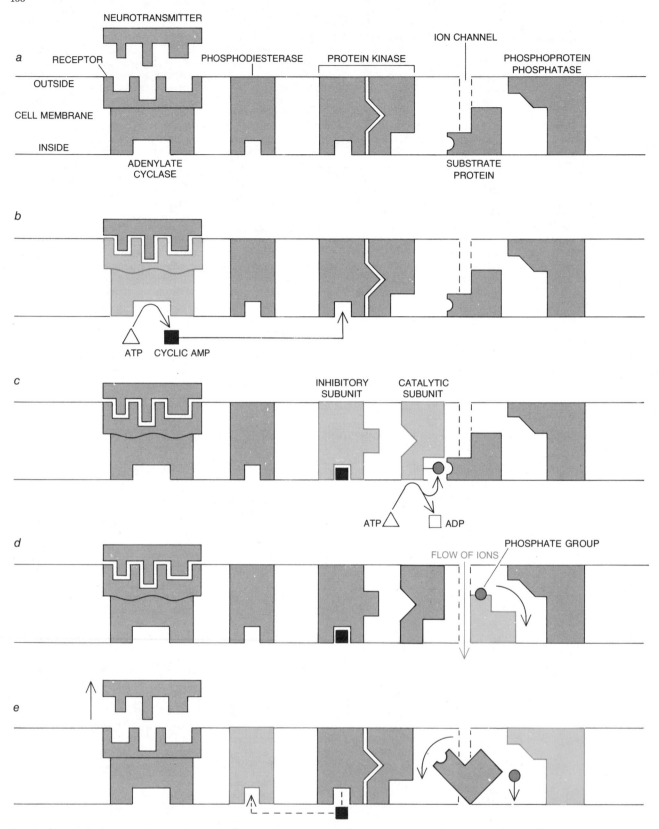

THEORETICAL MODEL explains how the increase in the level of cyclic AMP inside a receiving nerve cell can result in a transient change in the permeability of the cell membrane to ions, thereby altering the electrical excitability of the cell. In panel *a* the several molecular components that have been implicated in the process are shown in highly schematic form in their resting state. When an electrical impulse reaches the presynaptic terminal, neurotransmitter is released. It then crosses the synaptic space and binds to receptors on the receiving cell, activating adenylate cyclase to convert ATP into cyclic AMP (*b*). The cyclic AMP generated in this manner binds to the inhibitory subunit of protein kinase, causing it to dissociate from the catalytic subunit. Now activated, the catalytic subunit transfers a phosphate group from ATP to a substrate protein (*c*). The addition of phosphate changes the shape or position of the substrate protein, allowing certain ions to flow through existing pores in the membrane and altering the electrical excitability of the cell (*d*). Termination of the reaction begins when the neurotransmitter dissociates from the receptor, stopping further synthesis of cyclic AMP. Phosphodiesterase rapidly inactivates the remaining supply. Finally, phosphoprotein phosphatase removes phosphate group from the substrate protein (*e*).

clic AMP might therefore mediate the intracellular action of dopamine at certain synapses.

Further investigations by Yvonne Clement-Cormier and Kebabian in our laboratory and by Leslie L. Iversen and his co-workers at the University of Cambridge have largely confirmed that suggestion: among a large number of substances there is a remarkable parallel between the ability to act as an agonist or antagonist of the dopamine receptor and the ability to activate or inhibit the dopamine-sensitive adenylate cyclase. This correlation has since led to a new methodology for the rapid screening and development of drugs as potential dopamine receptor agonists (agents against Parkinson's disease) or antagonists (agents against schizophrenia). Whereas the traditional methods of measuring dopamine receptor activity involved behavioral tests that were time-consuming and often imprecise, the determination of the activity of the dopamine-sensitive adenylate cyclase in the presence of the drug under investigation provides a rapid and quantitative way of evaluating the drug's ability to either block or activate the dopamine receptor.

A link between cyclic AMP and synaptic transmission was also indicated when Floyd E. Bloom, Barry Hoffer and George Siggins, working at the National Institute of Mental Health, found physiological evidence that some of the actions of the neurotransmitter norepinephrine are mediated by cyclic AMP. At that time Bloom and his colleagues were studying the regulation by norepinephrine of neuronal activity in the cerebellum, which controls many of the automatic movements of the body, such as walking. The key elements that regulate such movements are large, elaborately branching neurons called Purkinje cells found in the cortex, or outer layer, of the cerebellum. Extending earlier anatomical work by Tomas Hokfelt and Kjell Fuxe at the Karolinska Institute in Stockholm, Bloom and his colleagues found that the locus coeruleus, a small cluster of norepinephrine-containing neurons buried deep in the brain stem, sends fine connections to the cortex of the cerebellum, and that stimulation of this pathway causes the firing rate of the Purkinje cells to decrease markedly. When they administered measured amounts of norepinephrine or cyclic AMP to individual Purkinje cells with a micropipette, they observed that the application of either compound slowed the firing rate of these cells in the same way that stimulation of the locus coeruleus did. Moreover, by means of a fluorescent-labeling technique that stains selectively for cyclic AMP they were able to show that either stimulation of the locus coeruleus or the direct application of norepinephrine causes a dramatic increase in the cyclic AMP content of the Purkinje cells. These and other results have suggested that the effects of norepinephrine on Purkinje-cell firing are mediated through the stimulation of a norepinephrine-sensitive adenylate cyclase and the resulting synthesis of cyclic AMP inside the cell.

Recent experiments in our laboratory have indicated that the role of cyclic AMP in the functioning of neurotransmitter receptors is by no means limited to the nervous system of vertebrates. For example, we have found in the thoracic ganglia of insects an enzyme that may mediate the effects of the neurotransmitter serotonin. This serotonin-sensitive adenylate cyclase is activated by very low concentrations of serotonin, and the effect of serotonin on the activity of the enzyme is specifically inhibited by drugs that are known to block serotonin receptors. Interestingly enough, one of the most potent of these blocking agents is the hallucinogen lysergic acid diethylamide (LSD). Our findings suggest that the serotonin receptor of neural tissue is intimately associated with a serotonin-sensitive adenylate cyclase and that some of the physiological effects of LSD may result from the inhibition of the enzyme.

At least five neurotransmitters have now been shown to stimulate specific neurotransmitter-sensitive adenylate cyclases: dopamine, norepinephrine, serotonin, histamine and octopamine. Moreover, recently acquired evidence suggests that a second cyclic nucleotide, cyclic guanosine monophosphate (cyclic GMP), may be involved in the effects of the neurotransmitter acetylcholine at certain synapses through the activation of guanylate cyclase, an enzyme that converts guanosine triphosphate (GTP) into cyclic GMP. Cyclic GMP may also be involved in mediating the effects of norepinephrine and histamine at certain receptors that are distinct from those associated with the cyclic AMP system.

It is worth noting that many of the behavioral drugs that affect neurotransmitter receptors produce effects resembling those that occur naturally in patients with mental or neurological diseases. For example, miners exposed to manganese poisoning or patients given antischizophrenic drugs exhibit a syndrome indistinguishable from naturally occurring Parkinson's disease, and LSD can produce hallucinations similar to those experienced by schizophrenics. These and other clinical observations raise the possibility that certain neurological and mental diseases may result from abnormalities in specific receptor-adenylate-cyclase systems. Such abnormalities might arise genetically through nonlethal mutations or be acquired through exposure to high levels of environmental toxins such as manganese.

Not all neurotransmitter receptors,

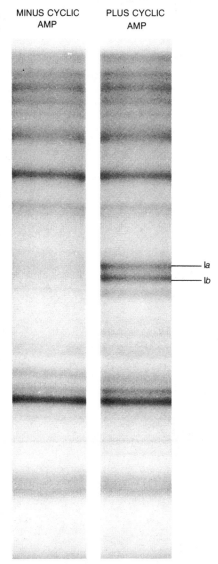

MINUS CYCLIC AMP   PLUS CYCLIC AMP

1a
1b

PHOSPHORYLATION of synaptic-membrane proteins in response to cyclic AMP is highly specific, as is shown in this experiment performed by Bruce K. Krueger, Javier Forn and Tetsufumi Ueda in the authors' laboratory. Synaptic membranes prepared from rat brain were incubated in a solution containing radioactive ATP in the presence or absence of added cyclic AMP, enabling molecules of protein kinase in the membrane to transfer a radioactive phosphate group from ATP to various substrate proteins. The phosphorylated proteins were then removed from the membrane with a detergent and separated from one another by placing a mixture of them at the top of a column of the gel-like substance polyacrylamide. Application of a high-voltage current caused the proteins to migrate downward and separate into a series of thin bands according to their size. By next placing the gels in a darkroom on top of X-ray film it was possible to detect which bands exposed the film and hence had incorporated radioactive phosphate. The print of an exposed film shown here reveals that although many proteins were phosphorylated by enzymes whose activity was independent of cyclic AMP, only two proteins were phosphorylated by a protein kinase whose activity was dependent on presence of cyclic AMP. The proteins are designated 1a (molecular weight of 86,000 daltons) and 1b (80,000 daltons).

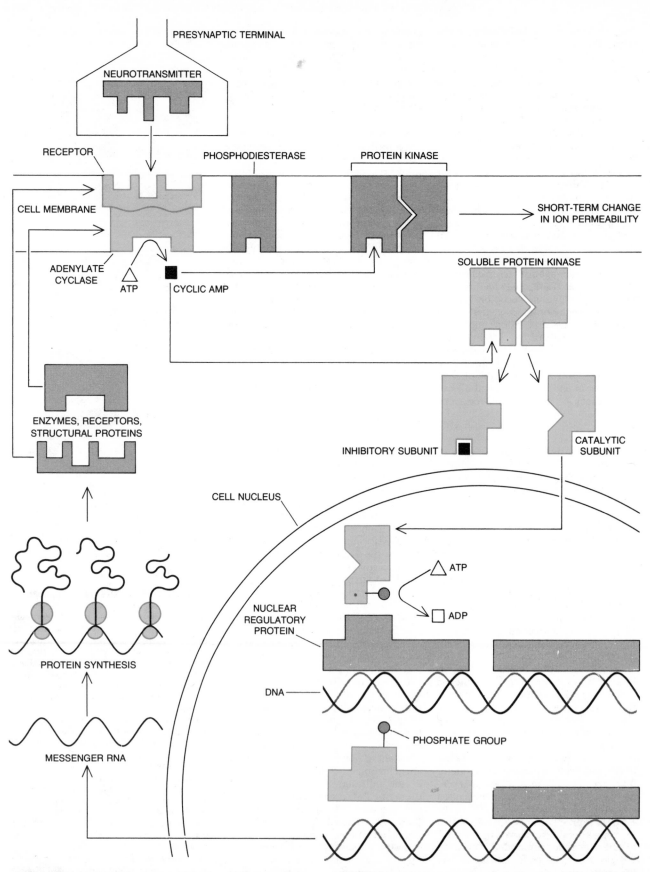

LONG-TERM EFFECTS of cyclic AMP on nerve-cell function are postulated to occur through the activation of a soluble protein kinase located in the cytoplasm. Once activated, this enzyme enters the cell nucleus, where it transfers a phosphate group from ATP to one of the nuclear regulatory proteins closely associated with the DNA of inactive genes. Phosphorylation alters the shape or binding characteristics of the regulatory protein in such a way that it dissociates from the DNA double helix, exposing the underlying stretch of DNA so that protein synthesis can occur. Proteins whose synthesis might be induced in this manner include neurotransmitter receptors, adenylate cyclases, structural proteins and enzymes involved in neurotransmitter synthesis or breakdown. In this way the cyclic AMP generated during the short-term process of synaptic transmission could produce long-term alterations in the electrical properties of the receiving cell.

however, have been linked to the synthesis of a cyclic nucleotide. For example, one of the best-studied synaptic mechanisms—the stimulation of the contraction of voluntary muscle through the release of acetylcholine at the junction between a nerve fiber and a muscle—appears to operate independently of the synthesis of a cyclic nucleotide [see "The Response to Acetylcholine," by Henry A. Lester; Offprint No. 1352]. This makes sense in view of the fact that the mediation of synaptic transmission by cyclic nucleotides involves a complex series of steps, which we shall discuss, that makes the process relatively long-lasting on the time scale of neuronal events. Those types of transmission that place a premium on speed, such as the contraction of voluntary muscle, therefore rely on faster receptor mechanisms.

So far we have described how certain neurotransmitters, by binding to a specific receptor, stimulate the production of cyclic AMP inside the receiving cell. The question remains: How does an increase in the level of cyclic AMP translate the message of the neurotransmitter into physiological action?

We know from the work of many neurobiologists over the past 20 years that a nerve cell responds to synaptic stimulation with a brief change in the permeability of the synaptic membrane to one or more kinds of ion. This change in permeability allows ions to flow across the membrane, generating an electric current and thereby altering the membrane's electric potential, or voltage. Depending on the ions that move and the direction of their movement, the change in electric potential induced by a neurotransmitter will make it either more or less likely that the cell will reach the threshold of excitation necessary for it to generate an impulse. In this respect a neuron acts much like an analogue computer, integrating the many hundreds of inhibitory and excitatory chemical messages that impinge on its surface at any given moment before deciding whether or not to fire.

In order to explore the possible role of cyclic AMP in mediating some of the changes in membrane permeability induced by neurotransmitters, we began several years ago a detailed investigation of the chain of biochemical events that occur inside a neuron following the binding of a neurotransmitter to its receptor and the activation of adenylate cyclase. Earlier experiments by Edwin G. Krebs and his colleagues at the University of Washington had provided some important clues. In their investigation of the mechanism by which adrenalin induces the conversion of glycogen into glucose in muscle cells, they found that the cyclic AMP generated inside the cells by the hormone-sensitive adenylate cyclase caused the transfer of a

phosphate group from ATP to the enzyme responsible for the initiation of glycogen breakdown. Somewhat later they discovered that the actual transfer of the phosphate group, the process called phosphorylation, was accomplished by the enzyme protein kinase. In biochemical nomenclature, kinase (more properly, phosphokinase) is a term reserved for enzymes that transfer a phosphate group from ATP to another molecule; for a protein kinase the other molecule is always a protein.

Cyclic AMP is thought to activate protein kinase by binding to an inhibitory subunit of the kinase in such a way as to change its shape and cause it to dissociate from the rest of the enzyme. The loss of the inhibitory component enhances the activity of the kinase, which then readily transfers a phosphate group to the enzyme controlling the pathway of glycogen breakdown. The addition of a phosphate group to this enzyme causes it to trigger a "cascade" of enzymatic reactions, leading ultimately to the breakdown of glycogen. Protein kinase therefore acts as the link between the cyclic AMP generated by the hormone and the activation of the biochemical pathway that accounts for the hormone's metabolic effects.

On the basis of this scheme we began looking for an analogous system in brain cells. Although glycogen breakdown is not a prominent effect of cyclic AMP in nervous tissue, we felt that a similar protein kinase could translate the change in cyclic AMP levels brought about by a neurotransmitter into a change in the permeability of the postsynaptic membrane to ions.

Within a relatively short time J.-F. Kuo and Eishichi Miyamoto, working in our laboratory, isolated a cyclic-AMP-dependent protein kinase from cattle brain. The enzyme was present in relatively large amounts in the brain tissue compared with most other tissues, and its activity was notably dependent on the presence of cyclic AMP. Furthermore, the concentration of cyclic AMP required to stimulate the enzyme to half its maximum activity was similar to the concentration of cyclic AMP normally found in brain tissue. This finding indicated that the increases in cyclic AMP levels known to be induced by various neurotransmitters would cause large changes in the activity of the cyclic-AMP-dependent protein kinase.

Other experiments demonstrated that the protein kinase could transfer a phosphate group to proteins other than those associated with the breakdown of glycogen. In fact, studies by Hiroo Maeno and Edward Johnson in our laboratory indicated that when brain tissue was homogenized, the proteins phosphorylated to the greatest extent were in the fractions of the homogenized tissue with the largest amounts of synaptic-membrane fragments, and that these fractions also

had the greatest concentration of protein kinase.

Thus it became evident that the synaptic membrane contains all the major elements for the neurotransmitter-induced transfer of a phosphate group to a substrate protein in the membrane: (1) a neurotransmitter-sensitive adenylate cyclase that generates cyclic AMP in response to a specific neurotransmitter, (2) a cyclic-AMP-dependent protein kinase that phosphorylates a substrate protein in the presence of cyclic AMP and (3) the membrane substrate protein that is phosphorylated by the protein kinase. The transfer of a phosphate group to such a protein could conceivably change the permeability of the membrane to ions, either directly by changing the configuration of the protein in order to open a channel that ions can flow through, or indirectly, for example by affecting the activity of an enzyme "pump" that physically transports ions across the membrane.

Further investigation showed that the synaptic-membrane fractions also contain the enzymatic machinery necessary for stopping the cyclic-AMP-dependent phosphorylation process and restoring the membrane to its resting state. These enzymes include not only phosphodiesterase, which degrades cyclic AMP to an inactive form of AMP, but also phosphoprotein phosphatase, which removes the phosphate group from proteins that have previously been phosphorylated by the cyclic-AMP-dependent protein kinase. Several of the components of this membrane-bound enzyme system have been shown to exist as a complex, thereby reducing the distance reaction products must travel from one enzyme to the next and enabling a phosphate group to be rapidly added to and removed from the substrate protein.

Following the discovery that fractions of homogenized brain tissue containing the largest amounts of synaptic membrane serve as excellent substrates for the cyclic-AMP-dependent protein kinase, Tetsufumi Ueda, Bruce K. Krueger and Javier Forn of our laboratory, together with Johnson and Maeno, attempted to isolate the specific protein or proteins that were being phosphorylated. Up to this point it had not been possible to tell whether a large percentage or only a very few of the dozens of proteins known to be present in the synaptic membrane were acting as substrates for phosphorylation. When Ueda and his co-workers incubated synaptic-membrane fractions in a solution containing radioactively labeled ATP in the presence or absence of cyclic AMP, they found that the phosphorylation of only two or three of the several dozen proteins in the membrane fraction was markedly increased by cyclic AMP. This result was gratifying, since it indicated that the effects of cyclic AMP on the phosphorylation of synaptic-membrane protein were specific and did not simply involve a general stimulation of cellular metabolism.

One of the synaptic-membrane proteins specifically phosphorylated by the cyclic-AMP-dependent protein kinase, designated Protein I, has recently been investigated in detail in our laboratory. Protein I, which has two molecular subunits, Ia and Ib, is localized almost exclusively in the synaptic region of nerve tissue and is apparently absent from those organelles of nerve cells (such as nuclei, mitochondria and ribosomes) that are not directly associated with synaptic transmission. Moreover, Protein I has not been found at all in any nonneural tissue (such as heart or liver) yet examined. It is also absent from the brain of fetal rats at stages of development before the formation of connections between nerve cells, and it appears

for the first time at the stage when synaptic complexes form.

The phosphorylation of Protein I by protein kinase in the synaptic membrane is extremely fast. In fact, in the shortest period that has yet been accurately studied—five seconds—the phosphorylation is already at the maximum level. The speed of this reaction is virtually a prerequisite to seriously considering the possibility that Protein I might be involved in the generation of the very brief changes in the permeability of the synaptic membrane to ions (lasting for a few hundred milliseconds or less) that give rise to postsynaptic potentials.

If protein phosphorylation mediated by cyclic AMP is indeed responsible for changes in the permeability of the synaptic membrane to ions, then there should be a correlation between the state of phosphorylation of a particular membrane protein or proteins and the state of ion permeability of the

cell membrane. The short duration of changes in the permeability of membranes in the nervous system has made it difficult to establish such a correlation within the limitations of present methodology. For this reason we have turned to some non-neuronal model systems, including the red blood cell of the turkey and the frog, to study such permeability changes in detail. Under appropriate conditions these cells respond to hormones such as adrenalin with an increase in the movement of sodium and potassium ions across the cell membrane. This increase, which is due to a change in membrane permeability, appears to be mediated by cyclic AMP.

Recently Stephen A. Rudolph of our laboratory has found that a single large membrane protein becomes phosphorylated whenever cyclic AMP or the adrenalin-related drug isoproterenol is added to the suspension of red blood cells. Furthermore, by simultaneously

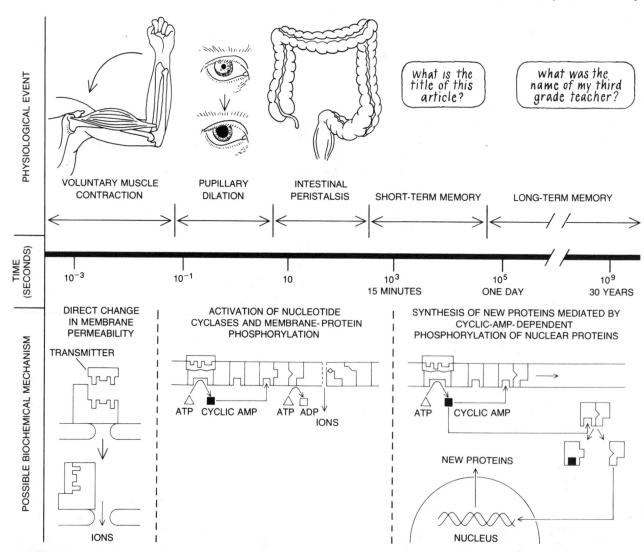

CONTINUUM OF SYNAPTIC EVENTS in the nervous system stretches from the very brief to the very long-lived. At the short end of the spectrum are processes, such as voluntary muscle contraction, that are initiated in the span of a few milliseconds by the direct action of a neurotransmitter to open an ion channel in the membrane. Events lasting from hundreds of milliseconds to minutes appear to be mediated indirectly through the neurotransmitter-induced synthesis of cyclic AMP, which initiates the phosphorylation of membrane proteins to produce a relatively slow change in ion permeability. Events ranging from hours to years in duration, such as memory, may involve the synthesis of new proteins directed by the cyclic-AMP-stimulated phosphorylation of proteins that regulate gene expression.

measuring the state of phosphorylation of this protein and the movement of sodium ions into the cell in the presence of isoproterenol he has found that the time required for the membrane protein to reach half its maximum level of phosphorylation coincides closely with the time required for the flow of sodium ions across the membrane to reach half its maximum rate.

The results of these and other experiments conducted with a variety of systems demonstrate a close correlation between the movement of ions across cell membranes and the cyclic-AMP-dependent phosphorylation of specific membrane proteins. It should be pointed out, however, that correlation does not always mean causality. There is at present no direct proof that phosphorylation is a necessary event for the observed changes in permeability; both events could conceivably be secondary effects of some other process. The definitive proof of a causal connection between membrane-protein phosphorylation and permeability changes remains one of the major challenges for experimentation. We hope it will eventually be possible to dissect out the individual molecular components responsible for controlling ion permeability, put them into synthetic membranes and determine whether prior cyclic-AMP-dependent phosphorylation of one or more of these components will result in permeability changes similar to those observed in intact cells.

Because of the complex nature of cyclic-AMP-mediated processes, involving several biochemical steps, these processes are best suited to the regulation of synaptic events that are relatively long-lasting. This may be the reason the neuronal pathways that appear to make use of cyclic nucleotides often play a modulatory role in the nervous system, regulating activity rather than initiating it. For example, the cyclic AMP formed in the cerebellum by the activation of norepinephrine fibers in the locus coeruleus tones down the "spontaneous" firing rate of the Purkinje neurons. In ganglia of the sympathetic nervous system the dopamine synapses mediated by cyclic AMP adjust the level of activity at other synapses not mediated by cyclic AMP. Even in its role in movement disorders such as Parkinson's disease the cyclic AMP formed in the caudate nucleus by the activation of dopamine-sensitive adenylate cyclase appears to regulate movements only after they have been initiated by signals from other areas of the brain.

Observed changes in membrane excitability seen at cyclic-AMP-mediated synapses in the cerebellum and in the sympathetic ganglion may last for hundreds of milliseconds or longer—a long time on the scale of neural events. Recent investigations by Eric R. Kandel of Columbia University College of Physicians and Surgeons, working with a ganglion in a mollusk, and by Benjamin Libet of the University of California School of Medicine at San Francisco, working with a ganglion in the sympathetic nervous system of the rabbit, have demonstrated events of even greater duration that appear to be related to cyclic AMP, some of them lasting for hours. Observations such as these support the possibility that synaptic events mediated by cyclic nucleotides could be the basis for certain long-term changes in the central nervous system of man.

This notion has been supported by evidence indicating that the phosphorylation of protein mediated by cyclic AMP may influence events in the nucleus of the cell. A number of investigators, starting with Thomas A. Langan of the University of Colorado School of Medicine, have shown that histones, positively charged proteins that bind to the negatively charged phosphate backbone of the double helix of DNA, are susceptible to phosphorylation by a cyclic-AMP-dependent protein kinase. When histones are intimately associated with DNA, they appear to inhibit the expression of the DNA's information content by blocking access to the enzymes that effect the transcription of DNA to RNA. Phosphorylation by protein kinase makes the charge of the histones more negative, thereby reducing their ability to bind to DNA.

From a mechanistic point of view the linkage between adenylate cyclase and protein kinase supplies a ready-made system for the transformation of short-term synaptic events into longer-lived biochemical changes. The cyclic AMP generated as a result of synaptic activity could conceivably activate a protein kinase, which would phosphorylate histone or some other nuclear regulatory protein and cause its removal from the DNA of inactive genes. The exposed genes would then be available for transcription into messenger RNA and ultimately translation into protein. Indeed, experiments in the laboratory of Erimino Costa at the National Institute of Mental Health suggest that cyclic AMP can induce the synthesis of tyrosine hydroxylase, an enzyme involved in the manufacture of dopamine and norepinephrine.

Thus the cyclic AMP system provides a mechanism by which the continued activation of a particular synapse could lead to the synthesis of new enzyme molecules or new receptor molecules, permanently altering the electrical properties of the receiving neuron. Whether such changes could constitute a molecular basis for information storage in the nervous system is hard to say, but it is certainly an attractive hypothesis. One can even speculate that the cyclic-AMP-dependent phosphorylation of synaptic-membrane proteins represents a type of short-term memory and that the phosphorylation of nuclear proteins and the synthesis of new protein molecules could represent a more permanent change—a long-term memory.

In sum, there exists in the brain a continuum of functional events that stretches from the brief to the very long-lived. At the short end of the scale are synaptic events, such as the contraction of voluntary muscle, that last for only a few milliseconds; at the long end are memories that can last for 50 years or more. On the basis of our present knowledge it seems possible that all but the very briefest of these events may involve cyclic-AMP-associated mechanisms.

Most of this discussion has emphasized the possible role of cyclic AMP in synapses and its importance in mediating the effects of many neurotransmitters and the actions of drugs that affect behavior. These areas have been a major focus of research on the role of cyclic nucleotides in the nervous system largely because of the conceptual and mechanistic analogies between the action of hormones and the transmission of nerve impulses. Mostly because of a comparative lack of evidence other roles for cyclic nucleotides in the nervous system have been somewhat underplayed. Considerable research over the past two or three years, both in our laboratory and elsewhere, suggests, however, that processes mediated by cyclic nucleotides are involved not only in the mechanism of changes in ion permeability induced by neurotransmitters but also in the regulation of a variety of other phenomena, including the activation of enzymes, the synthesis and release of neurotransmitters, intracellular movements, carbohydrate metabolism in the cerebrum and possibly even processes of growth and development. We shall not elaborate on these recent advances, but we should like to emphasize their potential importance to an overall understanding of the functioning of the nervous system.

In particular, it may be useful to view the synaptic and nonsynaptic actions of cyclic AMP not so much in isolation but rather as part of an integrating system. It may be that enough synaptic stimulation not only raises cyclic AMP levels sufficiently to alter the permeability of membranes but also initiates a logical sequence of events mediated by cyclic nucleotides. This sequence might include a decrease or an increase in the synthesis of a neurotransmitter in response to synaptic stimulation, an initiation of intracellular movements in order to transport newly synthesized products, the activation of carbohydrate metabolism to supply the necessary cellular energy requirements, and direct effects on the genetic material in the cell nucleus that may lead to long-term alterations of behavior, such as memory.

V

THE USE OF SEX HORMONES: ETHICAL AND POLITICAL ISSUES

THE USE OF SEX HORMONES: ETHICAL AND POLITICAL ISSUES

V

INTRODUCTION

The articles in Sections I–IV showed that hormone secretion is regulated by external and internal factors and examined the ways in which hormones act on the brain and other parts of the body. However, the study of hormones and reproductive behavior has far broader implications. Although any scientific endeavor has a potential impact on society, the study of reproduction is more obviously laden with social implications than most other fields of scientific inquiry. The papers in this section point to some ethical and political considerations that emerge as our understanding of sex hormones and behavior expands and as the pressure increases for wise use of this knowledge.

In many ways it is simpler to identify, analyze, and quantify a biological influence, such as a hormone, than a social influence, such as family expectations, on a behavior. However, social influences often override and obscure biological factors. Thus, even though the hormones of development and of adulthood may affect sex-typical behaviors (see Levine's article in Section II), social factors to which an individual is exposed during a lifetime may be even more important. The article by Jean Lipman-Blumen explores the influence of sex-role ideology on women's life goals. The evidence indicates that women are socialized at an early age to accept society's concept of appropriate behavior. Although Lipman-Blumen's study focuses on survey data from college students, there can be little doubt that the phenomenon described is a general one.

Advances in our understanding of how hormones work have made it possible to control fertility. Needless to say, appropriate use of this knowledge has been and continues to be a problem. Fredrick S. Jaffe's article traces the history of U.S. policy on contraception and analyzes the social, political, and economic concerns of our society that influence that policy.

The last article of this series deals with the ethics of experimentation with humans. The goal of much research is to improve living conditions for individuals and for society as a whole. Often the needs of individuals and the needs of people as a group are in conflict. Bernard Barber's article outlines the pressures on researchers, the needs of patients, and the goals of medicine and society and suggests guidelines for better serving each of these communities.

14

How Ideology Shapes
Women's Lives

by Jean Lipman-Blumen
January 1972

Data from a survey of college women reveal that a woman's life goals, particularly her educational and occupational aspirations, are guided by the type of sex-role ideology acquired in childhood

The "women's liberation" movement has brought to the fore the age-old question of what kinds of behavior are socially appropriate for women and men. It is often said that women tend to act on the basis of feelings and emotions rather than on the basis of reason. The motivating force behind female behavior is rarely seen as

being ideology. It is becoming increasingly apparent, however, that certain ideologies can predict the values and behavior of women with remarkable accuracy. These powerful systems of beliefs, which shape the destiny of women in ways never imagined by Freud, are transmitted implicitly rather than explicitly; they usually guide the behavior

of women silently and without their being consciously aware of it.

Such ideologies are largely based on a woman's concept of what kinds of behavior are appropriate to her role as a female. In the study I shall describe here female-role ideology referred primarily to a woman's system of beliefs regarding the appropriate behavior of women with

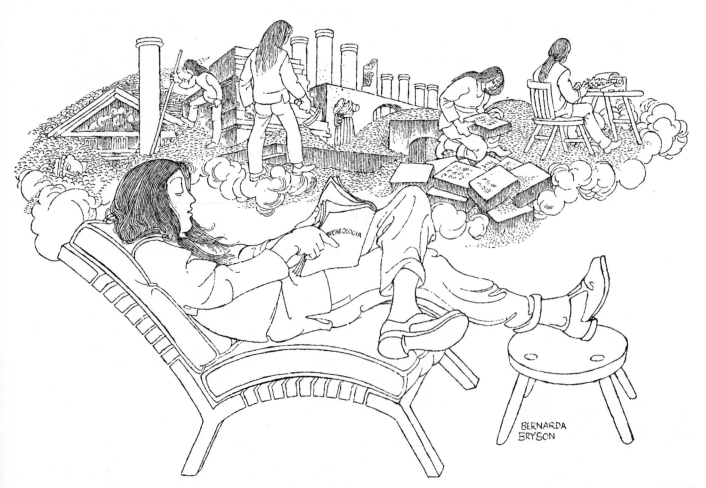

"CONTEMPORARY" VIEW of the female role, as defined in the survey, is based on the belief that women should be as free as men to pursue educational and occupational goals, that men and women should equally share responsibilities inside and outside the home.

respect to men. The study, which involved an extensive survey of the life plans of married women, was conducted under the auspices of the Radcliffe Institute in Cambridge, Mass., in 1968 (before the women's liberation movement had had a major impact). A detailed questionnaire was mailed to the wives of graduate students in the Boston area. Out of the 1,868 responses a subsample of 1,012 wives who had attended college was selected for analysis. The questionnaire inquired into early childhood experiences, academic achievements and plans, past and present family situations, personal values and life goals.

The age of the women who responded ranged from 18 to 54, with 23.4 years as the median. Forty-two percent of the women had been married one year or less, another 43 percent had been married from two to five years and 15 percent had been married more than five years. The mean number of years married was 3.2. Sixty percent of the women had no children, 21 percent had one child, 12 percent had two children, 5 percent had three children and 2 percent had four or more children. Since the women selected for analysis were all married to graduate students, their socioeconomic status was fairly homogeneous. Their original family backgrounds, however, were quite varied and in their diversity were presumably not unlike the backgrounds of the larger population of women who have attended college.

An index of female-role ideology was developed to encompass two major dimensions of the adult female role: an internal dimension, based on issues of task-sharing between husband and wife, and an external dimension, related to patterns of appropriate female behavior outside the home. Responses to a six-item scale were summed to obtain a female-role-ideology score. Although sex-role ideologies form a continuum, we grouped the respondents into two polar categories, which we labeled "traditional" and "contemporary." An oversimplified version of the traditional ideology is the belief that under ordinary circumstances women belong in the home, caring for children and carrying out domestic duties, whereas men are responsible for the financial support of the family. The contemporary ideology holds that the relationships between men and women are ideally egalitarian and that husbands and wives may share domestic, child-rearing and financial responsibilities. In our study sample 27

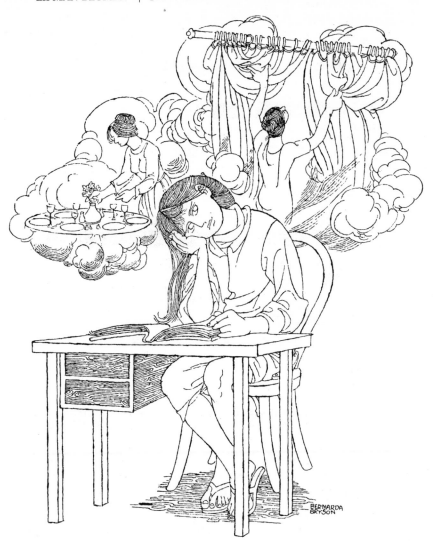

"TRADITIONAL" VIEW of the female role involves the belief that a woman's primary responsibilities are homemaking and child-rearing, that men are responsible for financial support of the family and that women with children should not expect to have a career.

percent of the women adhered to the traditional ideology and 73 percent held the contemporary view.

Studies by Ruth E. Hartley and others in the early 1960's have shown that by the age of five children have developed a sex-role ideology with well-defined notions of appropriate behavior for men and women. Because girls are presumably socialized at an early age to either the traditional or the contemporary sex-role ideology, the belief system is likely to shape much of their life pattern. Here a number of important questions arise. What kind of family do women with the contemporary or traditional ideologies come from? What adolescent relationships did they have with their parents? How is female-role ideology related to a woman's present life-style? How does it affect her life choices, particularly her educational and occupa-

tional aspirations? Are the contemporary and traditional ideologies associated with different hierarchies of values? Are married women with the contemporary viewpoint as happy with their life as women with the traditional viewpoint?

In America college education is regarded as a major avenue to career opportunities and a desirable style of life. Therefore it is not surprising that there is a strong relation between the educational aspirations of a college woman and her plans to pursue a professional career. What link is there, if any, between a woman's concept of her sex role and her educational plans?

In our study educational aspiration was measured by the response to the question: "What is the highest level of academic training that you expect to obtain?" As I have noted, all the women in the study sample had completed at

EDUCATIONAL ASPIRATION

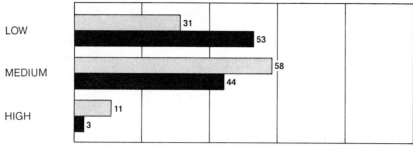

MODE OF ACHIEVEMENT

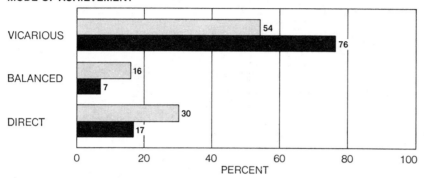

SEX-ROLE IDEOLOGY affects a woman's educational aspirations and how she seeks to satisfy her need for achievement outside the home. Women with a contemporary view (*gray bars*) have higher educational goals and are more likely to satisfy their achievement needs through their own efforts than women who hold a traditional view (*black bars*).

least part of a college program. The responses were grouped into three categories: low aspiration, medium aspiration and high aspiration. Women with low aspiration did not plan to seek a degree beyond the bachelor level; those with medium aspiration planned academic work up to and including a master's degree; those with high aspiration planned doctoral or postdoctoral studies.

Analysis of the data revealed that there was a strong interaction between a woman's concept of the female role and her educational aspiration. More than half of the women who held the traditional view of the female role did not plan to seek a degree beyond the bache-

lor's level, whereas a majority of the women with the contemporary viewpoint aspired to graduate studies, with 58 percent having medium aspiration and 11 percent having high aspiration. Only 3 percent of the women with the traditional viewpoint had high educational aspiration [*see illustration above*].

In order to gain a more precise understanding of how sex-role ideology is related to educational aspiration we examined a possible linking factor: mode of achievement. Mode of achievement is a measure of how a woman seeks to satisfy her need for achievement outside the home. There were three cate-

gories for mode of achievement: direct, balanced and vicarious. Women who preferred the direct mode felt it necessary to satisfy their achievement needs completely or predominantly through their own efforts; those who chose the balanced mode placed equal weight on their husband's accomplishments and on their own; those who selected the vicarious mode fulfilled their achievement needs either completely or predominantly through the accomplishments of their husband.

Since girls often are socialized in early childhood to satisfy their achievement needs passively by identification with the accomplishments of their father or their brothers, it is not surprising that they transfer this vicarious mode of achievement to their husband when they marry. The survey data show the strength of such socialization: a majority of all the women in the sample, both in the contemporary and in the traditional categories, sought to satisfy their achievement needs vicariously. As might be expected, those with the traditional ideology adhered much more to the vicarious mode, with 76 percent selecting this means of satisfying their achievement needs compared with 54 percent of those with the contemporary viewpoint. Almost a third of the college women with the contemporary ideology, but only a sixth of those with the traditional one, felt that they had to satisfy their achievement needs primarily through their own accomplishments. Relatively few seemed to prefer the balanced mode in which the accomplishments of husband and wife had equal weight.

There was a clear connection between mode of achievement and educational aspiration. Women who were passive, who sought vicarious satisfaction of their achievement needs, were more likely to express low educational aspiration, whereas balanced and direct achievers had higher educational aspirations. The relation between sex-role ideology and educational aspiration changed somewhat for vicarious achievers. Among those who held the contemporary view of female roles and were also vicarious achievers, educational aspiration was reduced so that they could not be distinguished from women in the traditional group in terms of expectations for doctoral or postdoctoral studies. For balanced and direct achievers there was an even stronger relation between sex-role ideology and educational aspiration, with the contemporary-ideology women 19 percent more likely to have plans for doctoral studies than the traditional-

MODE OF ACHIEVEMENT

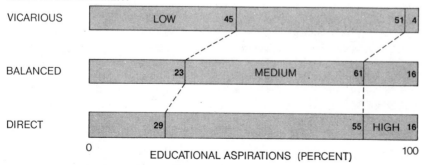

MODE OF ACHIEVEMENT and educational aspirations were closely linked. Vicarious achievers tended to have lower educational goals than did the balanced or direct achievers.

ideology women, who strongly tended not to have plans for further education.

In short, the relation between female-role ideology and educational aspiration is contingent on the way a woman has been socialized to meet her achievement needs outside the home. It is quite clear that the vicarious mode and the traditional view are linked and tend to predispose a woman to limit her educational goals. The balanced and direct modes of achievement are linked to the contemporary view of sex roles and tend to encourage high educational aspirations.

Since it appears that women are socialized at an early age to a female-role ideology, let us examine the family background of the respondents. Obvious socioeconomic indexes, such as parents' income, education or occupation, surprisingly had no bearing on the daughter's sex-role ideology. In fact, none of the usual socioeconomic characteristics of the family was related to female-role ideology. Women with the contemporary ideology were just as likely to come from homes with incomes of less than $3,500 as those with the traditional view were. Parents with a college education, including a doctoral degree, were just as likely to produce daughters with the traditional sex-role ideology as daughters with the contemporary one.

Another usually important factor, childhood religion, failed to show a statistically significant influence on sex-role ideology, although a Catholic upbringing tended to produce slightly more women with the traditional viewpoint than a Protestant or a Jewish upbringing did. And in spite of the common opinion that city dwellers are less bound by traditional attitudes than people raised in rural areas, women who came from rural homes were as likely to hold contemporary sex-role attitudes as women from urban and suburban areas were.

It is worth noting that homes disrupted by divorce, separation or death did not differ from intact homes in the proportion of traditional-ideology and contemporary-ideology women they produced. This holds true regardless of the age of the daughter when the home was disrupted. Moreover, having sisters or brothers, either younger or older, had no effect on sex-role ideology. Working mothers have been both praised and damned for the effects of their outside commitment on their children. In our sample whether or not a mother worked had no perceptible impact on her daughter's sex-role ideology. Nonworking mothers were just as likely as employed

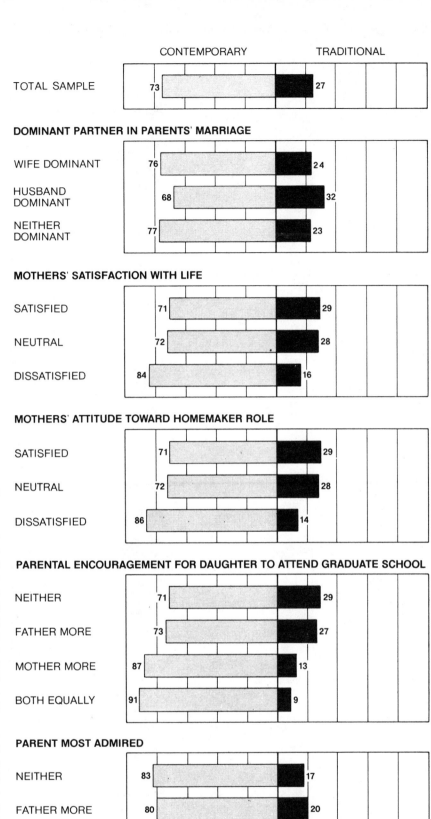

PARENTAL INFLUENCES on daughter's sex-role ideology (gray and black bars) were not expected variables such as income, education or religion but rather qualitative factors such as dominant parent, mothers' attitudes, encouraging parent and most admired parent.

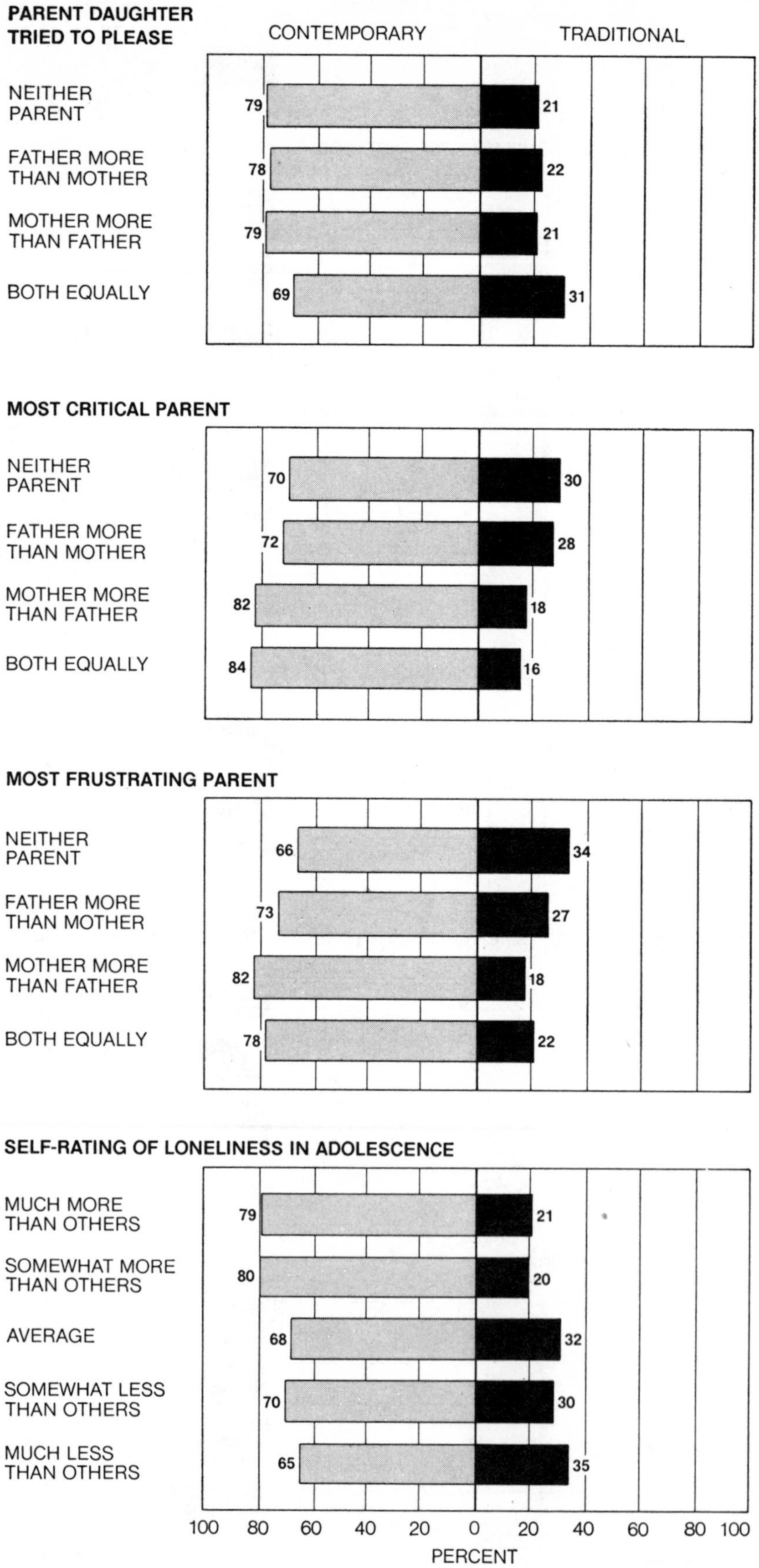

**PARENT DAUGHTER
TRIED TO PLEASE**

CONTEMPORARY   TRADITIONAL

NEITHER
PARENT   79 ▨ ■ 21

FATHER MORE
THAN MOTHER   78 ▨ ■ 22

MOTHER MORE
THAN FATHER   79 ▨ ■ 21

BOTH EQUALLY   69 ▨ ■ 31

MOST CRITICAL PARENT

NEITHER
PARENT   70 ▨ ■ 30

FATHER MORE
THAN MOTHER   72 ▨ ■ 28

MOTHER MORE
THAN FATHER   82 ▨ ■ 18

BOTH EQUALLY   84 ▨ ■ 16

MOST FRUSTRATING PARENT

NEITHER
PARENT   66 ▨ ■ 34

FATHER MORE
THAN MOTHER   73 ▨ ■ 27

MOTHER MORE
THAN FATHER   82 ▨ ■ 18

BOTH EQUALLY   78 ▨ ■ 22

SELF-RATING OF LONELINESS IN ADOLESCENCE

MUCH MORE
THAN OTHERS   79 ▨ ■ 21

SOMEWHAT MORE
THAN OTHERS   80 ▨ ■ 20

AVERAGE   68 ▨ ■ 32

SOMEWHAT LESS
THAN OTHERS   70 ▨ ■ 30

MUCH LESS
THAN OTHERS   65 ▨ ■ 35

100 80 60 40 20   0   20 40 60 80 100
PERCENT

OTHER PARENTAL FACTORS that influenced the daughter's sex-role ideology were parent daughter tried to please most, most critical parent and most frustrating parent. Women with a contemporary view tended to be lonelier than their peers in adolescence.

mothers to have daughters with the contemporary view of the female role.

In the light of these negative demographic findings, do childhood family variables contribute anything to the ideology of college women? If there is such an influence, we must seek the answer in more subtle factors such as the marital relationship between the parents. Women with a contemporary sex-role ideology tended to come from families in which most of the time neither parent was dominant or from families in which the mother was dominant. When the father was more dominant in the marriage, the tendency of the daughter to develop the traditional concept of the female role was enhanced.

An important predictor of a woman's female-role ideology is her perception of her mother's overall satisfaction with life. Dissatisfied mothers were more likely than satisfied ones to rear daughters with the contemporary view of the role of women, and satisfied mothers were more likely to have daughters with the traditional orientation. In traditional homes where the father was dominant, dissatisfied mothers were even more likely to raise daughters with the contemporary ideology. In homes where neither parent was dominant, dissatisfied mothers were not significantly more likely than satisfied ones to raise daughters with the contemporary view of female roles. Interestingly enough, daughters from contemporary homes who felt that their mothers were dissatisfied with their life did not turn to the traditional sex-role ideology as a means of avoiding dissatisfaction with their own life.

The homemaking responsibilities of a woman are perhaps among the most traditional features of married life. Does a mother's attitude toward homemaking influence her daughter's sex-role attitudes? The answer is yes. Mothers who were dissatisfied with homemaking had a greater tendency than satisfied homemakers to raise daughters with the contemporary view [see illustration on preceding page]. Daughters of mothers who were satisfied with household tasks or had a neutral attitude toward them had the greatest likelihood of holding the traditional view.

Were mothers who were dissatisfied with household work less satisfied with their life? Again the answer is a definite yes. Half of the mothers who were dissatisfied with homemaking tasks were dissatisfied in general with their life, but only 7 percent of mothers satisfied with homemaking were dissatisfied with their life. In addition, 85 percent of the mothers who enjoyed their homemaking role were satisfied with their life. Only 35 percent of the mothers who rejected homemaking found general satisfaction in their life. It may be that a mother who does not find household tasks satisfying and whose overall life satisfaction is low may encourage her daughter to seek a different life pattern. Higher education, particularly graduate school, represents a different way for a woman to allocate her time and energy. Is there, then, a connection between a mother's encouraging her daughter to go to graduate school and the daughter's concept of the female role? Apparently there is. A mother's encouragement enhanced the tendency toward the contemporary viewpoint more than a father's encouragement alone. When both parents equally encouraged their daughter to go to graduate school, however, the daughter was most likely to have the contemporary sex-role ideology.

Although sex-role ideology may be developed in early childhood, it is usually not until adolescence that a girl begins to apply her system of beliefs to her life pattern. At this stage her interaction with her parents presumably would help her to test and adjust the viability of the attitudes and beliefs that had been guiding her since childhood. Do daughters with the contemporary ideology have a pattern of development in adolescence that is different from the pattern of daughters with the traditional view of the female role? In a general way it appears to be so. Women who emerge with the contemporary ideology tend in adolescence to achieve a certain psychological distance from their family, to evolve a sense of separateness as individuals.

Admiration for a parent may be regarded as an index of willingness to remain an integral part of the family. In describing their relationships with their parents during adolescence, women with the contemporary ideology were the most likely to have rejected both parents as objects of admiration: 83 percent of the women who reported that they admired neither parent adhered to the contemporary female-role ideology. There was also a slight tendency for women who admired their fathers more than their mothers to hold the contemporary view, whereas women who admired their mothers more tended to favor traditional sex-role attitudes.

Efforts to please a parent provide another clue to a daughter's willingness to maintain a close sense of identification with that parent. Women who reported

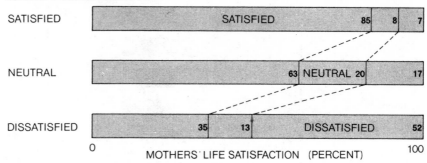

MOTHERS' ATTITUDE TOWARD HOMEMAKER ROLE

MOTHERS' SATISFACTION with life and homemaking were clearly related. Mothers perceived by daughters as satisfied homemakers were likely to be perceived as satisfied with life. Dissatisfied homemakers tended to be seen as being dissatisfied with life.

that they did not try to please either parent, who sought to keep their distance, were more likely to hold the contemporary view than women who tried to please both parents [see illustration on opposite page]. The amount of criticism from a parent is another indicator of the kind of rapport between daughter and parent. Of the women who reported

that they were constantly criticized by both parents, 84 percent held the contemporary view. Women with the contemporary viewpoint tended to have a critical mother, whereas women with the traditional viewpoint recalled having a critical father. Women with the contemporary ideology were frustrated most by their mother; those with the

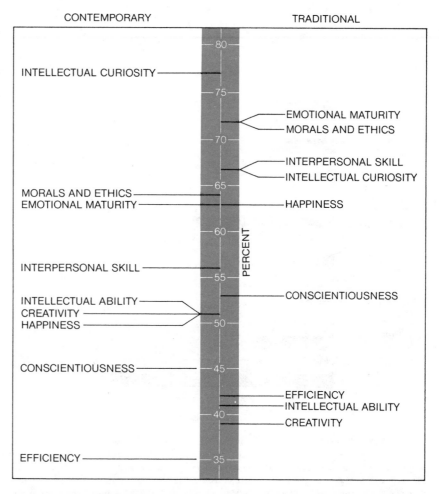

HIERARCHY OF VALUES of women with contemporary sex-role ideology differed from that of women with traditional views. Ranking is based on values rated as most important.

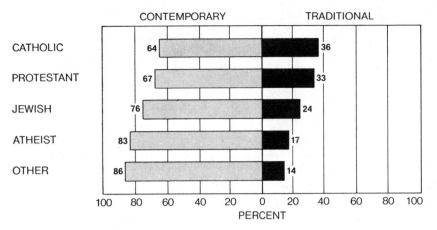

CATHOLIC 64 | 36
PROTESTANT 67 | 33
JEWISH 76 | 24
ATHEIST 83 | 17
OTHER 86 | 14

CONTEMPORARY   TRADITIONAL

PERCENT

PRESENT RELIGION (*above*) was related to sex-role ideology but childhood religion was not. Women with non-Christian beliefs favored the contemporary view of sex roles.

PRESENT RELIGION (NONCONVERTS)

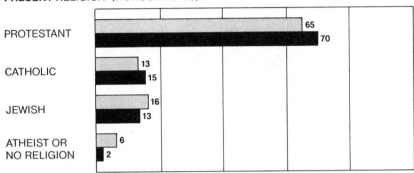

PROTESTANT 65 / 70
CATHOLIC 13 / 15
JEWISH 16 / 13
ATHEIST OR NO RELIGION 6 / 2

PRESENT RELIGION (CONVERTS)

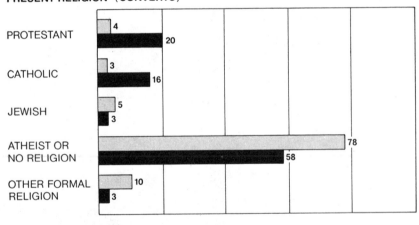

PROTESTANT 4 / 20
CATHOLIC 3 / 16
JEWISH 5 / 3
ATHEIST OR NO RELIGION 78 / 58
OTHER FORMAL RELIGION 10 / 3

RELIGIOUS CONVERSION

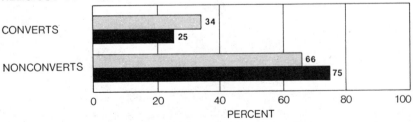

CONVERTS 34 / 25
NONCONVERTS 66 / 75

PERCENT

RELIGIOUS CONVERSION was a linking factor between childhood religion, present religion and sex-role ideology. For women who maintained their childhood religion (*top graph*) there was no statistically significant link between religion and sex-role ideology. For converts (*middle graph*) there was a strong association between religious views and sex-role views: converts with contemporary view (*gray*) moved away from Christianity more than converts with traditional (*black*) view of sex roles. Women who held a contemporary view were more likely to have converted from their childhood religion (*bottom graph*).

traditional viewpoint were more likely to say that neither parent frustrated them.

To feel that one's parent has been successful in life is to recognize and approve of the parent's overall life pattern. Adolescents who regard their parents as being successful are better able to accept their parents as role models and to pattern their own lives in a similar fashion. Rejection of the parental life pattern may force the adolescent to seek new approaches to the conduct of life. This is borne out in the data from the study: women with the contemporary ideology tended to regard both parents as being unsuccessful, and those with the traditional viewpoint tended to see both parents as being successful. The desire of an admiring daughter to please her parents and to tolerate their criticism and her inclination not to regard parental demands as being frustrating are consistent with the daughter's acceptance of her parents' life-style. It is not surprising that such daughters tend to see both parents as being successful.

Approval of parents by an adolescent may be important to family living in traditional terms, but a relatively unquestioning attitude toward familial values and life-styles may make it more difficult for a woman to break through to an alternative life-style as an adult. Reluctance to break with familiar patterns and values may have implications for a woman's ability to adapt to new and perhaps enriching experiences. Although the traditional viewpoint may ensure continuity and security, it may also lead in later life to dissatisfaction, particularly where a changing external environment may require flexibility in adapting to new conditions.

The reluctance to please parents, coupled with a decreased admiration for parents and a tendency to see them as frustrating and critical, are closely associated with the contemporary sex-role ideology. They may be the first steps in a woman's developing a sense of distance from the family in which she grew up. Gaining a sense of oneself as an individual is a necessary step toward enlarging one's sense of self-fulfillment. In a rapidly changing environment self-fulfillment may take on a new meaning that requires a new life-style for women, including new roles such as student and worker as well as the customary ones of wife and mother.

All psychological growth has certain costs, and it is relevant to ask at what price a contemporary ideology has been acquired. A sense of loneliness in adolescence may be considered one kind of short-term psychological price paid for developing new patterns of behavior. Women who held contemporary sex-role beliefs reported that they were lonelier than their peers in adolescence; women with the traditional viewpoint were less likely to be lonely than their peers. If the short-term effects of the contemporary sex-role ideology are painful, what about the long-term consequences? It appears that adult women with the contemporary sex-role ideology are just as happy with their present life as are women with the traditional viewpoint. Furthermore, there does not appear to be any difference in the anxiety levels of the two groups of women.

Differences in sex-role ideology might be expected to produce differences in value systems, and the hierarchy of values of the women in the contemporary category indeed differed from that of the women in the traditional group. The contemporary position placed the highest value on intellectual curiosity; the traditional one put emotional maturity, morals and ethics first [see bottom illustration on page 151]. Moreover, women with the traditional set of beliefs attached special meaning to interpersonal skills, happiness and conscientiousness.

For analytical purposes I have been stressing the striking contrasts between women with a contemporary sex-role ideology and women with a traditional ideology. It is equally enlightening, however, to look at the values these usually divergent groups share. Both rated honesty and understanding people as crucial qualities, and both depreciated perseverance, the ability to work under pressure, ambition, competitiveness, physical stamina and realism. Somewhat surprisingly, both groups gave low ratings to the qualities of self-confidence, enthusiasm, courage, physical attractiveness and sexuality.

I have noted that childhood religion was unexpectedly found to be unrelated to present sex-role ideology. In view of this finding it was surprising to discover that there was a strong association between the present religious affiliation of a woman and her attitude toward sex roles. Women who espoused atheism, who had no formal religion or who professed Judaism or Eastern religions clearly tended to favor the contemporary sex-role ideology. Adult Protestants and Catholics were more likely to hold the traditional viewpoint. This is all the more puzzling because there was also

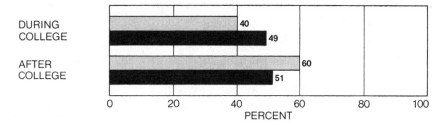

INFLUENCE OF SEX-ROLE IDEOLOGY on time of marriage was significant, with women holding a contemporary view more likely to complete their college studies before marrying.

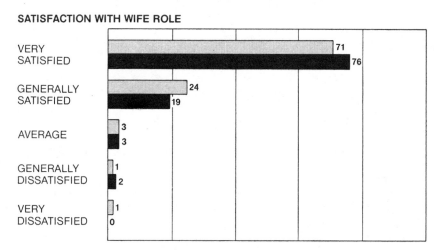

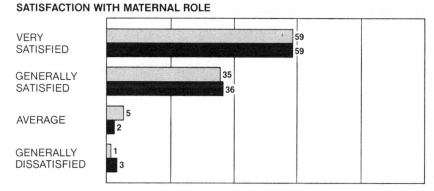

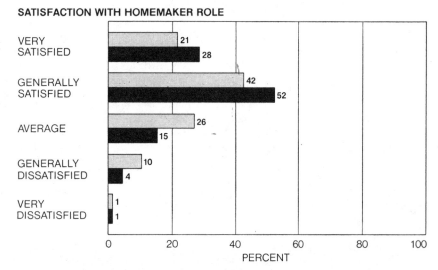

SIMILAR SATISFACTION profiles of women with contemporary and traditional views were found regarding wife and mother roles (top and middle graphs). Women with contemporary views, however, expressed less satisfaction about homemaking responsibilities.

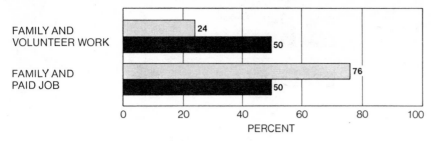

IDEAL LIFE ROLES differed for women with contemporary and traditional sex-role attitudes. Women with contemporary view (*gray*) favored family and paid employment, whereas women with traditional view (*black*) split equally between family and employment.

a distinct association between childhood religion and present religion.

The key to the puzzle appears to be religious conversion. For women who had maintained the religion they had had as children there was no link between sex-role ideology and present religion. For those women who had shifted their religious affiliation, however, there was a clear and most interesting connection between attitudes toward the female role and present religion [*see bottom illustration on page 152*].

In our analysis of the adolescent relationships these women had had with their parents we noted that as adolescents women with the contemporary viewpoint were in the process of disengaging themselves from the family patterns and values with which they had grown up. Women in the traditional category seemed more willing to accept the frame of reference provided by their parents and to continue to live within it. If this interpretation is correct, there should be some indirect confirmation of it in terms of rejection or continuance of childhood religion. More explicitly, rejection of childhood religion might serve as an index of the degree to which a woman has disengaged herself from her parents and family traditions. Women with the contemporary ideology therefore should be more likely than those with the traditional viewpoint to experience religious conversion. Data from the survey confirm this hypothesis: more than a third of the women with the contemporary ideology had moved away from their childhood religion, compared with only a fourth of the women in the traditional group. Women with the contemporary position who had rejected their childhood religion were more likely than those with the traditional view to turn to atheism or to have no formal religion; they were also considerably more likely than women with the traditional position to take up Eastern religions (in which, we might speculate, they sought for new meaning in their

life). Women in the traditional category who had converted were much more likely than women with the contemporary viewpoint to move toward the familiar religions of Protestantism and Catholicism.

It was interesting to examine whether or not women who attached great importance to intellectual qualities tended to act on these values in their daily life. One indicator is to see if women with the contemporary ideology were more likely than those with the traditional viewpoint to postpone marriage until the completion of their college studies, an action that would be consistent with placing a high value on intellectual activity. A look at the educational level of the respondents at the time of their marriage immediately brings out the fact that women with the contemporary ideology were indeed more likely than those with the traditional viewpoint to marry after the completion of their college studies. Women in the traditional group, who did not set such a high value on intellectual qualities, tended to marry while they were still in college.

It would appear that sex-role ideology is an important factor in predicting values. Does it also influence the degree of satisfaction women derive from informal activities with other women? Do women with the contemporary sex-role ideology derive less enjoyment from casual interaction with other women? This turns out to be the case. Women with the contemporary viewpoint said that they enjoyed activities such as chatting and card-playing much less than other women of their age; women in the traditional group tended to rate themselves as being average in this respect.

If these common female activities outside the home are less than exciting to women with the contemporary ideology, what about the three major roles of a married woman within the family: her conjugal role, her maternal role and her homemaker role? Women who saw the

relationship between the sexes in contemporary terms were just as likely to express satisfaction with their husband as women who took the more traditional view of marriage. Moreover, among the women in the sample who had children, mothers with the contemporary ideology were just as satisfied with their maternal role as were mothers in the traditional group. When it came to satisfaction with the role of homemaker, a different picture emerged. Women with the contemporary viewpoint were noticeably less enthusiastic about homemaking. Contrary to television advertisements for detergents and other household products, not all women find delight in cleaning house or washing clothes. Women with the contemporary position were not reluctant to convey their dislike for these household tasks. On the other hand, activities that allow more self-expression or creativity, such as cooking, entertaining, interior decorating, sewing and shopping, were equally acceptable to women in both categories.

The two groups of women have distinctly different concepts of the ideal life. For the woman in the traditional category the ideal life consists in devoting her energies to family and volunteer social activities. Fifty percent of the women in this group reported that their choice for the most satisfying way of life involves family and volunteer projects; only 24 percent of the women in the contemporary group gave this response. More than three-quarters of the women in the contemporary category said that the most satisfactory life-style is a combination of family and full-time or part-time employment.

Although it is clear that ideology affects life goals and choices, does it also produce differences in the self-concepts of women? Self-esteem, the acceptance of oneself as an individual, is an important component of one's self-image. How do the two groups in our survey compare in self-esteem? Curiously, the women in both groups have remarkably similar self-esteem profiles. Women in both categories express equal confidence in their competence as wife and mother. Their sense of competence regarding their ability as student, employee and community participant is also similar. Wives with the traditional viewpoint rate their ability to solve complex problems just as favorably as contemporary wives. The traditional and contemporary sex-role viewpoints lead to two distinct life patterns, but within each ideological position women are able to find fulfillment and meaning in their life.

15

Public Policy on Fertility Control

by Frederick S. Jaffe
July 1973

*In the U.S. over the past dozen years policy on
contraception has been almost entirely reversed. The
transformation reflects the concern of the community
with population size and poverty*

As recently as 1971 Federal law classified contraceptives among "obscene or pornographic materials," and until a few years ago the laws of many states restricted not only their sale but also the dissemination of information about them. In other words, public policy made it difficult for health professionals to dispense and for the public to obtain advice and materials for achieving effective contraception. Now most of the laws have been repealed and the Federal Government has (in the Department of Health, Education, and Welfare) an Office of Population Affairs, a National Center for Family Planning Services and a Center for Population Research. Clearly public policy on family planning has undergone a substantial change. How did the change come about, and what effects has it had? I shall discuss these questions from the viewpoint of a participant and an observer, since my principal responsibility with the Planned Parenthood Federation of America for more than 15 years has been in the area of public policy.

The change of policy did not transform the U.S. from a nation in which contraception was rarely practiced to one in which it is widespread; it has been widespread for a long time. What the change did do was to make it possible for increasing numbers of people to achieve their goals relating to size of family. As early as 1941, when the first large-scale study of attitudes and practices in family planning was made (in

Indianapolis by the Scripps Foundation for Research in Population Problems and the Milbank Memorial Fund), most white Protestant couples were found to practice some form of contraception at some point in their lives to limit and space births. In 1955, when a group from the Scripps Foundation and the University of Michigan made a national survey, whites of all religious persuasions reported the same pattern. Both surveys revealed significant socioeconomic differences, however, in the timing of the initiation of contraception, in employing the most effective methods and in success in controlling births. Many couples relied on the least effective schemes for contraception, which were folk methods or nonprescription methods. When nonwhite couples were sampled for the first time (in 1960, by the Scripps group), the findings were similar. In short, by 1960 most Americans had a favorable attitude toward contraception, but the effectiveness of the methods they used varied widely.

In 1936 the sociologist Norman E. Himes, in his book *Medical History of Contraception*, characterized the methods employed by large segments of the married population in the U.S. and western Europe as "amateur" and "back fence" contraception. It was, he said, "learned from friends, neighbors, childhood or adult acquaintances." According to Himes, the problem "is not shall we have conception control or no conception control, but rather shall we dif-

fuse the latest knowledge on scientific contraception or encourage by indifference and laissez-faire the use of quasi-unreliable, quasi-harmful methods with which many, including not a few of the otherwise enlightened, are in the habit of worrying along."

The problem as Himes stated it is precisely the issue that has been at stake in the evolution of public policy on family planning. The issue can be restated in ways that reveal more of its underlying social implications. Since there are significant differences in failure rates between the back-fence methods and the most effective techniques, whether or not the best methods are intentionally diffused as a matter of public policy depends on how important the society believes it is to prevent unwanted pregnancies and their social, economic, health and demographic consequences. Since there have been and still are socioeconomic differences in access to the best methods and therefore in ability to avoid contraceptive failures, the issue is also related to the society's broad policies on poverty and the prevention of dependency. Finally, since the most effective methods are the ones whose distribution is controlled by the medical profession and by health institutions, the issue becomes a test of the ability of the health system to diffuse scientific knowledge and practice—a process necessary to improve not only the control of fertility but also numerous other health practices.

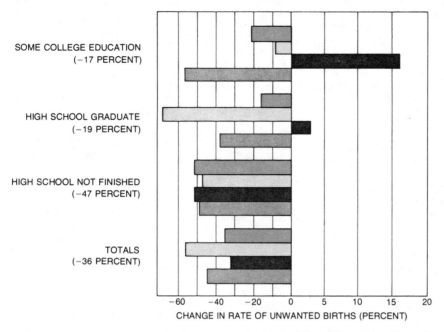

UNWANTED BIRTHS, as measured by a study done by the Office of Population Research of Princeton University, have declined among almost all groups since 1960. The percentage figures compare the rate of unwanted births in the period 1961 through 1965 with the rate from 1966 through 1970. Negative percentages indicate declines in the rate of unwanted births. Educational descriptions relate to wives. Bars represent whites (*dark color*), blacks (*light color*), whites who are not Catholic (*dark gray*) and white Catholics (*light gray*).

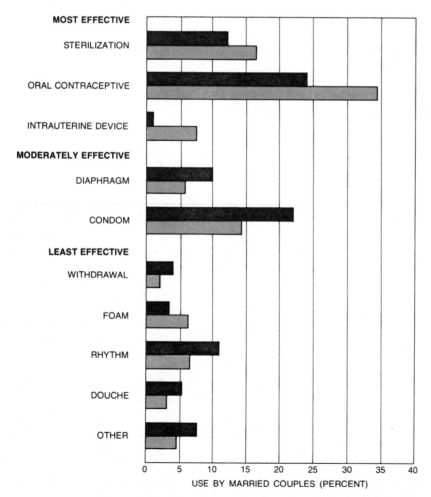

METHODS OF CONTRACEPTION employed by married couples are compared for 1965 (*gray*) and 1970 (*color*). These Princeton findings show a shift to more effective methods.

The Federal and state laws that made it difficult to dispense and obtain contraceptive advice and materials were often called Comstock laws, reflecting the far-reaching influence of the 19th-century movement personified by Anthony Comstock, who for many years beginning in 1873 was secretary of the New York Society for the Suppression of Vice. The laws, even though various court decisions helped to moderate their impact, had a chilling effect on public and professional attitudes and on the policies and practices of physicians and health institutions. For example, not until 1955 did a national magazine publish an article that for the first time named specific methods of contraception, and not until 1959 did a television network have a program that mentioned the subject. The constraints were most apparent in the administrative policies of Government hospitals and health agencies. Even for people who did not depend on publicly funded health agencies for medical care, however, public policy stigmatized contraceptive practice and created obstacles to obtaining medical contraception.

In the period from 1930 to 1950 Planned Parenthood and associated groups mounted unsuccessful efforts to repeal the restrictive laws. Paradoxically the shift in public policy began not with changes in law but with changes in administrative policies. A major turning point was reached in the late 1950's with a protracted and successful campaign by the same groups to reverse the long-standing but unwritten ban on contraceptive prescription in the municipal hospitals in New York City. (The prohibition was typical of most Government-operated health services at the time.) Although the campaign succeeded in its immediate objective of freeing hospital physicians to prescribe birth control, its major significance was in demonstrating how much public support there was for family planning.

In 1959, after a Presidential committee had recommended that the U.S. Government provide assistance on population programs to other nations requesting it, discussion of public policy on family planning became linked with discussion of the population problem. The ensuing debate was marked by the opposition of the Catholic bishops of the U.S. to the use of any public funds for birth-control programs at home or abroad and President Eisenhower's statement of opposition to a Government program. (He reversed his position four years later.) Officials of the Kennedy Administration expressed a much different view, describing in a series of speeches the Government's increasing concern over the impact of rapid population growth. The National Institutes of Health acknowledged a responsibility for supporting basic research in reproductive physiology that might lead to improved methods of fertility control. The work was assigned to the newly formed National Institute of Child Health and Human Development. (Public funds, however, played no part in the development of the oral contraceptive or the intrauterine device, which are the two methods that revolutionized contraceptive practice during the 1960's. Research on these methods was supported almost entirely by foundations, private philanthropists and industry.) By the end of 1963 attitudes in Washington had changed enough for Congress to adopt an amendment to the foreign-aid bill authorizing the use of assistance funds for "research into problems of population growth." In 1965 the National Academy of Sciences urged that family planning be made an integral part of domestic public medical programs and suggested that the appointment of an official "at a high national level" might facilitate Federal action. In the same year a Senate committee began a long series of hearings on the population problem.

The first major changes in law came at the state level in 1965 and 1966 when, with relatively little controversy, New York, Ohio, Massachusetts, Minne-

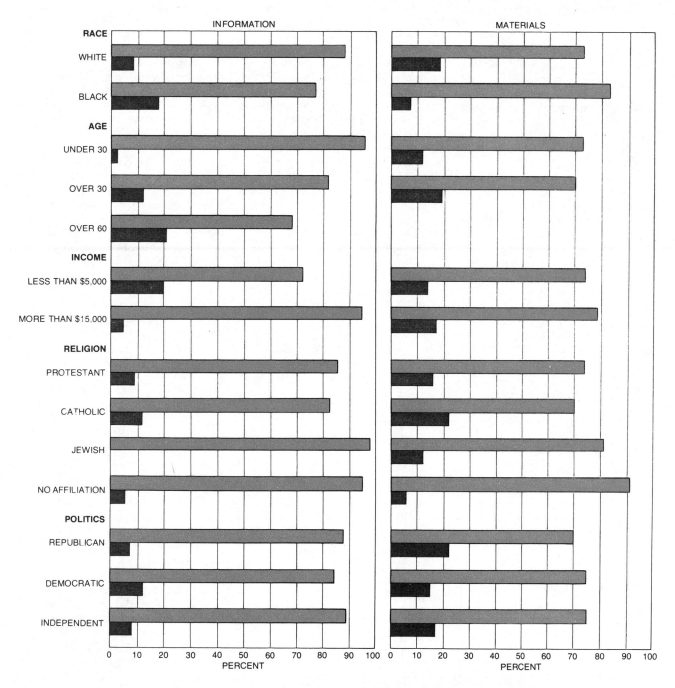

RESULTS OF POLL taken in 1971 by the Opinion Research Corporation for the U.S. Commission on Population Growth and the American Future are given. The chart shows the percentage of people in each category responding affirmatively (*color*) and negatively (*gray*) to a question about birth-control information and a question about birth-control materials. The information question was: "Do you think that information about birth control should or should not be made available by the Government to all men and women who want it?" The question on materials was whether or not the Government should make birth-control materials available.

sota and Missouri repealed certain Comstock-era restrictions on the dissemination of contraceptive information. Bills authorizing or encouraging public health departments or welfare agencies to provide family-planning services at public expense were adopted in California, Colorado, Florida, Georgia, Illinois, Iowa, Kansas, Michigan, Nevada, Oklahoma, Oregon and West Virginia. The U.S. Supreme Court, in *Griswold* v. *Connecticut*, struck down Connecticut's archaic statute—the only one in the country that prohibited the use of contraceptives—with a ruling that married couples have a constitutional right to practice contraception free of state interference. (Last year the court in effect extended the right to unmarried people.)

President Johnson referred in his State of the Union message of 1965 (and many times thereafter) to the importance of dealing with problems of population growth and providing family-planning services. The Department of Health, Education, and Welfare issued its first policy statement on family planning in 1966. The clearest statement of the objectives of U.S. domestic policy appeared the same year in the President's special message to Congress on health and education. The President cited family planning as one of four health problems requiring special attention. "We have a growing concern to foster the integrity of the family and the opportunity for each child," he said. "It is essential that all families have access to information and services that will allow freedom to choose the number and spacing of their children within the dictates of individual conscience."

The first Federal agency to move from words to action was the Office of Economic Opportunity, which as part of its antipoverty program began in 1965 to make grants to community-action agencies for family-planning projects. In the same year Federal maternity-care projects, which were designed primarily to reduce the incidence of mental retardation among children born to low-income women who were at high risk of bearing retarded infants, enabled some city health departments to start providing family-planning services on a limited basis.

Nonetheless, action tended to lag behind the change in expressed policy. The Federal role in biomedical research was implicitly acknowledged to be inadequate in 1965 when the advisory council of the National Institute of Child Health and Human Development admonished the agency to take the initiative in stimulating increased work on problems of human fertility, sterility and family planning. In 1967 an outside review of the Department of Health, Education, and Welfare found that none of the department's operating agencies "places high priority on family planning or is certain what precise functions it is expected to carry out in this field."

By 1967 Congress was beginning to prod the Federal agencies. In amendments to the Economic Opportunity Act family planning was designated for special emphasis in the antipoverty program. Congress also amended the Social Security Act to specify that at least 6 percent of the money appropriated for maternal- and child-health programs administered by the Department of Health, Education, and Welfare be devoted to family-planning service projects. The act also required the states to offer and provide family-planning services to all appropriate recipients of public assistance. Finally, Congress amended the Foreign Assistance Act to designate certain funds for family-planning and population programs overseas.

During the same period a number of state laws prohibiting abortion except to save the mother's life came under challenge. Colorado revised its abortion law in 1967, and 17 other states did so subsequently. In January of this year the U.S. Supreme Court changed the entire abortion picture by ruling that states could not interfere with decisions made by a woman and her physician during the first three months of pregnancy.

In 1968 President Johnson appointed a Committee on Population and Family Planning to assess the adequacy of the Federal program. In its report the committee recommended rapid increases in funding and strengthening of the administrative machinery for the three main parts of the Federal program: family-planning services at home; biomedical and behavioral research to improve methods of contraception and the understanding of population dynamics, and assistance to family-planning programs in developing countries. A year later President Nixon sent to Congress a population message, calling for more Federal effort in all these directions and asking for the establishment of a population commission. Legislation creating the commission was enacted in 1970. That same year Congress passed the Family Planning Services and Population Research Act, which put into effect a modified version of the recommendations of President Johnson's population committee. The act authorized $382 million for a three-year program of services and research.

In 1971, complying with a provision of the act, the Department of Health, Education, and Welfare submitted to Congress a five-year plan; it called for a program that would provide services to an estimated 6.6 million women of low or marginal income by 1975. A year later the Commission on Population Growth and the American Future presented its final report, which appears likely to have an influence on thinking in the field for many years to come. The report recommended a broad array of health, edu-

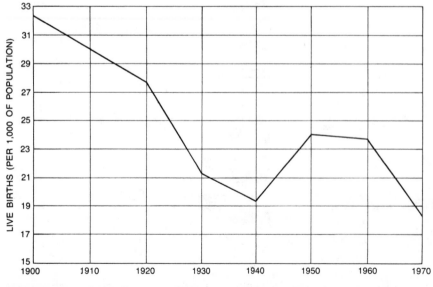

BIRTHRATE IN THE U.S. HAS DECLINED since 1900 except for the period following World War II. The development and rapid adoption of two of the three most effective methods of contraception, the contraceptive pill and the intrauterine device, have been factors in the recent decline. The third most effective method of contraception is sterilization.

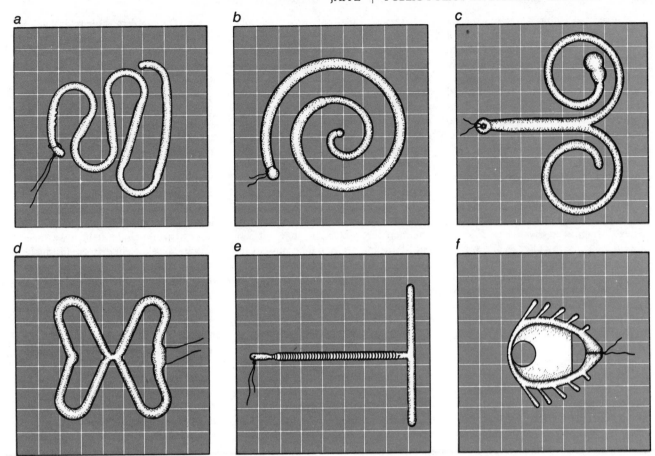

INTRAUTERINE DEVICES, which are among the most effective methods of birth control, include the types depicted here. They are the Lippes loop (*a*), the Margulies spiral (*b*), the double coil (*c*), the Birnberg bow (*d*), the copper *T* (*e*) and the Dalkon shield (*f*).

cation, economic and social programs to enable the U.S. to achieve a stabilized population in an orderly manner as rapidly as possible.

In sum, the change in public policy was expressed in numerous legislative and administrative actions at Federal, state and local levels. It was also expressed in an enormous expansion of organized family-planning programs serving people of low or marginal income. In 1960 no more than 150 public and voluntary health agencies, most of them affiliates of Planned Parenthood, operated such programs; they served about 150,000 women. By 1972 nearly 3,000 hospitals, health departments and voluntary agencies were providing services to an estimated 2.6 million women in two-thirds of the counties of the U.S. A decade ago hardly any public money was available for such services; in fiscal 1973 the Federal appropriation alone for family-planning project grants was $128 million. Federal support for research rose from close to nothing in 1962 to $40 million in fiscal 1973. Projecting the experience of the past few years, it appears feasible to achieve the Federal Government's stated goals in this area by 1975, provided that the amount of

Federal money available continues to rise. The future of the program is uncertain, however, as a result of the Administration's effort this year to cut down or eliminate support of many health and social programs, including family planning. It remains to be seen whether Congress will agree.

Whatever the outcome, the consequences of the changes that have already taken place can be measured by the increasing number of people of low or marginal income who have begun to use modern methods of fertility control, which is an aspect of medical care that was previously limited mainly to people of middle and high income. Periodic studies by the Office of Population Research at Princeton University show that between 1965 and 1970 the historic socioeconomic differences in patterns of contraceptive use were considerably reduced. Other studies indicate that fertility rates declined more rapidly in the latter part of the decade among poor and near-poor women than among women above the poverty level. Indirect effects of the policy change are less measurable but no less significant. By supporting the development of programs and facilitat-

ing public discussion of fertility control and population problems, Government actions have stimulated professional interest in family planning and the practice of effective birth control by people of all classes. As a result the change in public policy has begun to reverse the effects of the historic taboos that have surrounded contraception. The effects are suggested by the finding of the Princeton group that nearly three in five couples who practice contraception now employ the most effective methods (pills, intrauterine devices and sterilization) and that the incidence of unwanted pregnancy declined 36 percent between the first and the second half of the 1960's.

So much for the major changes. How were they brought about? Did the impetus come from within the health system or from outside it—from the political community, from citizens' groups and from the demands of individuals?

The question has no quick and easy answer. The list of people and groups that have worked to change public policy on family planning includes many physicians, health leaders and professional organizations. The health rationale for family planning, which is that having several children in rapid succession results in abnormally high rates of infant and maternal death and illness, was essentially formulated a generation ago and has been important in the policy debate. Unfortunately it has remained only a rationale. Most physicians did not perceive family planning as a medical activity and still do not, although the best methods of contraception now known and the new methods under investigation require close medical supervision.

In my view the health institutions and the health professionals have not collectively distinguished themselves in pressing for a change in policy or in responding to the opportunities created by the change. I believe the primary impetus for change has come from outside the health system in response to two principal concerns, which are directed respectively toward the rapid rate of growth of population and toward the problems of poverty. An essential precondition for the change was the technology represented by the pill and the intrauterine device, which made large-scale programs feasible for the first time. Key roles in the process of change were played by political leaders and by voluntary organizations such as Planned Parenthood.

It seems to me that three basic philosophical problems are involved in the sluggish response of the health system to the opportunities presented by the policy change on family planning. The first is the protracted debate over whether medical care should be delivered by categories or comprehensively. Family planning had the misfortune to come in from the cold when the watchword in health circles was "comprehensive." Although health leaders privately conceded the difficulty, if not the impossibility, of launching a new health service without a certain amount of specialized attention and protection, they felt compelled to oppose in public any special administrative arrangements or earmarked funding and to decry any form of "freestanding" (special purpose) clinic, which is the type of clinic serving a large proportion of the people who are involved in family-planning programs.

For years the essence of the argument for comprehensive service has been that it would provide the preventive care that is now so inadequately provided and that it would reduce the need for acute, episodic care. Few people argue against the desirability of such comprehensive services, but there are many differences of opinion on how to achieve

them. The problem is twofold, involving both restructuring the delivery of care and providing individuals with concrete opportunities to learn from experience the benefits of preventive services.

It is clear that little such learning has been achieved among the people who are able to pay for visits to private physicians; they continue to go to this or that physician or specialist for treatment of an existing illness. In contrast, a finding that emerged in the obstetrics and gynecology departments of some hospitals in the 1950's is of interest. It was that the introduction of family-planning services in postpartum clinics, which was necessary because the clinics were testing new contraceptive products, doubled the rate of postpartum return among ward patients. A fairly simple change yielded a considerable response from a group of patients who had previously been characterized by physicians and researchers as "unmotivated" to seek postpartum checkups.

On the basis of this experience and others Planned Parenthood suggested that if the family-planning service that low-income people appeared to need and want were offered, an opportunity would be created to provide them with other types of health care that they (like people of higher income) did not yet perceive as being needed, although health professionals had described the services as important. Data from computerized reporting systems for family-planning services show how the hypothesis has stood up. Of the estimated 2.6 million women served last year by organized family-planning programs, nine in 10 received pills or intrauterine devices, nine in 10 had annual pelvic examinations, eight in 10 had annual breast examinations and Pap tests, six in 10 had other laboratory procedures such as blood tests and screening for venereal disease and more than half had other medical examinations. In this instance a specialized approach has worked to achieve not only the primary purpose of the program but also other health goals: organized family-planning programs operated by a variety of health and other agencies have become the nation's largest providers of preventive health service to young women of low or marginal income.

The second philosophical issue is the related one of whether the focus of health policy should be on quality or on quantity. Family planning, whatever its broad social and health consequences, remains a relatively simple mass personal health service. The current health system offers few rewards for either individual practitioners or agencies to under-

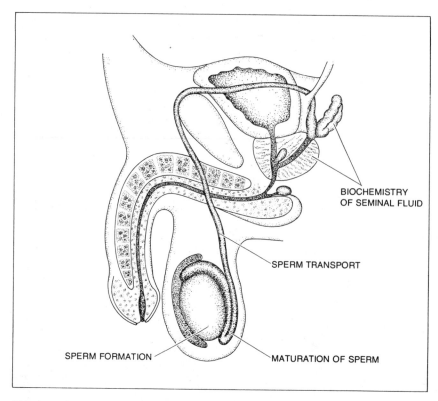

MALE REPRODUCTIVE SYSTEM is portrayed schematically to indicate points where the reproductive process is susceptible to control. The process can also be approached by measures directed at the output of the pituitary gland and the production or the effect of steroid hormones. Both pituitary and hormonal processes are under the control of the brain.

take seriously the task of delivering mass personal health services.

In the light of the information that has been emerging recently about the delivery of medical care in China by "barefoot doctors" and their role in (among other things) China's extensive family-planning efforts, I suggest that the slow response of the U.S. health system to the change in family-planning policy is related to the basic issue of whether a nation should choose to emphasize quality care for the few or basic core services for the many. In the U.S. the choice has been for the former policy, although the nation has the resources to provide everyone with at least a minimum standard of health care that meets basic preventive and curative needs.

The third philosophical issue is what I see as a fundamental misperception of the family-planning problem by many professionals in the fields of health and social service. It is expressed by such frequently voiced opinions as "Everyone in the U.S. who wants birth control can get it" and "The poor are not motivated to use birth control because they want large families." Yet over the past several years acceptance of family planning has constantly outpaced even the most optimistic assessments of what was possible. Similar arguments have been raised about abortion, yet in the three years since abortion was legalized in New York the ratio of abortions to live births, particularly among blacks and people of low income, has been far higher than anyone would have predicted. Now one hears the same arguments to explain why so few sexually active teen-agers appear to practice effective contraception, although it is only recently that any organized family-planning services have been made available to these young people.

Since many of these debates have involved services for low-income people, I believe a major reason for the widespread misperceptions has been the persistence of upper-class biases about poor people and upper-class ideologies about the reasons for their poverty. The academic community has had a role in reinforcing these biases. Much of the social research done since World War II has emphasized differences in attitudes among individuals and groups and deemphasized studies of how well or how badly social institutions function. The result has been a tendency to seek remedies for social problems by attempting to change or blame the victim rather than by modifying institutions.

David Mechanic of the University of

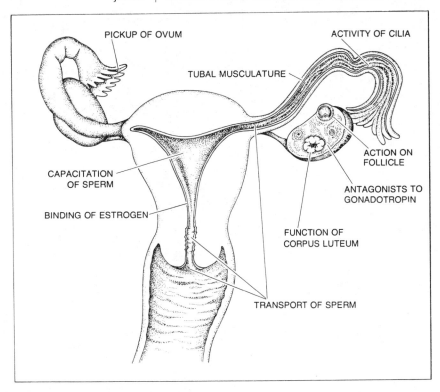

FEMALE REPRODUCTIVE SYSTEM offers a number of places where the reproductive process can be controlled. They include ovulation, transport of the egg, transport of sperm, fertilization and prevention of implantation. As is the case with the male reproductive system, pituitary and hormonal processes are also subject to a certain degree of control.

Wisconsin recently wrote: "While it is true that people's responses to health and illness are often conditioned responses to prior background and experience, the health services system has the capacity to modify such behavior patterns. It can foster dependency or encourage self-reliance. It can respect and enhance the dignity of persons or contribute to stigmatizing and humiliating them.... Barriers to medical and health care that are a product of the way health professionals and health care services function are more amenable to change than client attitudes and behavior. There is evidence that when cost and other barriers are removed from access to medical care, and a valuable service is offered, differential utilization of medical services by social class largely disappears."

That is the key hypothesis on which Planned Parenthood's approach to family planning has been based. Organized family-planning programs for people of low or marginal income have been growing at an average annual rate of 32 percent a year for five years. One can therefore argue that the family-planning experience offers a confirmation of the hypothesis and suggests its more general applicability.

In recent years there have been increasing demands for accountability in the way the health system functions. A variety of new ideas and approaches have emerged; they include the creation of provider agencies (such as free clinics) outside the health system, the concept of community control, the idea that health institutions can be and perhaps ought to be managed by professionals who are not physicians and the notion that the nation faces a health-care crisis that will require drastic changes in the mode of organizing, delivering and financing care [see "The Task of Medicine," by William H. Glazier; SCIENTIFIC AMERICAN, April]. Whatever the merits of these approaches, each one represents an attempt either to fashion a more rational and accountable system or to cope with deficits in the current system. The family-planning experience suggests that the health system can be made somewhat responsive to social goals, but it appears to lack the internal capacity to initiate social change or to generate the required modifications of institutional arrangements and practices. The achievement of such goals requires sustained, focused and systematic attention from outside the health system—a process in which political leaders and ordinary citizens can play a decisive role, particularly when their efforts can be informed by the judgments of even a few health professionals with technical skill and imagination.

16 The Ethics of Experimentation with Human Subjects

by Bernard Barber
February 1976

Research with human subjects has produced advances in medicine but also some instances of ethical abuses. Studies of the attitudes and practices of investigators suggest that better controls are required

The power, scope and funding of biomedical research have expanded enormously in the past 40 years. So also, inevitably, has clinical research with human subjects. That expansion has led in the past decade to widespread reflection on what is increasingly perceived as a new social problem: the abuse of human subjects of medical experimentation. In particular it is alleged that human subjects are not always protected from undue risk and do not always have the opportunity to voluntarily give their adequately informed consent to participation in experiments.

A social problem is defined in part by the concern it arouses, and this one has clearly aroused concern. Members of the medical profession itself led the way, with increasing numbers of journal articles, books and seminars on the issues. The public has become aroused, largely through popular accounts of dramatic incidents—genuine scandals in certain cases—involving the violation of the dignity and rights of patients. And the Federal Government has moved to protect human subjects, potential or actual. Beginning in 1966 the National Institutes of Health, the Food and Drug Administration and the Department of Health, Education, and Welfare have issued increasingly detailed regulations governing experimentation with human subjects in projects they support, which

means in most of the biomedical research done in the country. In 1974 a National Commission for the Protection of Human Subjects of Biomedical and Behavioral Research was established to advise the Department of Health, Education, and Welfare, and it is to be replaced by a long-term National Advisory Council that is to deal with the same issues.

The regulations, commissions and councils and the very fact of interference in medical activities by outsiders are viewed by many investigators as being onerous and even dangerous. On the other hand, many outsiders believe far more social control is required. The debate on the issue has been conducted without much reference to objective evidence. In 1970 our Research Group on Human Experimentation undertook two studies of investigators' attitudes and practices. On the basis of our results I would argue that there is indeed inadequate ethical concern among biomedical investigators, that it is reflected in excessively risky procedures and that better internal and external controls are essential.

There are two major reasons for the general recognition that experimentation with humans is a subject for concern, one of which I alluded to at the outset: the increased power, scope and funding of biomedical research. The oth-

er reason is a change in values: increased emphasis on equality, participation and the challenging of arbitrary authority.

It is easy to forget how new scientific medicine is. The revolutionary advances based on knowledge of physiology and biochemistry have come in the past 40 years, and they came from research. The basic work could be done with test-tube preparations and laboratory animals, but eventually human subjects had to be involved. Man is "the final test site," as Henry K. Beecher, a pioneer among physicians concerned about the ethics of research, once put it. Unfortunately there are no statistics on the number of people who are subjects in medical experiments or even on how many projects involve human subjects; the National Institutes of Health keeps records according to area of research (a disease or a physiological process, for example) rather than according to species of experimental subject; the NIH can say only that recently about a third of the projects it approves involve human subjects. It is clear, however, that the number of human subjects is larger than it used to be and that some small but significant minority of those subjects are involved in risky experiments. If more people have been put at more risk, then there is a rational basis for concern about the satisfactory balancing of risks and benefits, about adequate protection from unnecessary risk and about some groups being put at more risk than other groups.

Over and beyond this utilitarian basis for the new social concern with medical experimentation is the value factor, which arises from recent social changes. All over the world individuals have been demanding more equality of treatment and the right to be informed about and to participate in decisions affecting them and have been challenging the right of experts to make those decisions unilaterally. People who define themselves as being unequal, underprivileged or exploited are demanding better treatment and better protection, whether it is underdeveloped countries as against developed ones, blacks as against whites, women as against men, young as against old, patients as against doctors—or subjects as against investigators. This moral revolution of rising value-expectations has combined with the revolution in medicine to focus attention on the ethics of experimentation with human subjects.

Public awareness of the problem is too much the result of headlined scandals, but the scandals do illustrate some of the possible abuses. In the 1960's two respected cancer investigators who were studying the immune response to malignancies injected live cancer cells into a number of geriatric patients at the Jewish Hospital and Medical Center of Brooklyn without first obtaining the patients' informed consent. A few years later a leading virologist conducted an experiment at Willowbrook, a New York State institution for the severely retarded. Reasoning that a serious liver infection, hepatitis, was in effect endemic in the hospital anyway, he deliberately exposed some children to hepatitis virus in an attempt to achieve controlled conditions for testing a vaccine. The accusation was that the children's parents were not given enough information on which to base informed consent, and that in some cases consent was given perfunctorily by administrators of the institution.

More recently there was the exposure by the press of the ongoing syphilis experiment in Tuskegee, Ala. Since the 1930's a group of black subjects with syphilis had been kept under observation in an effort to study the course of the disease. That was not considered wrong in the 1930's, when the known treatments for the disease were only marginally effective, but by 1945 penicillin had become available as a safe and extremely effective cure for syphilis. Yet somehow the experiment was continued, and presumably some men died of the disease who could have been cured.

How significant are such scandals?

---

45. A researcher plans to study bone metabolism in children suffering from a serious bone disease. He intends to determine the degree of appropriation of calcium into the bone by using radioactive calcium. In order to make an adequate comparison, he intends to use some healthy children as controls, and he plans to obtain the consent of the parents of both groups of children after explaining to them the nature and purposes of the investigation and the short and long-term risks to their children. Evidence from animals and earlier studies in humans indicates that the size of the radioactive dose to be administered here would only very slightly (say, by 5-10 chances in a million) increase the probability of the subjects involved contracting leukemia or experiencing other problems in the long run. While there are no definitive data as yet on the incidence of leukemia in children, a number of doctors and statistical sources indicate that the rate is about 250/million in persons under 18 years of age. Assume for the purpose of this question that the incidence of the bone disease being discussed is about the same as that for leukemia in children under 18 years of age. The investigation, if successful, would add greatly to medical knowledge regarding this particular bone disease, but the administration of the radioactive calcium would not be of immediate therapeutic benefit for either group of children. The results of the investigation may, however, eventually benefit the group of children suffering from the bone disease. Please assume for the purposes of this question that there is no other method that would produce the data the researcher desires. The researcher is known to be highly competent in this area.

45A. Hypothetically assuming that you constitute an institutional review "committee of one," and that the proposed investigation has never been done before, please check the lowest probability that you would consider acceptable for your approval of the proposed investigation. (Check only one)

( ) 1.   If the chances are 1 in 10 that the investigation will lead to an important medical discovery.

( ) 2.   If the chances are 3 in 10 that the investigation will lead to an important medical discovery.

( ) 3.   If the chances are 5 in 10 that the investigation will lead to an important medical discovery.

( ) 4.   If the chances are 7 in 10 that the investigation will lead to an important medical discovery.

( ) 5.   If the chances are 9 in 10 that the investigation will lead to an important medical discovery.

( ) 6.   Place a check here if you feel that, as the proposal stands, the researcher should not attempt the investigation, no matter what the probability that an important medical discovery will result. (IF YOU CHECKED HERE, please explain): _____

_____

45B. Which of the above responses comes closest to what you feel the existing institutional review committee in your institution would make? ____ (Please write in the number of the response.)

45C. Which of the above responses comes closest to what you feel the majority of the researchers in your institution would make, acting in their role as researcher rather than as a "committee of one"? ____ (Please write in the number of the response.)

HYPOTHETICAL EXPERIMENT described here was one of six experiments submitted to investigators and administrators in hospitals and other research centers in a mailed questionnaire. In each case respondents were asked whether, under specified conditions, they would approve of the experiment. This proposal involved giving radioactive calcium to children with a bone disease and to a control group and measuring its uptake by bone.

44. It has been shown that the thymus has an important
bearing on the development and maintenance of immunity.
For this reason the researcher proposes an investigation
to determine the effect of thymus removal on the survival
of tissue transplants, a very timely and important problem.
In a sample of children and adolescents admitted for surgery to correct congenital heart lesions, he would randomly
select an experimental group for thymectomy. Though the
thymectomy will prolong the heart surgery by a few minutes,
there is otherwise extremely little additional surgical
risk from this procedure. At the conclusion of each heart
operation, a full-thickness skin graft, approximately one
cm. in diameter and obtained from an unrelated adult donor,
would be sutured in place on the chest wall of both the experimental and control groups. He would then compare the
survival of the skin grafts in each of the groups. It has
been shown in a number of investigations of neonatal rats
and other animals that those whose thymus had been removed
were much less likely to reject skin grafts. The possible
long-term immunological problems that might result are as
yet not completely known, but a number of studies in animals indicate significant immunological deficiencies after
thymectomy. Studies done in humans with myasthenia gravis,
some of whom had undergone thymectomy, have not definitely
demonstrated that the immunological abnormalities discovered
in these patients were the result of thymectomies. To quote
one authority: "There were no immunologic abnormalities
that could be attributed to the effect of thymectomy per se."
    The research will result in no therapeutic benefits for
the patients involved. The researcher plans to obtain the
consent of his potential patient-volunteers and/or their
parents after explaining the procedures involved in the investigation as well as the possible short-term surgical and
long-term immunological hazards for the subjects.

REMOVAL OF THYMUS GLAND during heart surgery was the experimental procedure proposed in another protocol in the questionnaire. Respondents were asked if they would approve of the experiment, given various probabilities that it would show thymectomy "considerably increases the probability of tissue-transplant survival in children and adolescents."

We do not know, because no one has been doing the kind of social bookkeeping about numbers of subjects, degree of risk, adequacy of consent and efficacy of protective mechanisms that would yield an overall view of experimentation with human beings and that might contradict the more extreme allegations of abuse elicited by the publicized scandals. In the absence of such intensive record keeping it remains for social research to fill the gap by sampling the total range of experimentation with human subjects. To that end our group conducted first a national mail survey of nearly 300 biomedical research institutions and then an intensive interview study of 350 individual investigators at two institutions.

Our national survey questionnaire was answered by 293 teaching and non-teaching hospitals and other research institutions that, our analysis showed, constituted a nationally representative sample of all such institutions. Those who filled out the questionnaire were generally themselves active researchers and members of their institution's review committee, set up to pass on research proposals. We asked the investigators to give us their response to six simulated proposals such as those that might come before a review committee. The proposals were detailed research protocols designed to measure the degree of the investigators' concern about informed consent and their willingness to approve of studies involving various levels of risk. We could be confident that the protocols were "hypothetical-actual" rather than "hypothetical-fantastic" because we constructed them with careful attention to the research literature, checked them with specialists and pretested them with a dozen chiefs of research at medical centers, who found them to be convincingly real.

One protocol described a study of chromosome breakage in users of hallucinogenic drugs; blood samples (for chromosomes) and urine samples (for evidence of drug use) were to be taken, at no risk but also without notification of the experimental purpose, from students routinely visiting the university health center. Another protocol proposed that the thymus gland, which is a component of the immune system, be removed unnecessarily from a random sample of children undergoing heart surgery; the objective was to learn the effect of the thymectomy on the survival of an experimental skin graft made at the same

time. The other protocols dealt with a random test of alternative treatments for a congenital heart defect in children; with an evaluation of the efficacy of a new drug for severe depression (placebos were given to some patients); with a study of lung function in patients kept under unnecessarily prolonged anesthesia after undergoing a routine hernia repair, and with an investigation of the effect of radioactive calcium on bone metabolism in children [see illustrations on this page and page 163].

The answers to the thymectomy, anesthesia and radioactive-calcium protocols in particular gave us measures of the respondents' attitudes toward the balancing of risks and benefits. A clear pattern emerged. In the case of the high-risk thymectomy, for example, 72 percent of the respondents said the project should not be approved no matter how high the probability was that it would establish the efficacy of thymectomy in promoting transplant survival. On the other hand, 28 percent of the respondents said they would approve the experiment; 6 percent said they would approve it even if the chance of significant results was no better than one in 10 [see illustration on next page]. Similarly, 54 percent were against doing the calcium study at all—but 14 percent said they would approve it even if the odds were only one in 10 that it would lead to an important medical discovery. Our basic finding was that whereas the majority of the investigators were what we called "strict" with regard to balancing risks against benefits, a significant minority were "permissive," that is, they were much more willing to accept an unsatisfactory risk-benefit ratio.

The same general pattern of a strict majority and a permissive minority emerged from our second study, in which we interviewed 350 investigators actively engaged in research with human subjects. The investigators were at institutions to which we gave the synthetic names University Hospital and Research Center and Community and Teaching Hospital. The institutions were picked (by a technique known as cluster analysis) as being representative of two kinds of medical center that do considerable amounts of research. The interviewees told us about 424 different studies involving human subjects, and for each study they estimated the risk for subjects, the potential benefit for subjects, the potential benefit for future patients and the potential scientific importance of the study. It was reassuring to find that the investigators considered that only 56 percent of the clinical investigations graded for risk and benefits involved any risk for the subjects. We went on, however, to cross-tabulate the estimated risks and benefits [see illustration on page 166], and we concluded that in 18 percent of the studies the risk was not adequately counterbalanced by the benefits. We called those studies the "less favorable" ones, and we proceeded to classify them further according to their potential benefits for other patients or for medical science. Even when these compensating justifications were taken into account, tabulation revealed a "least favorable" category of studies in which the poor immediate risk-benefit ratio was not compensated for by possible future benefits. These "least favorable" investigations constituted 8 percent of the investigations in our analysis.

The concept of informed consent is a troublesome one. The investigator wants to have enough subjects and is afraid of scaring them off. Patients are likely to be concerned about their own condition, may feel powerless with respect to the physician or hospital and often have difficulty understanding medical language or concepts. Even established medical procedures can have somewhat unpredictable consequences,

so that physicians feel there is a limit to how completely "informed" a patient can be. The fact remains that regulations of Government funding agencies and most institutions now require that the human subject of an experiment (or his guardian, in the case of small children and mentally incompetent patients) understand that something is being done (or some treatment is being withheld) for reasons other than immediate therapeutic ones; the subject or guardian must be informed of any risks and must give consent voluntarily.

With regard to informed consent, our questionnaires and interviews again revealed a minority with "permissive" views and practices, although that minority was smaller than it was for unfavorable risk-benefit ratios. For example, 23 percent of the questionnaire respondents said they would approve the chromosome-break proposal, which presented the informed-consent issue clearly and in effect by itself. The situation was more complex in the heart-defect protocol. Here other dubious elements competed with the fact that the investigator would not inform the parents that his decision whether or not to operate would be a random one, not based on therapeutic considerations. Only 12 percent of our respondents said they would approve

of the study without requiring any revisions, but only 65 percent specifically mentioned the lack of informed consent as a problem.

The best available research evidence on informed consent comes from a study conducted by Bradford H. Gray, who was then a graduate student at Yale University, at a distinguished university hospital and research center (not the one in our interview study). With the consent of the responsible investigator, Gray interviewed 51 women who were the subjects in a study of the effects of a new labor-inducing drug. Although the women had signed a consent form, often in the hectic course of the admitting procedure or in the labor room itself, 20 of them (39 percent) learned only from Gray's interview, which was held after the drug infusion had been started or even after the delivery, that they were the subjects of research. Among those who did know, most of them did not understand at least one aspect of the study: that there might be hazards, that it was a double-blind experiment, that they would be subjected to special monitoring and test procedures or that they were not required to participate; four of the women said they would have refused to participate if they had known there was any choice. Many of the women had been

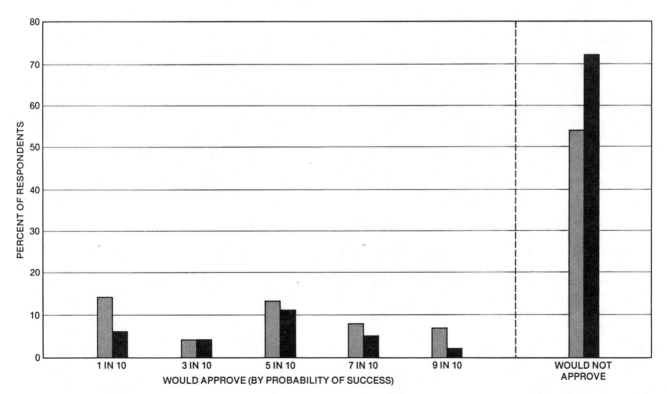

REACTION OF RESPONDENTS to the two hypothetical-experiment questions illustrated on the preceding two pages is shown: the calcium study (light gray bars) and the experimental removal of the thymus gland for a skin-transplant study (dark gray). "As

the proposal stands," 54 percent of the respondents would refuse to approve the calcium study and 72 percent would refuse to approve the thymectomy, regardless of the probability of success. Substantial minorities were much more "permissive," however.

THERAPEUTIC BENEFIT FOR SUBJECTS	RISK		
	NONE	VERY LITTLE	SOME, MODERATE OR LARGE
MINOR, LITTLE OR NONE	11	14	2
SOME	14	12	2
GREAT	10	19	7

RISKS AND BENEFITS were cross-tabulated for some 400 current research projects reported by investigators in two hospitals. Studies falling on or below the diagonal were considered to have risks for subjects that were more or less counterbalanced by benefits for subjects. (In 9 percent of the studies respondents reported no risk and were not asked about benefits.) Studies above the diagonal (*colored boxes*) were classified as "less favorable" for their subjects: they contained risks for subjects and, according to the investigators, offered relatively low benefits. These cases, 18 percent of the total, were further subdivided (in a table not reproduced here) according to benefit for others or for science. Studies that were low in those justifications (8 percent of total) were called "least favorable."

referred for the study by their private physician, but instead of being informed that an experimental drug was to be administered they were told that it would be a "new" drug; they trusted their doctor and assumed that "new" meant "better."

How does it happen that the treatment of human subjects is sometimes less than ethical, even in some of the most respected university-hospital centers? We think the abuses can be traced to defects in the training of physicians and in the screening and monitoring of research by review committees, and also to a fundamental tension between investigation and therapy. We have data bearing on each of these causative factors.

It is in medical school that the profession's central and most serious concerns are presumably given time and place and that its basic knowledge and values are instilled. Yet the evidence from our interviews shows that there is not much training in research ethics in medical school. Of the more than 300 investigators who responded to questions in this area, only 13 percent reported they had been exposed in medical school to part of a course, a seminar or even a single lecture devoted to the ethical issues involved in experimentation with human subjects; only one respondent said he had taken an entire course dealing with the issues. Another 13 percent reported that the subject had come to their attention when, as students, they did practice procedures on one another; for 24 percent it was in the course of experiments with animals; 34 percent remembered discussion of ethical issues in specific

research projects. One or more of these learning experiences were reported by 43 percent of the respondents—but the remaining 57 percent reported not a single such experience. The figures were about the same whether the investigators were graduates of elite U.S. medical schools, other U.S. schools or foreign schools. The figures were a little better, however, for those who had graduated since 1950 than for older investigators.

What little ethics training there is is apparently not very effective: the investigators who reported having learned something about research ethics were only slightly less permissive in response to protocols presenting the risk-benefit issue than those who reported no such experiences. It would appear that both the amount and the quality of medical-school training in the ethics of research could be improved. In this connection it is worth remembering that the many physicians who are not engaged in investigation at all also need some background in experimentation ethics, if only so they can evaluate requests that they direct their patients toward a colleague's research project.

Scientific "peer review" is a keystone of scientific inquiry, operating implicitly in many ways and explicitly in the case of professional journals, grant-awarding committees and many institutional reviewing boards such as the "tissue committees" that assess the results of surgery in hospitals. Ethical peer review of experimentation with human beings should be the counterpart of scientific peer re-

view, but until the mid-1960's such activity received limited support among biomedical researchers. Even after 1966, when the NIH mandated ethical peer review for all its grantees, effective review did not become universal. Our questionnaire went to hospitals and other research centers that had filed with the NIH formal assurances that the required institutional review committee had been established, but 10 percent of the respondents said their institution's committee reviewed only proposals for outside funds and 5 percent reported that only formal proposals to the NIH were reviewed. The two institutions in our interview study were among the 85 percent that stated they were reviewing all research proposals, and yet 8 percent of our interviewees volunteered the information that at least one of their own investigations with human subjects had not been reviewed.

How effective are the review committees in handling the protocols that do come before them? Our questionnaire respondents told us that in 34 percent of the institutions the committees had never required any revisions, rejected any proposals or had any proposals withdrawn in anticipation of rejection for ethical reasons; 31 percent reported revisions, 32 percent outright rejections and 19 percent withdrawals. Either some of these committees have very few ethical problems coming before them or they are ineffective. Gray's study in an institution with an active and strong committee suggests that they are ineffective rather than underworked. The committee whose performance he examined found relatively few proposals that did not need some kind of modification, and he thinks "a record of few actions by committees is an indication that their members are indifferent or that their standards are loose."

The peer-review groups seemed weak in other ways. In some institutions there was no face-to-face discussion among the reviewers. Only 22 percent of the committees had members from outside the institution, something that was then recommended and has since been mandated by the Department of Health, Education, and Welfare. In practically none of the institutions was there continuous monitoring of studies that were approved, although this was even then required by Government regulations. In general ethical peer review is hampered by the fact that each committee operates in isolation and must consider every new issue on its own and without benefit of precedent. A case-reporting system, such as operates in the law, would make that unnecessary and would promote both equity among institutions and high standards. The major weakness in the system is the lack of keen interest in and support of the review committees on the part of most working biomedical investigators. Research is their business; research is their mission and predominant interest, not applied ethics or active advocacy of patients' rights.

Most biomedical investigators are, however, interested in taking care of patients and making them well. As a result medical institutions and individual investigators operate today with two powerful sets of values and goals. On the one hand there is the pursuit and advancement of scientific knowledge. On the other there is the provision of humane and effective therapy for patients. Through a broad range of complex interactions these two sets of values and goals are harmonious, even complementary and mutually reinforcing. Occasionally, however, scientific research and humane therapy can be in conflict. When that happens, there is sometimes a tendency to choose the pursuit of knowledge at the expense of the ethical treatment of patients. An irreducible minimum of conflict may be inevitable. The ethical task now is to come as close as possible to that minimum—and to resolve unavoidable conflict in favor of humane therapy.

There is evidence that the enhanced excitement attending scientific achievement and the rewards bestowed on it in recent decades have skewed the decision-making process in many cases of conflict. As our data show, the medical schools have been largely indifferent to training their students in the ethics of research. Moreover, their record in peer review has been inferior to that of other institutions. Answers to our questionnaire showed they were less likely than other research centers to have set up a review committee before the NIH required one, less likely to have one that met the first NIH guidelines in 1966, less likely to have a committee that reviews all clinical research and less likely to include on their committee medical or nonmedical members from outside the institution. Medical schools, the Association of American Medical Colleges and professional associations of clinical investigators have been much quicker to seek research funds or to protest funding cuts than to organize seriously for the purpose of studying the ethics of research and making policy in that area.

The same emphasis on the pursuit of knowledge rather than on ethics is apparent among individual biomedical investigators. Ethical concern for the subjects of their research is not a major factor when they select their collaborators; at least it is not often mentioned as a characteristic they look for in collaborators. Scientific ability is a major concern. When we asked our 350 interview subjects, "What three characteristics do you most want to know about another researcher before entering into a collaborative relationship with him?" 86 percent of the respondents mentioned scientific ability, 45 percent mentioned motivation to work hard and 43 percent mentioned personality. Only 6 percent of them listed anything we could classify as "ethical concern for research subjects."

The tension between investigation and ethical concern is perhaps best illustrated by indications that the struggle for scientific priority and recognition exerts pressure on ethical considerations. Our data show that the social structure of competition and reward is one of the sources of permissive behavior in experimentation with human subjects; the relatively unsuccessful scientist, striving for recognition, was most likely to be permissive both in his approval of hypothetical protocols and in his own investigative work. We divided our respondents into four categories based on the number of papers they had published and the number of times their work had been cited by other workers; the frequency of citation has been shown to be a good measure of scientific excellence. We called the most-cited investigators the "high quality" scientists and those who had published a great deal but were never cited the "extreme mass-producer" scientists. It was the extreme mass-producers who were most often engaged in investigations with less favorable risk-benefit ratios, who approved of the protocols with poorer risk-benefit ratios and who least often expressed awareness of the importance of consent. Caught up in the socially structured competitive system of science, unsuccessful in it but still pursuing the prize of peer recognition, they appear to be more likely to overvalue scientific work as against humane therapy.

It is not only the mass-producers, contending for recognition among peers in their discipline, who are apt to be more permissive. We also weighed the rank achieved by each worker within his own institution against various measures of his effectiveness compared with that of his colleagues. We found that the "underrewarded" investigators tended to be the more permissive. There is also a quite different kind of medical investigator who we think is likely to be pushed toward permissive practices by scientific competition: some of the professionally esteemed, highly successful medical scientists who are engaged in intense competition for priority and recognition in well-publicized areas of research. There are not many of those people, and they did not emerge in our sample, although some workers who refused to be interviewed may belong in that category. In the absence of real data we can only point to such evidence as published discussions concerning the worldwide heart-transplant competition of a few years ago, which raised questions about the premature exposure of human subjects to what were then still experimental procedures.

Given the fact that there are ethical defects in current medical-research standards and practices, do the resulting

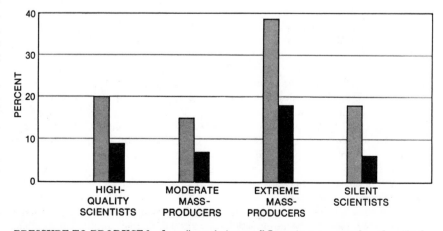

PRESSURE TO PRODUCE leads to "permissiveness." Investigators were classed as "high-quality scientists" (most cited), "moderate mass-producers" (many papers, few citations), "extreme mass-producers" (many papers, no citations) or "silent scientists" (few papers and citations). Extreme mass-producers were twice as likely as high-quality scientists to have a role in one of the less favorable (*light gray*) or least favorable (*dark gray*) studies.

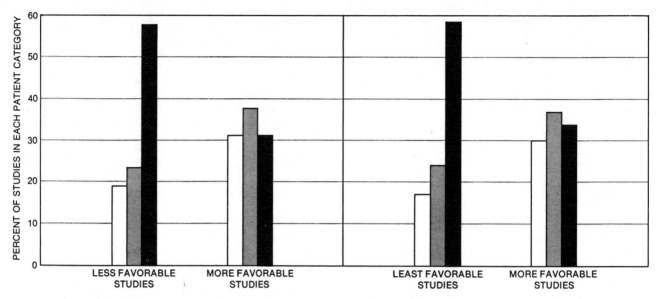

DIFFERENTIAL TREATMENT of various patient categories is evident when studies identified as having the less favorable or the least favorable risk-benefit ratios were classified according to whether fewer than 50 percent of their subjects were ward or clinic patients (*white bars*), between 50 and 75 percent were (*light gray*) or more than 75 percent were (*dark gray*). The less favorable studies were almost twice as likely to have subjects a large majority of whom were ward or clinic patients (*dark gray bars*) as the more favorable studies (*left*). About the same thing was true of studies that had been identified as having least favorable ratios (*right*).

abuses strike particularly, as is often alleged, at certain social groups: at the poor, at children and at institutionalized patients (prisoners in particular)?

The evidence from our interviews with 350 investigators indicates that the poorer patients in hospitals are indeed at a disadvantage as subjects of research. For each of the 424 studies our respondents reported, they told us whether fewer than 50 percent, between 50 and 75 percent or more than 75 percent of the subjects were ward or clinic patients (as opposed to patients in private or semiprivate rooms and under the care of their own physician). We found first of all that ward and clinic patients were more likely to be subjects of experiments. Moreover, when we examined the cases we had previously identified as having "less favorable" and "least favorable" risk-benefit ratios, we found that both categories were almost twice as likely to involve subjects more than three-quarters of whom were ward and clinic patients as the studies with the more favorable ratios were.

The ward and clinic patients are, of course, vulnerable to that kind of discrimination. They can most readily be channeled into an experimental group by admitting physicians and clerks without interference from a personal physician. They tend to be less knowledgeable about hospitals, more readily intimidated and less likely to understand what they are told about an experimental project, and therefore less likely to be able to withhold their consent or to give genu-

inely informed consent. In sum, they are the least likely to be able to protect themselves.

Many institutionalized patients are poor and perhaps incompetent, and they may feel completely dependent on the institution's administrators and physicians. Prisoners are a special case: they are institutionalized in an implicitly coercive situation, so that genuinely informed consent may be a logical impossibility. On the other hand, a prison population is by definition a good source of experimental and control subjects living under controllable conditions, and there have been instances where prison studies have been conducted humanely, with good scientific results and apparently with good effect on the prisoners' morale. Experimentation with prisoners is nevertheless subject to grave abuses. Last summer the head of the Food and Drug Administration told a Senate committee that a review of experimentation in 19 prisons revealed abuses ranging from unprofessional supervision of drug tests to inadequate medical care and follow-up treatment.

Children constitute still another special group. Small children cannot give consent for their own participation in experiments; older children, who could, are often not asked. As the Willowbrook incident demonstrated, parents are not always adequately protective of their children's interests. In the case of institutionalized patients, prisoners and children, new regulations of the Department of Health, Education, and Welfare call

for special protective committees and procedures. These will only be effective, however, in a context of better ethical training for investigators and more effective peer review.

The ethical problems that attend medical research with human subjects are representative of an entire class of problems created by the impact of professionals and professional power on the general public and on public policy. In the area of research with human subjects the medical investigators are not alone; there is a tendency in other fields too for humane concerns to be left at the laboratory door. Psychologists and sociologists have often been accused of circumventing the requirement for consent and of applying unethical manipulative techniques in their investigations of human behavior, and neither profession has welcomed scrutiny from outsiders or restrictive regulation. The issue goes beyond research ethics, however. Many professions now command knowledge that has great potential usefulness for human welfare but bestows power that can be abused. Because professional power is largely based on knowledge that has not yet diffused to the general public it must to a considerable degree be self-regulated, but because professional power is of such major public consequence it must also be subject to significant public control. The medical-research profession does not have a proud record of self-regulation or acceptance of public controls.

BIBLIOGRAPHIES

I ENVIRONMENTAL REGULATION OF SEX HORMONES

1. The Effects of Light on the Human Body

PREVENTION OF HYPERBILIRUBINEMIA OF PREMATURITY BY PHOTOTHERAPY. J. F. Lucey, M. Ferreiro and J. Hewitt in *Pediatrics*, Vol. 41, pages 1047–1056; 1968.

NATURAL AND SYNTHETIC SOURCES OF CIRCULATING 25-HYDROXYVITAMIN D IN MAN. John G. Haddad and Theodore J. Hahn in *Nature*, Vol. 244, No. 5417, pages 515–516; August 24, 1973.

THE EFFECTS OF LIGHT ON MAN AND OTHER MAMMALS. Richard J. Wurtman in *Annual Review of Physiology*, Vol. 37, pages 467–483; 1975.

DAILY RHYTHM IN HUMAN URINARY MELATONIN. H. J. Lynch, R. J. Wurtman, M. A. Moskowitz, M. C. Archer and M. H. Ho in *Science*, Vol. 187, No. 4172, pages 169–171; January 17, 1975.

2. Nonvisual Light Reception

ON TEMPORAL ORGANIZATION IN LIVING SYSTEMS. Colin S. Pittendrigh in *The Harvey Lectures, Series 56*. Academic Press, 1961.

THE ROLE OF THE EYE AND OF THE HYPOTHALAMUS IN THE PHOTOSTIMULATION OF GONADS IN THE DUCK. J. Benoit in *Annals of the New York Academy of Sciences*, Vol. 117, Art. 1, pages 204–216; September 10, 1964.

BIOCHRONOMETRY. Edited by M. Menaker. National Academy of Sciences, 1971.

RHYTHMS, REPRODUCTION, AND PHOTORECEPTION. Michael Menaker in *Biology of Reproduction*, Vol. 4, No. 3, pages 295–308; June, 1971.

3. The Reproductive Behavior of Ring Doves

CONTROL OF BEHAVIOR CYCLES IN REPRODUCTION. Daniel S. Lehrman in *Social Behavior and Organization among Vertebrates*, edited by William Etkin. The University of Chicago Press, 1964.

HORMONAL REGULATION OF PARENTAL BEHAVIOR IN BIRDS AND INFRAHUMAN MAMMALS. Daniel S. Lehrman in *Sex and Internal Secretions*. Edited by William C. Young. Williams & Wilkins Company, 1961.

INTERACTION OF HORMONAL AND EXPERIMENTAL INFLUENCES ON DEVELOPMENT OF BEHAVIOR. Daniel S. Lehrman in *Roots of Behavior*, edited by E. L. Bliss. Harper & Row, Publishers, 1962.

4. The Social Order of Japanese Macaques

PRIMATE SOCIETIES: GROUP TECHNIQUES OF ECOLOGICAL ADAPTATION. Hans Kummer. Aldine Publishing Company, 1971.

THE SOCIAL BEHAVIOR OF MONKEYS. Thelma Rowell. Penguin Books, 1972.

BIOLOGICAL BASES OF HUMAN SOCIAL BEHAVIOR. Robert A. Hinde. McGraw-Hill Book Company, 1974.

CONCEPTUAL AND METHODOLOGICAL PROBLEMS ASSOCIATED WITH THE STUDY OF AGGRESSIVE BEHAVIOR IN PRIMATES UNDER SEMINATURAL CONDITIONS. G. Gray Eaton in *The Neuropsychology of Aggression*, edited by Richard E. Whalen. Plenum Press, 1974.

MALE DOMINANCE AND AGGRESSION IN JAPANESE MACAQUE REPRODUCTION. G. Gray Eaton in *Reproductive Behavior*, edited by William Montagna and William A. Sadler. Plenum Press, 1974.

II INTERNAL REGULATION OF SEX HORMONES

5. Hormones

HORMONES AND BEHAVIOR. Frank A. Beach. Paul B. Hoeber, Inc., 1948.

THE HORMONES IN HUMAN REPRODUCTION. George W. Corner. Princeton University Press, 1943.

THE HORMONES: PHYSIOLOGY, CHEMISTRY AND APPLICATIONS. Edited by Gregory Pincus and Kenneth V. Thimann. Academic Press, Inc., 1955.

HORMONES IN REPRODUCTION. *British Medical Bulletin,* Vol. 11, No. 2; May, 1955.

RECENT PROGRESS IN HORMONE RESEARCH: Vol. 12. Edited by Gregory Pincus. Academic Press, Inc., 1956.

6. The Hormones of the Hypothalamus

NEURAL CONTROL OF THE PITUITARY GLAND. G. W. Harris. The Williams & Wilkins Company, 1955.

THE HYPOTHALAMUS: PROCEEDINGS OF THE WORKSHOP CONFERENCE ON INTEGRATION OF ENDOCRINE AND NON-ENDOCRINE MECHANISMS IN THE HYPOTHALAMUS. Edited by L. Martini, M. Motta and F. Fraschini. Academic Press, 1970.

CHARACTERIZATION OF OVINE HYPOTHALAMIC HYPOPHYSIOTROPIC TSH-RELEASING FACTOR. Roger Burgus, Thomas F. Dunn, Dominic Desiderio, Darrell N. Ward, Wylie Vale and Roger Guillemin in *Nature,* Vol. 226, No. 5243, pages 321–325; April 25, 1970

STRUCTURE OF THE PORCINE LH- AND FSH-RELEASING HORMONE, I: THE PROPOSED AMINO ACID SEQUENCE. H. Matsuo, Y. Baba, R. M. G. Nair, A. Arimura and A. V. Schally in *Biochemical and Biophysical Research Communications,* Vol. 43, No. 6, pages 1334–1339; June 18, 1971.

SYNTHETIC POLYPEPTIDE ANTAGONISTS OF THE HYPOTHALAMIC LUTEINIZING HORMONE RELEASING FACTOR. Wylie Vale, Geoffrey Grant, Jean Rivier, Michael Monahan, Max Amoss, Richard Blackwell, Roger Burgus and Roger Guillemin in *Science,* Vol. 176, No. 4037, pages 933–934; May 26, 1972.

SYNTHETIC LUTEINIZING HORMONE-RELEASING FACTOR: A POTENT STIMULATOR OF GONADOTROPIN RELEASE IN MAN. S. S. C. Yen, R. Rebar, G. Vandenberg, F. Naftolin, Y. Ehara, S. Engblom, K. J. Ryan, K. Benirschke, J. Rivier, M. Amoss and R. Guillemin in *The Journal of Clinical Endocrinology and Metabolism,* Vol. 34, No. 6, pages 1108–1111; June, 1972.

7. The Physiology of Human Reproduction

GERM CELLS AND FERTILIZATION. Edited by C. R. Austin and R. V. Short. Cambridge University Press, 1972.

GONADOTROPINS. Edited by B. B. Saxena, C. G. Beling and H. M. Gandy. Wiley-Interscience, 1972.

HORMONES IN REPRODUCTION. Edited by C. R. Austin and R. V. Short. Cambridge University Press, 1972.

CONTRACEPTIVE RESEARCH: A MALE CHAUVINIST PLOT? Sheldon J. Segal in *Family Planning Perspectives,* Vol. 4, No. 3, pages 21–25; July, 1972.

THE REGULATION OF MAMMALIAN REPRODUCTION. Edited by Sheldon J. Segal, Ruth Crozier, Philip A. Corfman and Peter G. Condliffe. Charles C Thomas, Publisher, 1973.

8. Sex Differences in the Brain

HORMONES AND SEXUAL BEHAVIOR. William C. Young, Robert W. Goy and Charles H. Phoenix in *Science,* Vol. 143, No. 3603, pages 212–218; January 17, 1964.

SEX HORMONES, BRAIN DEVELOPMENT AND BRAIN FUNCTION. Geoffrey W. Harris in *Endocrinology,* Vol. 75, No. 4, pages 627–651; October, 1964.

SEXUAL DIFFERENTIATION OF THE BRAIN AND ITS EXPERIMENTAL CONTROL. G. W. Harris and S. Levine in *The Journal of Physiology,* Vol. 181, No. 2, pages 379–400; November, 1965.

III TARGETS FOR STEROID HORMONE ACTION

9. Hormones and Genes

EFFECT OF ACTINOMYCIN AND INSULIN ON THE METABOLISM OF ISOLATED RAT DIAPHRAGM. Ira G. Wool and Arthur N. Moyer in *Biochimica et Biophysica Acta,* Vol. 91, No. 2, pages 248–256; October 16, 1964.

ON THE MECHANISM OF ACTION OF ALDOSTERONE ON SODIUM TRANSPORT: THE ROLE OF RNA SYNTHESIS. George A. Porter, Rita Bogoroch and Isidore S. Edelman in *Proceedings of the National Academy of Sciences,* Vol. 52, No. 6, pages 1326–1333; December, 1964.

PREVENTION OF HORMONE ACTION BY LOCAL APPLICATION OF ACTINOMYCIN. D. G. P. Talwar and Sheldon J. Segal in *Proceedings of the National Academy of Sciences*, Vol. 50, No. 1, pages 226–230; July 15, 1963.

SELECTIVE ALTERATIONS OF MAMMALIAN MESSENGER-RNA SYNTHESIS: EVIDENCE FOR DIFFERENTIAL ACTION OF HORMONES ON GENE TRANSCRIPTION. Chev Kidson and K. S. Kirby in *Nature*, Vol. 203, No. 4945, pages 599–603; August 8, 1964.

TRANSFER RIBONUCLEIC ACIDS. E. N. Carlsen, G. J. Trelle and O. A. Schjeide in *Nature*, Vol. 202, No. 4936, pages 984–986; June 6, 1964.

10. The Receptors of Steroid Hormones

RECEPTORS FOR REPRODUCTIVE HORMONES. Edited by Bert W. O'Malley and Anthony R. Means. Plenum Press, 1973.

STEROID-CELL INTERACTION. R. J. B. King and W. I. P. Mainwaring. University Park Press, 1974.

THE ROLE OF ESTROPHILIN IN ESTROGEN ACTION. Elwood V. Jensen, Suresh Mohla, Thomas A. Gorell and Eugene R. De Sombre in *Vitamins and Hormones*, Vol. 32, pages 89–127; 1974.

FEMALE STEROID HORMONES AND TARGET CELL NUCLEI. Bert W. O'Malley and Anthony R. Means in *Science*, Vol. 183, No. 4125, pages 610–620; February 15, 1974.

11. Interactions between Hormones and Nerve Tissue

HORMONES AND BEHAVIOR: A STUDY OF INTERRELATIONSHIPS BETWEEN ENDOCRINE SECRETIONS AND PATTERNS OF OVERT RESPONSE. Frank A. Beach. Paul B. Hoeber, Inc., 1948.

EARLY HORMONAL INFLUENCES ON THE DEVELOPMENT OF SEXUAL AND SEX-RELATED BEHAVIOR. Robert W. Goy in *The Neurosciences: Second Study Program*, edited by Francis O. Schmitt. The Rockefeller University Press, 1970.

GENERAL ENDOCRINOLOGY. C. Donnell Turner and Joseph T. Bagnara. W. B. Saunders Company, 1971.

NEUROPHYSIOLOGICAL ANALYSIS OF MATING BEHAVIOR RESPONSE AND HORMONE-SENSITIVE REFLEXES. Donald Pfaff, Catherine Lewis, Carl Diakow and Melvyn Keiner in *Progress in Physiological Psychology: Vol. 5*, edited by E. Stellar and J. M. Sprague. Academic Press, 1973.

CHEMICAL STUDIES OF THE BRAIN AS A STEROID HORMONE TARGET TISSUE. Bruce S. McEwen, Carl J. Denef, John L. Gerlach and Linda Plapinger in *The Neurosciences: Third Study Program*, edited by Francis O. Schmitt and Frederic G. Worden. The MIT Press, 1974.

IV   HORMONES AND NEUROTRANSMITTERS

12. Neurotransmitters

THE UPTAKE AND STORAGE OF NORADRENALINE IN SYMPATHETIC NERVES. L. L. Iversen. Cambridge University Press, 1967.

BIOGENIC AMINES AND EMOTION. Joseph J. Schildkraut and Seymour S. Kety in *Science*, Vol. 156, No. 3771, pages 21–30; April 7, 1967.

BIOCHEMESTRY OF CATECHOLAMINES. Perry B. Molinoff and Julius Axelrod in *Annual Review of Biochemstry*, Vol. 40, pages 465–500; 1971.

NORADRENALINE: FATE AND CONTROL OF ITS BIOSYNTHESIS. Julius Axelrod in *Science*, Vol. 173, No. 3997, pages 598–606; August 13, 1971.

THE PINEAL GLAND: A NEUROCHEMICAL TRANSDUCER. Julius Axelrod in *Science*, Vol. 184, pages 1341–1348; June 28, 1974.

13. "Second Messengers" in the Brain

CYCLIC AMP. G. Alan Robison, Reginald W. Butcher and Earl W. Sutherland. Academic Press, 1971.

METABOLISM AND FUNCTIONS OF CYCLIC AMP IN NERVE. George I. Drummond and Yvonne Ma in *Progress in Neurobiology*. Vol. 2, Part 2, pages 119–176; 1973.

THE ROLE OF CYCLIC NUCLEOTIDES IN CENTRAL SYNAPTIC FUNCTION. Floyd E. Bloom in *Reviews of Physiology, Biochemistry and Pharmacology*. Vol. 74, pages 1–103; 1975.

POSSIBLE ROLE FOR CYCLIC NUCLEOTIDES AND PHOSPHORYLATED MEMBRANE PROTEINS IN POSTSYNAPTIC ACTIONS OF NEUROTRANSMITTERS. Paul Greengard in *Nature*, Vol. 260, No. 5547, pages 101–108; March 11, 1976.

CYCLIC NUCLEOTIDES IN THE NERVOUS SYSTEM. John W. Daly. Plenum Press, 1977.

CYCLIC NUCLEOTIDES AND NERVOUS SYSTEM FUNCTION. James A. Nathanson in *Physiological Reviews*, Vol. 57, pages 157–256; 1977.

V THE USE OF SEX HORMONES: ETHICAL AND POLITICAL ISSUES

14. How Ideology Shapes Women's Lives

FAMILY, SOCIALIZATION AND INTERACTION PROCESS. Talcott Parsons and Robert F. Bales. The Free Press of Glencoe, 1955.

CHILDREN'S CONCEPTS OF MALE AND FEMALE ROLES. Ruth E. Hartley in *Merrill-Palmer Quarterly*, Vol. 6, No. 2, pages 83–92; January, 1960.

THE DEVELOPMENT OF SEX DIFFERENCES. Edited by Eleanor E. Maccoby. Stanford University Press, 1966.

15. Public Policy on Fertility Control

FAMILY PLANNING, PUBLIC POLICY AND INTERVENTION STRATEGY. F. S. Jaffe in *Journal of Social Issues*, Vol. 23, No. 4, pages 145–163; July, 1967.

REPRODUCTION IN THE UNITED STATES: 1965. Norman B. Ryder and Charles F. Westoff. Princeton University Press, 1971.

REPORT OF THE SECRETARY OF HEALTH, EDUCATION, AND WELFARE SUBMITTING A FIVE-YEAR PLAN FOR FAMILY PLANNING SERVICES AND POPULATION RESEARCH PROGRAMS. Senate Committee on Labor and Public Welfare. October, 1971.

THE FUTURE OF FEDERAL SUPPORT FOR FAMILY PLANNING SERVICES AND POPULATION RESEARCH. Jeannie I. Rosoff in *Family Planning Perspectives*, Vol. 5, No. 1, pages 7–18; Winter, 1973.

16. The Ethics of Experimentation with Human Subjects

EXPERIMENTATION WITH HUMAN SUBJECTS. Edited by Paul A. Freund. George Braziller, Inc., 1970.

EXPERIMENTATION WITH HUMAN BEINGS: THE AUTHORITY OF INVESTIGATOR, SUBJECT, PROFESSIONS, AND STATE IN THE HUMAN EXPERIMENTATION PROCESS. Jay Katz. Russell Sage Foundation, 1972.

RESEARCH ON HUMAN SUBJECTS: PROBLEMS OF SOCIAL CONTROL IN MEDICAL EXPERIMENTATION. Bernard Barber, John J. Lally, Julia Loughlin Makarushka and Daniel Sullivan. Russell Sage Foundation, 1973.

HUMAN SUBJECTS IN MEDICAL EXPERIMENTATION. Bradford H. Gray. Wiley-Interscience, 1975.

INDEX